THE HANDBOOK OF
CANCER
IMMUNOLOGY

HANDBOOK OF CANCER IMMUNOLOGY

Volume 5
Immunotherapy

THE HANDBOOK OF
CANCER
IMMUNOLOGY

Edited by
Harold Waters
**Smithsonian Science
Information Exchange**

Garland STPM Press
New York & London

Library of Congress Cataloging in Publication Data
Main entry under title:

Immunotherapy.

   (The Handbook of cancer immunology; v. 5)
   Includes bibliographies and index.
   1. Cancer—Immunological aspects.   2.   Immunotherapy
I. Waters, Harold, 1942–   II.   Series.
[DNLM: 1. Immunotherapy—Handbooks.   2.   Neoplasms—
Therapy—Handbooks.   QZ200 H235 v. 5]
RC268.3.H35   vol. 5 [RC271.I45]   616.9′94′061 77-25702
ISBN 0-8240-7004-6

Printed in the United States of America

CONTENTS

PREFACE

Rationale for immunotherapy is based on observations from the last century, namely, that cancer patients would frequently superimpose infectious disease processes on their neoplastic states. Every once in a while one or two of these patients would survive the infection, considered amazing enough at the time, but then some would go on to survive their well-diagnosed cancers as well. Now we find ourselves trying to duplicate these results of accident by injecting cancer patients and their animal counterparts with cow bacteria, special reticuloendothelial cells, programmed nucleic acids, and many items and agents in between.

Clinical immunotherapy clearly started as a shotgun approach, but now we find that some of the pellets are continuing on their own self-propelled trajectories. Some of them even appear to be coming awfully close to the mark and will undoubtedly zero in even closer as we learn more about the basics of neoplasia and immunology.

This volume takes a broad look at immunotherapy. Future volumes will reflect continued advances in this most promising area and will focus ever more finely in providing further details of clinical and experimental immunology.

—Harold Waters
Washington, D.C.
April, 1978

CHAPTER 1

ANTIBODY, LYMPHOCYTE, AND TUMOR CELL INTERACTIONS

Ronald B. Faanes

Memorial Sloan-Kettering
Cancer Center
Rye, New York 10580

Investigators have established in both *in vivo* and *in vitro* systems that animals and humans can mount an immune response against neoplastic cells. It appears from the available evidence that antitumor responses are extremely complex. This complexity, however, may be a reflection of our limited knowledge and failure to approach the host-tumor interaction as a dynamic system.

There is ample evidence which indicates that tumor-bearing hosts produce cytolytic lymphocytes and antitumor antibodies (see Refs. 24, 54, 146). Although infiltration of leukocytes into the tumor mass is evident (12, 51, 123a, 125), there is no cytological evidence which indicates that the presence of these immunological parameters actively suppresses tumor growth in vivo; therefore, whether the host's immunological response plays a role in modifying or controlling neoplasia is not clearly understood (30, 66, 118–120, 144).

The role of the immunological response in neoplastic disease is a difficult question to approach experimentally. We are dealing with the dynamic interaction of at least four biologically active parameters, each subject to its individual physiological perturbations: (1) The tumor cell, whose surface until recently was considered a fixed landscape, is now realized to present a topography which is constantly changing. Myriads of biochemical alterations occurring during neoplastic transformation certainly cannot be excluded, but will not be discussed in this chapter. (2) Lymphocytes are known to require macromolecular synthesis to obtain the differentiated state necessary for activity (90) and are subject to feedback and circadian regulation (43, 45, 93, 103a, 148). It is presently being realized that membrane mobility is also required for recognition and destruction of the tumor cell by cytolytic lymphocytes (33, 58, 140, 154). (3) Tumor-specific antibody production is also subject to circadian and feedback control (43, 93, 148, 103a, 151). (4) Finally, the homeostasis of the host itself must cope with the additional burden of tumor growth and its secretions.

THE ROLE OF ANTIBODY IN NEOPLASTIC DISEASE

Serum factors arising during the course of neoplastic progression which passively induce unresponsiveness to the respective foreign tissue have been known for many years. Kaliss (68) formulated the theory of immunological enhancement to explain the phenomenon of serum-augmented tumor proliferation (see Refs. 23, 41, 54). The original concept that serum antibody could abrogate the cytotoxic effects of lymphocytes by binding to tumor cell surfaces was based on studies showing that the factor responsible for enhancement in serum from tumor-bearing mice was removed by antimouse 7S immunoglobulin (53).

Numerous theories have since been proposed to explain the

mechanism of antibody inhibition of host responses; however, no real agreement has been reached in understanding how specific antibody nullifies an effective immune response. Resulting from the lack of understanding, these theories have been categorized into central and peripheral inhibition (68) to describe the probable step in lymphoid cell differentiation which is impaired. Peripheral inhibition has been subdivided into efferent and afferent inhibition. Presently, efferent inhibition can be defined with precision; in this case, specifically immune lymphocytes compete with antibody for antigens on the tumor cell surface and, as a consequence, the tumor is protected from lymphoid cell destruction. Greater difficulty is encountered when attempting to define afferent inhibition. It may result from sequestration of antigen or inhibition by the antigen-antibody complex. A classical example of such enhancement comes from the early work of Snell et al. (138) in mice. It was shown that lymph nodes draining the site of a grafted tumor were less reactive to the tumor if the mice were injected with immune serum prepared against the tumor prior to tumor transplantation.

The description of central blockade awaits further investigations. It is presumed in this case that antibodies act directly on the immunologically competent cells and specifically decrease their immunological reactivity. In many cases it is difficult to distinguish between central and afferent inhibition. Initially, it was felt that serum abrogation of the development of lymphocyte-mediated cytolysis (LMC)* was simply a result of antibody binding to cell surface antigens (efferent blockade) and sterically interfering with lymphoid cell interaction. The evidence is fairly conclusive that antibody must initially combine with antigen before inhibition of development or expression of the actual cytolytic event takes place. The class of immunoglobulin responsible for in vivo enhancement and in vitro blocking has been extensively characterized and investigators agree that IgG$_1$ and IgG$_2$ 7S immunoglobulins are responsible (38, 64, 65, 69, 122, 142). Antibodies which block in vitro assays for cellular immunity have been found to be associated with and can be eluted from resected tumors (6, 122, 137, 143). Also, the specificity of the antibody-blocking phenomenon correlates very well both in vivo and in vitro. It appears, therefore, that in vitro models for studying efferent blockade have their counterpart in vivo.

The role of efferent blockade in neoplastic disease requires further discussion. The blocking obtained by alloantiserum and by antitumor antibody is not static. Target cells do not remain protected from LMC if excess antibody is washed away (137). In the case of allogeneic reactions, immune lymphocytes will exert their cytolytic activity in the presence of

*Abbreviations are collected and explained at the end of the chapter.

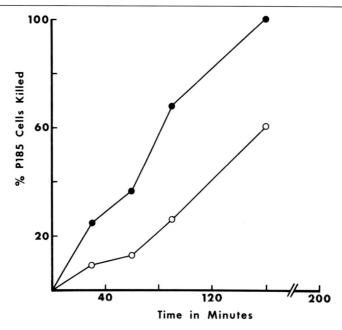

Fig. 1.   Escape from isoantiserum inhibition of lymphocyte-mediated target cell lysis. 1×10^5 ^{51}Cr-labeled murine P-815 mastocytoma cells were incubated with 1×10^6 immune PEC in 10% anti-P-815 isoantiserum (○) or 10% NMS (●). Percent P-815 cells killed was calculated from the amount of ^{51}Cr released into the culture supernatant.

excess antisera (39) (Fig. 1). In this experiment, murine P-815 mastocytoma cells (H-2^d) were preincubated in 10% hyperimmune serum before being mixed with immune spleen cells. Initially, the isoantiserum (IS) exerts a significant block of LMC compared to P-815 cells incubated in normal mouse serum (NMS). However, after 60 min, the immune lymphocytes began to lyse the P-815 target cells. IS was in excess in this experiment because supernatants from the reaction mixtures blocked a second LMC reaction. This escape from IS inhibition of LMC does not take place at 0°C (Table 1), indicating that target cells play an active role in this phenomenon.

We (38), as have others (5, 28, 29, 156), monitored antibody bound to cells *in vitro* and found that adsorbed immunoglobulin is rapidly released into the culture media when incubation is carried out at 37C. The amount of IgG released is related to the amount adsorbed to the cell surface (28, 38). The molecular weight of the released IgG molecule is not significantly altered according to G-200 chromatography (28); however, when

Table 1. Effect of temperature on the escape of lymphocyte-mediated target cell lysis from IS inhibition

Incubation Temperature	% P-815 Cells Killed	
	NMS	IS
4 C	64%	13%
37 C	78%	30%

Note: 1×10^5 P-815 cells were incubated with 10% NMS or IS at 0 C for 20 min. The antibody-coated cells were washed and incubated at the respective temperatures for 60 min at which time immune peritoneal cells were added. Percent P-815 cells killed was determined 90 min after mixtures were incubated at 37 C.

[131]I-IgG was incubated with ^{125}I-lactoperoxidase-labeled (102) P-815 cells at 37C, the released [131]IgG chromatographed with ^{125}I, indicating that a low-molecular-weight surface component was shed (unpublished data). Leonard (84), using immunofluorescence, has described the shedding of cell surface fragments from guinea pig hepatoma cells.

Liepins (personal communication) has studied the changes in surface morphology of murine P-815 cells exposed to isoantiserum using scanning electron microscopy (SEM). Figure 2a shows mastocytoma cells incubated in normal mouse serum. The scanning micrograph in Fig. 2b shows the significant surface protrusions which occur on cells incubated in the presence of antibody. These surface protrusions or "blebs" are similar to the membrane boiling phenomenon described in cells undergoing mitosis (117). The intriguing finding in Figure 2b is that the blebs appear to pinch-off the P-815 cell forming a "mini"-cell. Nowotney et al. (109) have described a factor obtained from the ascitic fluid of TA3-bearing mice which promotes in vivo growth of the respective tumor. Electron microscopy of this factor shows it to be membrane in nature.

Cytophilic antibodies and/or classical opsonins are known to promote phagocytosis of tumor cells (10, 11, 121). Several investigators (26, 27, 83) have reported that macrophages exert their cytotoxicity through "piece-meal cytophagocytosis." Perhaps their observation is not showing the actual cytolytic event but the ingestion of readily released antibody-induced membrane vesicles, which is only a false target. This could ex-

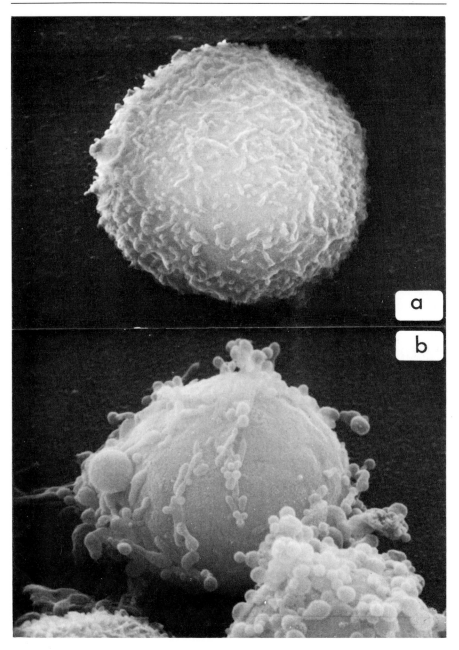

Fig. 2. (a) P-815 mastocytoma cells incubated at 37°C in the presence of NMS. No modifications in the cell surface morphology occur. (× 12,000.) (b) P-815 mastocytoma cells incubated at 37 C in hyperimmune serum. P-815 cells show loss of microvilli and budding of membrane vesicles which occur after one hour at 37 C. (× 11,700.)

plain the several instances where macrophages are only cytostatic to tumor cells (77, 78, 108, 111). These data readily suggest that tumor cells, when confronted with antibody, have the capacity to release whole segments of their membrane in the form of a "mini-cell" which can act as a screen from the hosts' defense. Davey et al. (31) have provided evidence which proposes that there may be a quantitative relationship between the lability of membrane components and the capacity of the tumor to metastasize. Pertinent to this issue, Shearer et al. (44, 131–134) have shown that several tumor cell lines significantly increase their rate of proliferation when exposed to antibody directed toward their cell surface.

Recently, several investigators (34, 35, 123, 153) have presented evidence that coating of tumor cells with antibody occurs in vivo. Progressive growth of the polyoma virus-induced tumors results in detectable increases in the concentration of cytotoxic antibody on the tumor cell surface (18, 122). The accumulation of antibody on the polyoma cell surface correlated with antibody levels in the serum.

Dorval et al. (34, 35) have shown that antibody adsorbed to tumor cells in vivo is rapidly released from cell surfaces when cells were cultured at 37C in vitro. We have found (unpublished data) that antibody bound to P-815 cells in vitro which is not released at 0C is released at 37C in the presence of inhibitory concentrations of cyanide, iodoacetamide, and cytochalasin-B. We have found that 35% of the antibody released at 37C and suspected to be bound to cell-surface components will rebind to fresh P-815 cells. The latter finding is contradictory to that observed with cells whose surface is coated in vivo with antibody. In light of these findings the significance of adsorbed antibody-release from cells incubated at 37C has yet to be delineated. Technically it is not feasible to investigate the actual significance of in vivo-bound antibody; however, an abundance of in vitro evidence indicates that in vivo-bound IgG dramatically reduces the efficiency of the host defense against the tumor (54). Antibody-induced defoliation of surface antigens has been a suspected mechanism of tumor-cell evasion of host defense and was originally thought to be an explanation for "antigenic modulation" (16, 110).

Recent evidence in the case of antigenic modulation of the TL antigen on thymus-derived leukemia indicates that the TL antigen remains on the cell surface (37, 157). It appears that the antibody alters the conformation in such a manner that it does not allow the expression of complement-mediated cytolysis when the antibody is combined with antigen. Lerner et al. (85) have reported that incubation of Moloney virus-transformed lymphocytes with anti-Moloney virus antibody at 37C prior to the addition of complement results in nonsusceptibility of the transformed cells to complement cytotoxicity. In these experiments it was demonstrated that the necessary steps for complement activation were accomplished, but the cytotoxic event was not initiated. Lesley and Hyman (86) and Knopf et al.

(75) have determined that a third to a half of the surface-bound antibody is internalized (presumably with antigen) and believe that this accounts for the development of insensitivity to complement in their studies. Braslowsky et al. (18) have presented in vitro evidence that complement insensitive cells occur in vivo. In these studies the sensitivity to complement-mediated cytotoxicity of antibody-coated tumor cells removed from tumor-bearing mice decreases during growth of the tumor in vivo.

We have shown (155, 155a) that surface antigens of murine DBA/2J P815-mastocytoma cells are modified when the tumor is grown in BALB/c mice, despite the fact that both strains share the same major histocompatibility complex (MHC). The modification occurring on P-815 cells is detected by a reduced susceptibility to LMC. The altered susceptibility was not attributed to modification of antigens in the MHC because BALB/c-grown mastocytoma and DBA-grown mastocytoma have the same capacity to adsorb anti-H-2^d antibody. The antigenic changes occurring on P-815 cells are readily reversible suggesting antigenic modulation (16, 110). The differences in susceptibility between the two cell types must reside in antigens outside the MHC. Because of the rapid reversal of the phenomenon we think that antibodies against minor histocompatibility antigens are blocking the recognition by cytolytic lymphocytes (155a).

Because of the impermanence of antibody bound to tumor-cell surfaces, efferent blockade as an explanation for antibody-induced enhancement seems unlikely. More likely, antibody-induced release of factors from tumor cells causes a blockade at the effector-cell level (central blockade) (105). As to whether effector-cell function or its production is the site of the blocking-factor activity is presently not understood.

Factors arising in the serum of tumor-bearing animals and humans which suppress immune responses (6–9, 108a, 136) against the respective tumor are poorly defined. It is currently thought that antigen-antibody complexes comprise the major portion of these serum-blocking factors (7–9, 53, 54). It appears that serum-blocking factors arise through host/tumor interaction and are not an accumulation of cell components from the progressive death or senescence of antibody-coated cells. In support of the above, Thompson et al. (145) have reported that serum-blocking factors are absent in immunosuppressed animals.

Antibody/Lymphocyte Interaction in Tumor Cell Cytotoxicity

Cell surface-bound antibody can initiate killing of a tumor cell in a complement independent fashion. This immune phenomenon is characterized by an in vitro reaction in which nonsensitized lymphocytes lyse IgG-coated target cells. Many synonyms and abbreviations have been used to describe this system, including antibody-dependent cell-mediated cytotoxicity (ADCMC, ADCC, or ACMC), antibody-dependent lymphocyte-mediated cytotoxicity (antibody-dependent LMC, ADLMC), antibody-mediated cell-dependent immune lympholysis (ABCIL), and lymphocyte-dependent antibody assay (LDA assay). ADCC has to date been demonstrated by in vitro methods only and has recently been fully reviewed (23, 46, 96, 114, 146); however, preliminary results by Carlson and Terres (22) suggest that this activity occurs in vivo. In brief, the effector cell, called a K cell, appears to be either a lymphocyte or a nonphagocytic, nonglass-adherent monocyte (20, 50, 96, 112, 113, 159). The K cell is nonimmunoglobulin-bearing (50) and thymus-independent (17, 52, 79, 149), but has a receptor for a site on the Fc portion of IgG (47, 80, 107). It is present in normal human and animal peripheral blood, lymph nodes, and spleens, but in varying numbers. The antibody that is capable of inducing K-cell cytotoxicity is IgG (98, 99, 112, 150), and indirect evidence suggests that all four human IgG subclasses are active (81, 100).

The first step in the reaction is the binding of antibody to the target cell which, presumably, results in a conformational alteration of the Fc portion of the IgG molecule, such that it is recognized and bound by the K cell via its Fc receptor (47, 80, 107, 126). ADCC lysis appears in all the assays so far examined to be identical to that produced by sensitized T cells (139). The assay is a highly sensitive method of detecting antibody, and activity can be detected in some sera to dilutions as high as 10^{-11} (113).

As yet, there are no reports which indicate the role, if any, that the above described, antibody-induced cell-surface modification plays in the efficiency of ADCC immunity. But MacLennan (97) has shown that ADCC is readily inhibited by antigen-antibody complexes. Other investigations (127, 152) have revealed that this reaction is readily inhibited by other serum immunoglobulins. Its role as an in vivo defense mechanism is currently being questioned. It appears, therefore, that the humoral response in this case works in favor of the tumor. A paradox has evolved, however, with regard to the role of immune complexes in regulating the development of host defense. Several investigators have suggested that immune complexes suppress both the humoral and cellular immune response (9, 33a, 48), while others have reported stimulation (32, 40, 59, 89, 106, 160). In fact, Uhr and Möller (148) reported that the development of delayed-type hypersensitivity (DTH) was facilitated by antigen-antibody complex. Liew and Parish (89) have shown that suppression of antibody formation was accompanied by a concomitant increase in DTH. These results, in addition to those reported by Mackaness and Lagrange (95), suggest that an inverse relationship often exists between DTH and the humoral immune response. In isolated instances, passively administered immune sera have been reported to suppress rather than enhance tumor growth (3, 135, 147, 160). The underlying mechanism for these observations is not understood.

Using an assay system which measures "pure" T-cell immune responses (24, 25, 92), we have shown that passive administration of IS with allogeneic tumor cells modulates the induction of LMC activity (40). The factor in IS is likely to be specific antibody induced by immunization: (1) both in vivo-augmenting and in vitro-blocking activities are present in IS; (2) both activities are removed by absorption with specific cells; (3) demonstration of the augmentation effect requires injection of tumor cells plus IS together. The augmentation effects were best manifested when mice were immunized with low doses of tumor cells.

The IS-augmented induction of LMC activity is similar to the enhanced development of plaque-forming cells (PFC) when mice received antiserum and sheep red-blood cells (SRBC) together (32, 32a, 59). These studies demonstrated that 19S antibodies may stimulate PFC formation, whereas 7S antibodies usually suppressed. Our experimental results suggest that the augmenting factor in immune serum was 19S antibody, because the activity appears within 10 days after a primary injection and fractionates with the 19S fraction in G-200 chromatography.

Development of in vivo augmenting activity, after immunization, occurs before significant levels of 7S antibody-blocking activity occurs in the serum. It appears that either the humoral or cellular immune response is subject to regulation by the level of 7S vs. 19S antibody production and the consequent formation of the antigen-antibody complex.

The exact role of passively administered antibody in augmenting T cell responses is not understood at present. Our experimental evidence is unique in revealing that the antigen-antibody complex has a profound effect on the development of LMC activity. We have found, as have others (see reviews 45, 94, 116, 148), that antibody and antigen must combine in optimal proportions to achieve the observed effects on LMC activities. Although the influence of IgG-immune complex vs. IgM-immune complex on the development of immune responses has yet to be delineated, our data indicate that IgM-immune complex augments the development of LMC, while the IgG-immune complex works in an opposing fashion.

Playfair (116) has postulated that antigen binding, augmentation of antibody production, and suppression of antibody production can be mediated by passively acquired Ig on the surface of T cells, which suggests that Ig can attach to T cells with or without being complexed with antigen. In fact, Hudson and Sprent (63) have recently shown that IgM-antibody is specifically adsorbed to H-2-activated mouse T lymphocytes.

These observations tempt us to postulate the following hypothesis. Inbred "normal" mice are now known to contain significant amounts of natural antibody (74); therefore, they may contain low levels of allo-activated T cells. The passive administration of IgM with antigen negates the animal's requirement to produce an endogenous supply. Macrophages recognize the IgM-antigen complex and, through their digestion, produce processed IgM-antigen complexes, which adsorb to the omnipresent, activated T cells initiating clonal expansion of the specific, cytotoxic T cell.

Lymphocyte Tumor Cell Interaction Independent of Antibody

Concomitant with the development of a humoral response to nucleated antigens, thymus-derived lymphocytes differentiate into cytolytic, small lymphocytes (see Ref. 24). Govaerts (49), in 1960, was the first to describe the lytic activity of immune lymphocytes when he observed that thoracic duct lymphocytes from dogs which had rejected kidney allografts caused lysis of donor cells in vitro. There have since been extensive investigations in the area of lymphocyte-mediated cytolysis. Presently there are several types of effector cells which have the capacity for lysing a large number of target cells (2, 23, 24, 71–73, 82, 87, 115). Within a lymphocyte population, the thymus-derived killer T cell has been shown to be the active lymphoid cell in rejection of allogeneic cells (see review 24). This thymus-derived cell has therefore, been most extensively studied. The killer T cell is theta positive (25, 92) and has recently been shown to bear Ly2,3 antigens (21).

Sensitized T lymphocytes capable of producing LMC in vitro can be isolated from tumor-bearing hosts (62) or generated by immunizing an animal with an incompatible graft (see reviews 13, 24). Spleen, lymph node, and peripheral blood lymphocytes are convenient sources of cytotoxic effector lymphocytes. It is important with respect to tumor immunology to study effector lymphocytes infiltrating the tumor or site of graft rejection. Several investigators (13, 123a) have identified and characterized the cytotoxic cells arising at the site of graft rejection. The effector cell is a nonadherent, small to medium size lymphocyte. This corroborates with the results of Cerottini et al. (24) and others who have studied the killer T cell in other systems.

The exact mechanism of T lymphocyte destruction of target cells is presently not well understood (4, 13, 56). T-cell-mediated destruction is almost certainly independent of antitarget antibody. Initial contact of killer cell and target cell appears to be a random event. The nature of this contact and the recognition structure on the lymphocyte and target cell remain to be defined. The evidence suggests that in the mouse the antigen receptors on the T cell are associated with the serologically defined H-2 antigens of the MHC (70). Subsequent to random contact, specific lymphocyte target cell recognition is initiated. Movement within the lymphocyte membrane appears necessary during the early phase of killing as suppression with membrane-active agents such as cytochalasin B or DMSO is readily observed (58, 140, 154). Following specific contact, the permeability or osmotic barrier of the target cell begins to deteriorate as a rapid efflux of low-molecular-weight molecules ensues (57, 103, 124).

Several investigators (88, 88a, 123b) have purified PEC by using $1 \times g$ sedimentation velocity (104) to remove nonspecific, contaminating lymphocytes so that direct visualization of the lytic reaction could be studied with SEM. By using the standard ^{51}Cr-release assay as described by Brunner et al. (19) to monitor cell lysis, we were able to observe T-cell cytotoxicity in the same preparation. During stages of LMC preceding significant ^{51}Cr-release, cytolytic lymphocytes adhered to P-815 cells by means of interdigitation of surface microvilli without detectable changes in the surface morphology of either cell (Fig. 3a). The formation of a uropod by sensitized lymphocytes has been implicated in the attachment process (1, 76) and is thought to represent the activation of lymphocytes (14). We, as well as Sanderson (124), have not observed such a structural modification of the lymphocyte at any stage of LMC.

The only evidence of target cell damage prior to detectable ^{51}Cr-release was obtained at the TEM level. P-815 cells in contact with lymphocytes showed degeneration of their mitochondria (Fig. 4a and b); whereas, adhering lymphocytes showed no evidence of mitochondria disruption, thus providing an internal control for our preparation. P-815-cell degeneration at the mitochondrial level is significantly suppressed when anti-P-815 antibody is present in the reaction mixture (unpublished observations).

Upon the initiation of ^{51}Cr-release, and presumably target-cell lysis, some target cells undergo drastic changes in surface morphology, which consist of the loss of surface microvilli and the appearance of blebs throughout their surface, i.e., zeiosis or "boiling" (124) (Fig. 3b). The size of these blebs varied from cell to cell but occurred only on target cells with adhering lymphocytes. The fact that some mastocytoma cells formed blebs, which pinched off from the surface producing spherical structures which in turn interacted with neighboring lymphocytes, raises again the possibility that this process may represent an escape mechanism of tumor cells from further damage by killer T cells similar to that observed with antibody. The shedding of cytoplasmic fragments of degenerating target cells ("clasmatosis") has been reported by Biberfeld et al. (14), but it is not clear whether or not these fragments were fully separated from the cell since his observations were based on thin sections.

We defined lysed cells as those which have lost their three-

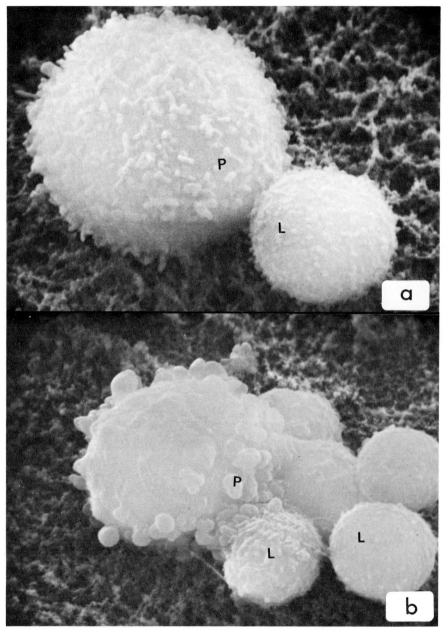

Fig. 3. (a) P-815 mastocytoma cells exposed to lymphocytes immunized against a different alloantigen (i.e., EL-4 cells). No alteration in surface morphology occurs. (× 11,500.) (b) P-815 mastocytoma cells exposed to specifically immunized lymphocytes. Blebs or surface protrusions on P-815 target cells are induced by sensitized lymphocytes. (× 7800.)

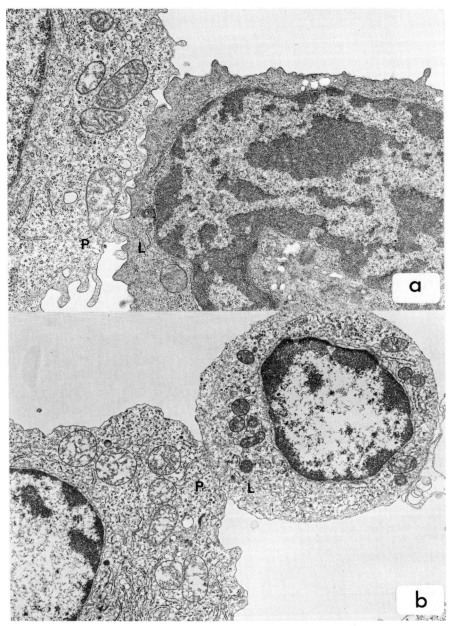

Fig. 4. (a) TEM of a specifically immunized lymphocyte adhering to a P-815 target cell at a stage preceding ^{51}Cr-release. Note that some of the target cell mitochondria appear damaged, while killer cell mitochondria remain intact. (× 13,200.) (b) TEM of the LMC reaction during the period of ^{51}Cr-release. The damage of the target cell mitochondria becomes rather extensive. Again note that the lymphocyte mitochondria appear structurally intact. (× 8800.)

dimensional structure and appeared as collapsed, flattened cells on the supporting coverslip (Fig. 5). This cell morphology was apparent only during the final stages of the LMC process when ^{51}Cr-release was above 50%. Lymphocytes remained attached to these collapsed structures and never showed a loss of their three-dimensional morphology. Neither blebbing nor collapse of target cells occurred in control experiments where nonspecifically immune lymphocytes, i.e., lymphocytes immunized against a different alloantigen, were substituted for specific killer T cells. Regardless of the fact that control lymphocytes were capable of adhering to nonspecific targets, they caused neither ^{51}Cr-release, blebbing, nor final collapse of the target cells. Our observations are in agreement with the cinematographic studies of Sanderson (124) who has reported that zeiosis or "boiling" of target cells occurs only in the presence of sensitized lymphocytes.

Our TEM observations were in agreement with those obtained by SEM, in that adhesion of killer T cells to target cells occurred without alteration in the surface morphology of either cell. Contrary to the reports of Biberfeld and Johansson (15) and Adelstein et al. (1), killer T cells did not form uropods or cytoplasmic extensions directed toward the target

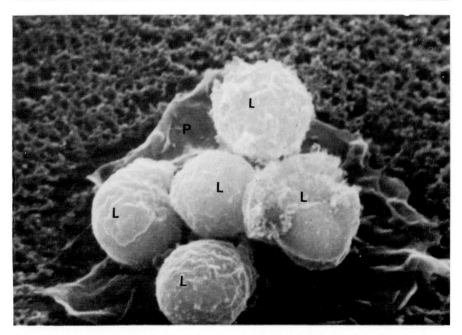

Fig. 5. Immunized lymphocytes remain attached to the lysed or collapsed P-815 target mastocytoma cell.

cell. At the TEM level the contact zone between the two cells consisted of interdigitation of the surface membranes similar to that observed with the SEM, but without the formation of specialized intercellular junctions. The latter observation is in agreement with those of Biberfeld and Johansson (15), but is contradictory to the equidensitometric studies of Koren et al. (76), which were interpreted to show the existence of membrane discontinuities in the contact zone. Fluorescein transfer between killer and target cells has also suggested the existence of permeable junctions between interacting cells (128); however, work by Kalina and Berke (67) was unable to support this hypothesis. Although the ultrastructure failed to reveal membrane specialization in the contact area, other methods suggest its existence.

That the first evidence of cellular damage is at the mitochondrial level is of interest, as these organelles are the primary sites of ATP formation (101), and damage to their structural integrity, particularly the inner mitochondrial membrane, could severely limit the availability of this high-energy metabolite to the cell. ATP has been proposed to function as a cardinal absorbent of water on cellular proteins, i.e., the "association induction hypothesis." Disruption of the respiratory and oxidative phosphorylation process by metabolic inhibitors results in an increase of the total free water of the cell (91). Interestingly, ATP has been found to be released by target cells before ^{86}Rb and ^{51}Cr (56).

The cytolytic events induced by specifically immune lymphocytes may, therefore, be carried out via disruption of the functional and structural integrity of target cell mitochondria. This causes an imbalance in the intracellular ATP pool and results in an increase of free cellular water, which leads to a final disruption of the cell, as suggested by Ferluga and Allison (42). The failure of maintaining an osmotic balance may result in the alteration of the target cell surface morphology recognized by bleb formation. This formation of blebs which occurs on the entire free surface of the target cell is compatible with the proposed sequence of events leading to an osmotic imbalance and disruption of the target cell.

Leukocytes other than killer T cells have been observed to infiltrate tumor masses and have been separated from resected tumors (62, 87, 123a, 130). The number of macrophages at the tumor foci is often greatly underestimated because many of them may not be recognized readily in histological sections. The importance of macrophages at the tumor foci is not well understood at present. A correlation with metastatic potential has been reported (36); 90% of the animals having greater than 50% macrophages in their sarcomas could be cured by resecting the tumors. However, under comparable conditions, 90% of the animals with their sarcomas containing less than 10% macrophages died of metastasis. Mice depleted of T cells had greatly reduced concentrations of macrophages in their tumors, which suggests a cell-cell collaboration within the tumor. Macrophages have been shown to be nonspecifically cytotoxic for tumor cells (77, 108), but whether their presence within the tumor results in active tumor destruction or provides an environment for lymphocyte collaboration is not known. (For a further discussion of macrophages in neoplastic disease, see recent comprehensive treatises (2, 87, 108, 111, 158).)

A second cytotoxic cell which is described as being nonthymus-derived has been reported (60, 61, 71–73, 115, 129). This killing activity present in the cells of normal mice is extremely low and is effective only on selected tumor lines. The natural killer cell appears within 8 weeks after birth and then declines rapidly. Nude and thymectomized mice are good sources of this killer cell.

The role, if any, these cell-mediated antitumor reactions play in controlling neoplastic disease is currently being extensively investigated. Each appears to have its limitations, which in the eyes of the investigators seem to be a significant restriction in the contribution of that reaction to the host's defense. Additional confusion arises in assessing what *in vitro* assays measure with respect to the antitumor status of the host. The long-term assays (55, 141) quantitate the potential for a lymphoid cell populations' ability to inhibit growth, while short-term assays (24) quantitate the immediate potential for tumor cell destruction by the host. A different cell is suspected to account for the effect measured in each assay system (82, 140a).

ACKNOWLEDGMENTS

The author wishes to express his appreciation to Patricia Higgins for her editing of this manuscript, to Drs. Y. S. Choi, D. F. Kiszkiss and E. Hahn for their critical reviews, and to Dr. A. Liepins for the electron micrographs. This study was supported by research grants CA-08748, CA-16271, CA-17049, and CA-17404 from the National Cancer Institute, National Institutues of Health, Bethesda, Maryland.

ABBREVIATIONS

ADCC   Antibody-dependent cell-mediated cytotoxicity
ATP   Adenosine triphosphate
B cells   Bursa or bone-marrow derived
DMSO   Dimethyl sulfoxide
DTH   Delayed type hypersensitivity
IS   Isoantiserum
LMC   Lymphocyte-mediated cytotoxicity
MHC   Major histocompatibility complex

NMS   Normal mouse serum
PEC   Peritoneal exudate cells
PFC   Plaque-forming cells
SEM   Scanning electron microscopy
SRBC   Sheep red blood cells
T cells   Thymus-derived
TEM   Transmission electron microscopy
TL   Thymus leukemia

REFERENCES

1. Adelstein, E. H., Barrett, B., and Senhauser, D. A. 1976. Ultrastructure of lymphocyte tumor cell interaction with localization of cell bound antibody by ferritin labeling. Cancer Res. 36: 302–308.

2. Alexander, P. 1976. The functions of the macrophage in malignant disease. Ann. Rev. Med. 27: 207–224.

3. Alexander, P., Connell, D. I., and Midulska, Z. B. 1966. Treatment of murine leukemia with spleen cells or sera from allogeneic mice immunized against the tumor. Cancer Res. 26: 1508–1515.

4. Allison, A. C., and Ferluga, J. 1976. How lymphocytes kill tumor cells. N. Engl. J. Med. 295: 165–167.

5. Amos, D. B., Cohen, I., and Klein, W. J., Jr. 1970. Mechanism of immunologic enhancement. Transplant. Proc. 2: 68–75.

6. Bansal, S. C., Hargreaves, R., and Sjögren, H. O. 1972. Facilitation of polyoma tumor growth in rats by blocking sera and tumor eluate. Int. J. Cancer 9: 97–108.

7. Baldwin, R. W. 1976. Role of immunosurveillance against chemically induced rat tumors. Transplant. Rev. 28: 62–74.

8. Baldwin, R. W., and Price, M. R. 1976. Tumor antigens and tumor-host relationships. Ann. Rev. Med. 27: 151–163.

9. Baldwin, R. W., and Robins, R. A. 1976. Factors interfering with immunological resection of tumors. Brit. Med. Bull. 32: 118–123.

10. Bennett, B. 1965. Phagocytosis of mouse tumor cells in vitro by various homologous and heterologous cells. J. Immunol. 95: 80–85.

11. Bennett, B., Old, L. J., and Boyse, E. A. 1964. The phagocytosis of tumor cells in vitro. Transplantation 2: 183–202.

12. Berg, J. W. 1971. Morphological evidence for immune response to breast cancer: A historical review. Cancer 28: 1453–1456.

13. Berke, G., and Amos, D. B. 1973. Mechanism of lymphocyte-mediated cytolysis. The LMC cycle and its role in transplantation immunity. Transplant. Rev. 17: 71–107.

14. Biberfeld, P., Biberfeld, G., Perlmann, P., and Holm, G. 1973. Cytological observations on the cytotoxic interaction between lymphocytes and antibody-coated monolayer cells. Cell. Immunol. 7: 60–72.

15. Biberfeld, P., and Johansson, A. 1975. Contact areas of cytotoxic lymphocytes and target cells. Exp. Cell Res. 94: 79–87.

16. Boyse, E. A., Stockert, E., and Old, L. J. 1967. Modification of the antigenic structure of the cell membrane by thymus-leukemia antibody. *Proc. Natl. Acad. Sci. USA* 58: 954–957.

17. Briton, S., Perlmann, H., and Perlmann, P. 1973. Thymus-dependent and thymus independent effector functions of mouse lymphoid cells. Comparison of cytotoxicity and primary antibody formation *in vitro. Cell. Immunol.* 8: 420–434.

18. Braslowsky, G., Ran, M., and Witz, I. P. 1976. Tumor bound immunoglobulins: The relationship between the *in vivo* coating of tumor cells by potentially cytotoxic antitumor antibodies and the expression of immune complex receptors. *Int. J. Cancer* 18: 116–121.

19. Brunner, K. T., Mauel, J., Rudolf, H., and Chapuis, B. 1970. Studies of allograft immunity in mice. I. Induction, development and *in vitro* assay of cellular immunity. *Immunology* 18: 501–515.

20. Campbell, A. C., MacLennan, I. C. M., Snaith, M. L., and Barnett, I. G. 1972. Selective deficiency of cytotoxic B lymphocytes in man. *Clin. Exp. Immunol.* 12: 1–8.

21. Cantor, H., and Boyse, E. A. 1975. Functional subclasses of T lymphocytes bearing different Ly antigens. I. The generation of functionally distinct T-cell subclasses is a differentiative process independent of antigen. *J. Exp. Med.* 141: 1376–1389.

22. Carlson, G. A., and Terres, G. 1976. Antibody-induced killing *in vivo* of L1210/MTX-R cells quantitated in passively immunized mice with ^{131}I-iododeoxyuridine-labeled cells and whole body measurement of retained radioactivity. *J. Immunol.* 117: 822–829.

23. Carpenter, C. B., d'Apice, A. J. F., and Abbas, A. K. 1976. The role of antibodies in the rejection and enhancement of organ grafts. *Adv. Immunol.* 22: 1–65.

24. Cerottini, J., and Brunner, K. T. 1974. Cell mediated cytotoxicity, allograft rejection, and tumor immunity. *Adv. Immunol.* 18: 67–137.

25. Cerottini, J. C., Nordin, A. A., and Brunner, K. T. 1970. Specific *in vitro* cytotoxicity of thymus-derived lymphocytes sensitized to alloantigens. *Nature (Lond.)* 228: 1308–1309.

26. Chambers, V. C., and Weiser, R. S. 1969. The ultrastructure of target cells and immune macrophages during their interaction *in vitro. Cancer Res.* 29: 301–317.

27. Chambers, V. C., and Weiser, R. S. 1971. The ultrastructure of target L-cells and immune macrophages during their interaction *in vivo. Cancer Res.* 31: 2059–2066.

28. Chang, S., Stockert, E., Boyse, E. A., Hämmerling, U., and Old, L. J. 1971. Spontaneous release of cytotoxic alloantibody from viable cells sensitized in excess antibody. *Immunology* 21: 829–838.

29. Cone, R. E., Bernoco, D., Ceppellini, R., Dorval, G., and Jacot-Guillarmod, H. 1976. Reversible modifications of cell membrane structures induced by antibodies against transplantation antigens of man, in V. P. Eijsvoogel, D. Roos, W. P. Zeijlemaker (eds.), *Leukocyte Membrane Determinants Regulating Immune Reactivity.* Academic Press, New York.

30. Currie, G. 1976. Immunological aspects of host resistance to the development and growth of cancer. *Biochem. Biophys. Acta* 458: 135–165.

31. Davey, G. C., Currie, G. A., and Alexander, P. 1976. Spontaneous shedding and antibody induced modulation of histocompatibility antigens on murine lymphomata: Correlation with metastic capacity. Brit. J. Cancer 33: 9–14.

32. Dennert, G. 1971. The mechanism of antibody-induced stimulation and inhibition of the immune response. J. Immunol. 106: 951–955.

32a. Diamantstein, T., and Naher, H. 1978. Specific immune response enhancing factor in serum of immunized mice. Nature (Lond.) 271: 257–259.

33. Diener, E., and Paetkau, V. H. 1972. Antigen recognition: Early surface-receptor phenomena induced by binding of a tritium-labeled antigen. Proc. Natl. Acad. Sci. USA 69: 2364–2368.

33a. Diener, E., and Feldman, M. 1970. Antibody-mediated suppression of the immune response in vitro. II. A new approach to the phenomenon of immunological tolerance. J. Exp. Med. 132: 31–43.

34. Dorval, G., Witz, I. P., Klein, E., and Wigzell, H. 1976. Tumor-bound immunoglobulins: An in vivo phenomenon of masked specificity. J. Natl. Cancer Inst. 56: 523–527.

35. Dorval, G., Witz, I. P., Klein, E., and Wigzell, H. 1976. Tumor-bound immunoglobulins. I. Further analysis of the characteristics of binding of immunoglobulins to in vivo grown tumor cells. Int. J. Cancer 17: 109–119.

36. Eccles, S. A., Alexander, P. 1974. Macrophage content of tumors in relation to metastatic spread and host immune reaction. Nature 250: 667–669.

37. Esmon, N. L., and Little, J. R. 1976. An indirect radioimmunoassay for thymus leukemia (TL) antigens. J. Immunol. 117: 911–917.

38. Faanes, R. B., and Choi, Y. S. 1974. Interaction of isoantibody and cytotoxic lymphocytes with allogeneic tumor cells. J. Immunol. 113: 279–288.

39. Faanes, R. B., Choi, Y. S., and Good, R. A. 1973. Escape from isoantiserum inhibition of lymphocyte mediated cytotoxicity. J. Exp. Med. 137: 171–182.

40. Faanes, R. B., Walker, M., and Choi, Y. S. 1976. Isoantiserum augmented development of lymphocyte mediated cytotoxicity. J. Exp. Med. 144: 1284–1293.

41. Feldman, J. D. 1972. Immunological enhancement: A Study of blocking antibodies. Adv. Immunol. 15: 167–214.

42. Ferluga, J., and Allison, A. C. 1974. Observations on the mechanism by which T-lymphocytes exert cytotoxic effects. Nature 250: 673–675.

43. Fernandes, G., Halberg, F., Yunis, E. J., and Good, R. A. 1976. Circadian rhythmic plaque-forming cell response of spleens from mice immunized with SRBC. J. Immunol. 117: 962–966.

44. Fink, M. P., Parker, C. W., and Shearer, W. T. 1975. Antibody stimulation of tumor growth in T-cell depleted mice. Nature 255: 404–405.

45. Fitch, F. W. 1975. Selective suppression of immune responses. Regulation of antibody formation and cell-mediated immunity by antibody. Prog. Allergy 19: 195–244.

46. Forman, J., and Möller, G. 1973. The effector cell in antibody-induced cell mediated immunity. Transplant. Rev. 17: 108–149.

47. Gelfand, E. W., Resch, K., and Prester, M. 1972. Antibody-mediated target cell lysis by nonimmune cells. Characterization of the antibody and effector cell populations. Eur. J. Immunol. 2: 419–424.

48. Gorczynski, R., Kotiainen, S., Mitchison, N. A., and Tigelaar, R. E. 1974.

Antigen-antibody complexes as blocking factors on the T lymphocyte surface, in G. M. Edelman (ed.), Cellular Selection and Regulation in the Immune Response, pp. 143–154. Raven Press, New York.

49. Govaerts, A. 1960. Cellular antibodies in kidney homotransplantation. J. Immunol. 85: 516–522.

50. Greenberg, A. H., Hudson, L., Shen, L., and Roitt, I. M. 1973. Antibody-dependent cell-mediated cytotoxicity due to a "null" lymphoid cell. Nature New Biol. 242: 111–113.

51. Hamlin, I. M. 1968. Possible host resistance in carcinoma of the breast: A histological study. Brit. J. Cancer 22: 382–401.

52. Harding, B., Pudifin, D. J., Gotch, F., and MacLennan, I. C. M. 1971. Cytotoxic lymphocytes from rats depleted of thymus processed cells. Nature New Biol. 232: 80–81.

53. Hellström, I., and Hellström, K. E. 1969. Studies on cellular immunity and its serum-mediated inhibition in Moloney virus-induced mouse sarcomas. Int. J. Cancer 4: 587–600.

54. Hellström, K. E., and Hellström, I. 1970. Immunological enhancement as studied by cell culture techniques. Ann. Rev. Microbiol. 24: 373–398.

55. Hellström, I., and Hellström, K. E. 1971. Colony inhibition and cytotoxicity assays, in B. R. Bloom and P. R. Glade (eds.), In Vitro Methods in Cell-Mediated Immunity, pp. 409–414. Academic Press, New York.

56. Henney, C. S. 1973. On the mechanism of T-cell mediated cytolysis. Transplant. Rev. 17: 37–70.

57. Henney, C. S. 1973. Studies on the mechanism of lymphocyte-mediated cytolysis. II. The use of various target cell markers to study cytolytic events. J. Immunol. 110: 73–84.

58. Henney, C. S., and Bubbers, J. E. 1973. Studies on the mechanism of lymphocyte-mediated cytocysis. I. The role of divalent cations in cytolysis by T lymphocytes. J. Immunol. 110: 63–72.

59. Henry, C., and Jerne, N. K. 1968. Competition of 19S and 7S antigen receptors in the regulation of the primary immune response. J. Exp. Med. 128: 133–152.

60. Herberman, R. B., Nunn, M. E., Holden, H. T., and Laurin, D. H. 1975. Natural cytotoxic reactivity of mouse lymphoid cells against syngeneic and allogeneic tumors. II. Characterization of effector cells. Int. J. Cancer 16: 230–239.

61. Herberman, R. B., Nunn, M. E., and Laurin, D. H. 1975. Natural cytotoxic reactivity of mouse lymphoid cells against syngeneic and allogeneic tumors. I. Distribution of reactivity and specificity. Int. J. Cancer 16: 216–229.

62. Holden, H. T., Haskill, J. S., Kirchner, H., and Herberman, R. B. 1976. Two functionally distinct anti-tumor effector cells isolated from primary murine sarcoma virus-induced tumors. J. Immunol. 117: 440–446.

63. Hudson, L., and Sprent, J. 1976. Specific adsorption of IgM antibody on H-2 activated mouse T-lymphocytes. J. Exp. Med. 143: 444–449.

64. Jansen, J. J. J., Koene, R. A. P., Kamp, G. J., Tamboer, W. P. M., and Wijdeveld, P. G. A. B. 1975. Isolation of pure IgG. Subclasses from mouse alloantiserum and their activity in enhancement and hyperacute rejection of skin allografts. J. Immunol. 115: 387–391.

65. Jansen, J. L. J., Koene, R. A. P., Kamp, G. J. V., Hagemann, J. F. H. M., and Wijdeveld, P. G. A. B. 1975. Hyperacute rejection and enhancement of mouse skin grafts by antibodies with a distinct specificity. J. Immunol. 115: 392–394.

66. JeeJeebhoy, H. F. 1975. The role of the immune response in oncogenesis. In Vitro 11: 166–171.

67. Kalina, M., and Berke, G. 1976. Contact regions of cytotoxic T lymphocytes-target cell conjugates. Cell. Immunol. 25: 41–51.

68. Kaliss, N. 1969. Immunological enhancement. Int. Rev. Exp. Pathol. 8: 242–273.

69. Kaliss, N., Sinclair, N. R. St. C., and Cantrell, J. L. 1976. Immunological enhancement of a murine tumor allograft by passive alloantibody IgG and F(ab')$_2$. Eur. J. Immunol. 6: 38–42.

70. Katz, D. H., and Benacerraf, B. 1972. Regulatory influence of activated T-cells on B-cell responses to antigen. Adv. Immunol. 15: 2–94.

71. Kiessling, R., Klein, E., Pross, H., and Wigzell, H. 1975. "Natural" killer cells in the mouse. II. Cytotoxic cells with specificity for mouse Moloney leukemia cells. Characteristics of the killer cell. Eur. J. Immunol. 5: 117–121.

72. Kiessling, R., Klein, E., and Wigzell, H. 1975. "Natural" killer cells in the mouse. I. Cytotoxic cells with specificity for mouse Moloney leukemia cells. Specificity and distribution according to genotype. Eur. J. Immunol. 5: 112–117.

73. Kiessling, R., Petranyi, G., Klein, G., and Wigzell, H. 1975. Genetic variation of in vitro cytolytic activity and in vivo rejection potential of non-immunized semi-syngeneic mice against a mouse lymphoma line. Int. J. Cancer 15: 933–940.

74. Klein, P. A. 1975. Anomalous reactions of mouse alloantisera with cultured tumor cells. I. Demonstration of widespread occurrence using reference typing sera. J. Immunol. 115: 1254–1260.

75. Knopf, P. M., Destree, A., and Hyman, R. 1973. Antibody induced changes in expression of immunoglobulin surface antigen. Eur. J. Immunol. 3: 251–259.

76. Koren, H. S., Ax, W., and Freund-Moelbert, E. E. 1973. Morphological observations on the contact-induced lysis of target cells. Eur. J. Immunol. 3: 32–37.

77. Krahenbuhl, J., and Remington, J. S. 1974. The role of activated macrophages in specific and nonspecific cytostasis of tumor cells. J. Immunol. 113: 507–516.

78. Krahenbuhl, J. L., Lambert, L. H., and Remington, J. S. 1976. The effects of activated macrophages on tumor target cells: Escape from cytostasis. Cell. Immunol. 25: 279–293.

79. Lamon, E. W., Skurzak, H. M., Klein, E., and Wigzell, H. 1972. In vitro cytotoxicity by a nonthymus-processed lymphocyte population with specificity for a virally determined tumor cell surface antigen. J. Exp. Med. 136: 1072–1079.

80. Larsson, A., and Perlmann, P. 1972. Study of Fab and F(ab')$_2$ from rabbit IgG for capacity to induce lymphocyte-mediated target cell destruction in vitro. Int. Arch. Allergy 43: 80–88.

81. Larsson, A., Perlmann, P., and Natvig, J. B. 1973. Cytotoxicity of human lymphocytes induced by rabbit antibodies to chicken erythrocytes. Inhibition by normal IgG and by human myeloma proteins of different IgG subclasses. Immunology 25: 675–686.

82. Leclerc, J. C., Gomard, E., Plata, F., and Levy, J. P. 1973. Cell-mediated immune reaction against tumors induced by oncornaviruses. II. Nature of the effector cells in tumor-cell cytolysis. Int. J. Cancer 11: 426–432.

83. Lejeune, F., Evans, R. 1972. Ultrastructural cytochemical and biochemical changes occurring during syngeneic macrophage lymphoma interaction in vitro. Eur. J. Cancer 8: 549–555.

84. Leonard, E. J. 1973. Cell surface antigen movement: Induction in hepatoma cells by antitumor antibody. J. Immunol. 110: 1167–1169.

85. Lerner, R. A., Oldstone, M. B. A., and Cooper, N. R. 1971. Cell cycle-dependent immune lysis of Moloney virus-transformed lymphocytes: Presence of viral antigen, accessibility to antibody, and complement activation. Proc. Natl. Acad. Sci. USA 68: 2584–2588.

86. Lesley, J., and Hyman, R. 1974. Antibody induced changes in expression of the H-2 antigen. Eur. J. Immunol. 4: 732–739.

87. Levy, M. H., and Wheelock, E. F. 1974. The role of macrophages in defense against neoplastic disease. Adv. Cancer Res. 20: 131–163.

88. Liepins, A., Faanes, R. B., Choi, Y. S., and de Harven, E. 1977. Ultrastructural changes during T-lymphocyte-mediated cytolysis. Cell. Immunol. 28: 109–124.

89. Liew, F. Y., and Parish, C. R. 1972. Regulation of the immune response by antibody. I. Suppression of antibody formation and concomitant enhancement of cell-mediated immunity by passive antibody. Cell. Immunol. 4: 66–85.

90. Lindahl-Kiessling, K., and Osoba, D. 1974. Lymphocyte Recognition and Effector Mechanisms. Academic Press, New York.

91. Ling, G. N., and Walton, C. L. 1976. What retains water in living cells. Science 191: 293–295.

92. Lonai, P., Clark, W. R., and Feldman, M. 1971. Participation of θ-bearing cells in an in vitro assay of transplantation immunity. Nature (Lond.) 229: 566–567.

93. Luce, G. G. 1971. Body Time. Pantheon Books, New York.

94. Lustig, H. J., and Bianco, C. 1976. Antibody-mediated cell cytotoxicity in a defined system: Regulation by antigen, antibody and complement. J. Immunol. 116: 253–260.

95. Mackaness, G. B., and Lagrange, P. H. 1974. Restoration of cell mediated immunity to animals blocked by a humoral response. J. Exp. Med. 140: 865–870.

96. MacLennan, I. C. M. 1972. Antibody in the induction and inhibition of lymphocyte cytotoxicity. Transplant. Rev. 13: 67–90.

97. MacLennan, I. C. M. 1972. Competition for receptors for immunoglobulin on cytotoxic lymphocytes. Clin. Exp. Immunol. 10: 275–283.

98. MacLennan, I. C., and Howard, A. 1972. Evidence for correlation between the antigenic specificity and charge of IgG. A study of antibody-inducing lymphocyte mediated cell damage. Immunology 20: 1043–1049.

99. MacLennan, I. C. M., Loewi, G., and Harding, B. 1970. The role of immunoglobulins in lymphocyte-mediated cell damage in vitro. I. Comparison of the effects of target cell specific antibody and normal serum factors on cellular damage by immune and non-immune lymphocytes. Immunology 18: 397–404.

100. MacLennan, I. C. M., Howard, A., Gotch, F. M., and Quie, P. G. 1973.

Effector activating determinants on IgG. I. The distribution and factors influencing the display of complement, neutrophil and cytotoxic B-cell determinants on human IgG sub-classes. *Immunology* 25: 459–469.

101. Mahler, H. R. 1973. Mitochondria: Molecular biology, genetics, and development, in *Addison Wesley Module in Biology, No. 1.* Addison Wesley Publishing Co., Reading, Mass.   /

102. Marchalonis, J. J., Cone, R. E., and Santer, V. 1971. Enzymic iodination. A probe for accessible surface proteins of normal and neoplastic lymphocytes. *Biochem. J.* 124: 921–927.

103. Martz, E., Burakoff, S. J., and Benacerraf, B. 1974. Interruption of the sequential release of small and large molecules from tumor cells by low temperature during cytolysis mediated by immune T-cells or complement. *Proc. Natl. Acad. Sci. USA* 71: 177–181.

103a. McGovern, J. P., Smolensky, M. H., Reinberg, A. 1977. Chronobiology in allergy and immunology charges. C. Thomas Pub.

104. Miller, R. G. 1973, in R. Pain, and B. S. Smith (ed.), *New Techniques in Biophysics and Cell Biology 1.* Wiley, London.

105. Mitchell, M. S. 1972. Central inhibition of cellular immunity to leukemia L1210 by isoantibody. *Cancer Res.* 32: 825–831.

106. Möller, G. 1969. Induction of DNA synthesis in normal human lymphocyte cultures by antigen-antibody complexes. *Clin. Exp. Immunol.* 4: 65–82.

107. Möller, G., and Suehag, S. E. 1972. Specificity of lymphocyte-mediated cytotoxicity induced by *in vitro* antibody-coated target cells. *Cell. Immunol.* 4: 1–19.

108. Nelson, D. S. (ed.). 1976. *Immunobiology of the Macrophage.* Academic Press, New York.

108a. Nepom, J. T., Hellström, I., and Hellström, K. E. (1977). Antigen-specific purification of blocking factors from sera of mice with chemically induced tumors. *Proc. Natl. Acad. Sci. U.S.A.* 71: 177–181.

109. Nowotny, A., Grohsman, J., Abdelnoor, A., Rote, N., Yang, C., and Waltersdorff, R. 1974. Escape of TA3 tumors from allogeneic immune rejection: Theory and experiments. *Eur. J. Immunol.* 4: 73–78.

110. Old, L. J., Stockert, E., Boyse, E. A., and Kim, J. H. 1968. Antigenic modulation loss of TL antigen from cells exposed to TL antibody. Study of the phenomena *in vitro. J. Exp. Med.* 127: 523–539.

111. Olivotto, M., and Bomford, R. 1974. *In vitro* inhibition of tumor cell growth and DNA synthesis by peritoneal and lung macrophages from mice injected with *Corynebacterium parvum. Int. J. Cancer* 13: 478–488.

112. Penfold, P. L., Greenberg, A. H., and Roitt, I. M. 1976. Characteristics of the effector cells mediating cytotoxicity against antibody-coated target cells. III. Ultrastructural studies. *Clin. Exp. Immunol.* 23: 91–97.

113. Perlmann, P., and Perlmann, H. 1970. Contractual lysis of antibody-coated chicken erythrocytes by purified lymphocytes. *Cell. Immunol.* 1: 300–315.

114. Perlmann, P., Perlmann, H., and Wigzell, H. 1972. Lymphocyte mediated cytotoxicity in vitro. Induction and inhibition by humoral antibody and nature of effector cells. *Transplant. Rev.* 13: 91–114.

115. Petranyi, G. G., Kiessling, R., and Klein, G. 1975. Genetic control of natural killer lymphocytes in the mouse. *Immunogenetics* 2: 53–61.

116. Playfair, J. H. L. 1974. The role of antibody in T-cell responses. *Clin. Exp. Immunol.* 17: 1–18.

117. Porter, K., Prescott, D., and Frye, J. 1973. Changes in surface morphology of Chinese hamster ovary cells during the cell cycle. *J. Cell Biol.* 57: 815–836.

118. Prehn, R. T. 1976. Do tumors grow because of the immune response of the host. *Transplant. Rev.* 28: 34–42.

119. Prehn, R. T. 1976. Tumor progression and homeostasis. *Adv. Cancer Res.* 23: 203–236.

120. Prehn, R. T., and Lappe, M. A. 1971. An immunostimulation theory of tumor development. *Transplant. Rev.* 7: 26–54.

121. Ptak, W., and Hanczakowska, M. 1975. Alloantibody-induced cytotoxicity of macrophages. *J. Immunol.* 115: 796–799.

122. Ran, M., and Witz, I. P. 1972. Tumor associated immunoglobulin enhancement of syngeneic tumors by IgG_2-containing tumor eluates. *Int. J. Cancer* 9: 242–247.

123. Ran, M., Klein, G., and Witz, I. P. 1976. Tumor-bound immunoglobulins. Evidence for the in vivo coating of tumor cells by potentially cytotoxic antitumor antibodies. *Int. J. Cancer* 17: 90–97.

123a. Russell, S. W., Gillespie, G. Y., Hansen, C. B., and Cochrane, C. G. (1976). Inflammatory cells in solid murine neoplasms. II. Cell types found throughout the course of moloney sarcoma regression or progression. *Int. J. Cancer* 18: 331–338.

123b. Ryser, J. E., Sordat, B., Cerottini, J. C., and Brunner, K. T. (1977). Mechanism of target cell lysis by cytolytic I lymphocytes. 1. Characterization of specific lymphocyte-target cell conjugates separated by velocity sedimentation. E. J. Immunol. 7: 110–117.

124. Sanderson, C. J. 1976. The mechanism of T-cell mediated cytotoxicity. II. Morphological studies of cell death by time-lapse microcinematography. *Proc. R. Soc. Biol.* 192: 241–255.

125. Schoorl, R., de la Rivière, A. B., von dem Borne, A. E. G., Kg., and Feltkamp-Vroom, T. M. 1976. Identification of T and B lymphocytes in human breast cancer with immunohistochemical techniques. *Amer. J. Pathol.* 84: 529–542.

126. Scornik, J. C. 1974. Antibody dependent cell-mediated cytotoxicity. II. Early interactions between effector and target cells. *J. Immunol.* 113: 1519–1532.

127. Scornik, J. C., Cosenza, H., Lee, W., Köhler, H., and Rowley, D. 1974. Antibody dependent cell-mediated cytotoxicity. I. Differentiation from antibody independent cytoxicity by normal IgG. *J. Immunol.* 113: 1510–1517.

128. Sellin, D., Wallach, D. F. H., and Fischer, H. 1971. Intercellular communication in cell-mediated cytotoxicity fluorscein transfer between H-2D target cells and H-2B lymphocytes in vitro. *Eur. J. Immunol.* 1: 453–458.

129. Sendo, F., Aoki, T., Boyse, E. A., and Buafo, C. K. 1975. Natural occurrence of lymphocytes showing cytotoxic activity to BALB/c radiation induced leukemia RL o 1 cells. *J. Natl. Cancer Inst.* 55: 603–609.

130. Senika, A., De Giorgi, L., and Cevy, J. P. 1974. Cell-mediated antitumor immunity in oncornavirus-induced tumors: specific cytostasis of tumor cells by spleen and lymph node cells. *Int. J. Cancer* 14: 386–395.

131. Shearer, W. T., Philpott, G. W., and Parker, C. W. 1973. Stimulation of cells by antibody. *Science* 182: 1357–1359.

132. Shearer, W. T., Philpott, G. W., and Parker, C. W. 1974. Humoral immunostimulation. I. Increased uptake of ^{125}I-iododeoxy-uridine and ^{3}H-thymidine into TNP-cells treated with anti-TNP antibody. *J. Exp. Med.* 139: 367–379.

133. Shearer, W. T., Atkinson, J. P., Frank, M. N., and Parker, C. W. 1975. Humoral stimulation. IV. Role of complement. *J. Exp. Med.* 141: 736–752.

134. Shearer, W. T., Philpott, G. W., and Parker, C. W. 1975. Humoral immunostimulation. II. Increased nucleoside incorporation, DNA synthesis and cell growth in L-cells treated with anti-L cell antibody. *Cell. Immunol.* 17: 447–462.

135. Shin, H. S., Kaliss, N., and Borenstein, D. 1972. Antibody-mediated suppression of grafted lymphoma cells. I. Participation of a host factor(s) other than complement. *Proc. Soc. Exp. Biol. Med.* 139: 684–689.

136. Sjögren, H. O. 1973. Blocking and unblocking of cell-mediated tumor immunity, in H. Busch (ed.), *Methods in Cancer Research*, Vol. 10, pp. 19–34. Academic Press, New York.

137. Sjögren, H. O., Hellström, I., Bansal, S. C., Warner, G. A., and Hellström, K. E. 1972. Elution of "blocking factors" from human tumors, capable of abrogating tumor-cell destruction by specifically immune lymphocytes. *Int. J. Cancer* 9: 274–283.

138. Snell, G. D., Winn, H. J., Stimpfling, J. H., and Parker, S. J. 1960. Depression by antibody of the immune response to homografts and its role in immunological enhancement. *J. Exp. Med.* 112: 293–314.

139. Strom, T. B., Tilney, N. L., Carpenter, C. B., and Busch, G. J. 1973. Identity and cytotoxic capacity of cells infiltrating renal allografts. *N. Engl. J. Med.* 292: 1257–1263.

140. Stulting, R. D., Berke, G., and Hiemstra, K. 1973. Evaluation of the effects of cytochalasin B on lymphocyte-mediated cytolysis. *Transplantation* 16: 684–686.

140a. Stutman, O., Shen, F. W., and Boyse, E. A. (1977). LY phenotype of T cells cytotoxic for syngeneic mouse mammary tumors: evidence for T cell interactions. *Proc. Natl. Acad. Sci. U.S.A.* 74: 5667–5671.

141. Takasugi, M., and Klein, E. 1971. The methodology of microassay for cell-mediated immunity (CMI), in B. R. Bloom and P. R. Glade (eds.), *In Vitro Methods in Cell-Mediated Immunity*, pp. 415–422. Academic Press, New York.

142. Takasugi, M., and Klein, E. 1971. The role of blocking antibodies in immunological enhancement. *Immunology* 21: 675–684.

143. Tamerius, J., Nepom, J., Hellström, I., and Hellström, K. E. 1976. Tumor-associated blocking factors: Isolation from sera of tumor-bearing mice. *J. Immunol.* 116: 724–730.

144. Thomas, L. 1959. Mechanisms involved in tissue damage by the endotoxins of gram negative bacteria, in H. S. Lawrence (ed.), *Cellular and Humoral Aspects of the Hypersensitive States*, p. 451. Hoeber-Harper, New York.

145. Thompson, D. M. P., Steele, K., and Alexander, P. 1973. The presence of tumor-specific membrane antigen in the serum of rats with chemically induced sarcomata. Brit. J. Cancer 27: 27–47.

146. Ting, C., and Heberman, R. B. 1976. Humoral host defense mechanisms against tumors. Int. Rev. Exp. Pathol. 15: 93–152.

147. Tsoi, M., and Weiser, R. A. 1968. Mechanism of immunity to sarcoma. I. Allografts in the C57/K_s mouse. II. Passive transfer studies with immune serum in x-irradiated hosts. J. Natl. Cancer Inst. 40: 31–36.

148. Uhr, J. W., and Möller, G. 1968. Regulatory effect of antibody on the immune response. Adv. Immunol. 8: 81–127.

149. van Boxel, J. A., Stobo, J. D., Paul, W. E., and Green, I. 1972. Antibody-dependent lymphoid cell-mediated cytotoxicity: No requirement for thymus-derived lymphocytes. Science 175: 194–196.

150. Wasserman, J., Packalén, T., and Perlmann, P. 1971. Antibody-induced lysis of thyroglobulin-coated chicken erythrocytes by lymphocytes of nonimmunized guinea pigs. Int. Arch. Allergy 41: 910–919.

151. Weigle, W. O. 1975. Cyclical production of antibody as a regulatory mechanism in the immune response. Adv. Immunol. 21: 87–111.

152. Wisloff, F., Michaelsen, T. E., Froland, S. S. 1974. Inhibition of antibody-dependent human lymphocyte-mediated cytotoxicity by immunoglobulin classes IgG subclasses, and IgG fragments. Scand. J. Immunol. 3: 29–38.

153. Witz, I. P. 1973. The biological significance of tumor bound immunoglobulins. Curr. Top. Microbiol. Immunol. 61: 151–171.

154. Wolberg, G., Hiemstra, K., Burge, R. J., and Singler, R. C. 1973. Reversible inhibition of lymphocyte-mediated cytolysis by dimethyl sulfoxide (DMSO). J. Immunol. 111: 1435–1443.

155. Wolf, J. E., Faanes, R. B., and Choi, Y. S. Antigenic changes of DBA/2J mastocytoma cells when grown in the BALB/c mouse. (1977. J. Natl. Canc. Inst. 58: 1407–1412.)

155a. Wolf, J. E., Faanes, R. B., and Chol, Y. S. The existence of antibodies against minor histocompatibility antigens (unpublished observation).

156. Yefenof, E., Witz, I. P., and Klein, E. 1976. Interaction of antibody and cell surface localized antigen. Int. J. Cancer 17: 633–639.

157. Yu, A., and Cohen, E. P. 1974. Studies on the effect of specific antisera on the metabolism of cellular antigens. II. The synthesis and degradation of TL antigens of mouse cells in the presence of TL antiserum. J. Immunol. 112: 1296–1307.

158. Zembala, M., Ptak, W., and Hanczakowska, M. 1973. The role of macrophages in the cytotoxic killing of tumor cells in vitro. Immunology 25: 631–644.

159. Zighelboim, J., Bonavida, B., and Fahey, J. L. 1973. Evidence for several cell populations active in antibody dependent cellular cytotoxicity. J. Immunol. 111: 1737–1742.

160. Zighelboim, J., Bonavida, B., and Fahey, J. L. 1974. Antibody-mediated in vivo suppression of EL-4 leukemia in a syngeneic host. J. Natl. Cancer Inst. 52: 879–881.

CHAPTER 2

RADIOLABELED ANTITUMOR ANTIBODIES

David Pressman

Department of Immunology Research
Roswell Park Memorial Institute
Buffalo, New York 14263

The development of the use of radiolabeled antitumor antibodies as possible diagnostic and therapeutic agents in the control of cancer is traced historically and various problems involved in the development are discussed.

In view of the current interest in the use of radioiodinated antibodies to carry diagnostic or therapeutic amounts of radioactivity to tumors or to carry therapeutic amounts of toxic agents to tumors, I am taking this opportunity to trace the development of these fields and some of the impact of these studies on other fields.

Since the turn of the century attempts have been made to use antisera prepared against malignant tissues in the treatment of cancer. Thus, in 1895 J. Hericourt and Charles Richet (who was Nobel Laureate in Medicine and Physiology in 1913 for his work in anaphylaxis), following their 1888 report (32) that antisera prepared against infectious agents were effective in combating the corresponding diseases, reasoned that such antisera prepared against cancerous tissue might be effective in combating cancer (33). They prepared antisera against a human osteogenic sarcoma in an ass and two dogs by injecting them with the gauze filtrate of the homogenate of the tumor and bleeding the animals 6, 7, and 12 days afterwards to obtain the sera. These sera were used effectively in reducing two different tumors, one a fibrosarcoma of the chest wall, proven to be a fibrosarcoma on microscopic section, and the other a cancer of the stomach. In both cases they reported good results with a reduction in tumor volume. Subsequently they reported results for over 50 cases treated similarly by themselves or their colleagues with excellent results in general (34). They reported alleviation of pain, reduction of ulceration, decreased volume of the tumor and retardation of the course of the disease. Normal serum was ineffective in the case so treated.

Since then many investigators have made studies on the treatment of cancer in humans or in animals with heterologous antitumor antisera. In spite of glowing reports, a general therapy did not develop. The failure of investigators to obtain consistent positive results may have been due to one or more reasons: (a) The serum contained no antibodies which would react with any part of the tissue. This is unlikely, since antibodies of some sort can usually be obtained by such a procedure. (b) The sera contained antibodies which cross-reacted with other tissues and were completely taken up by the other tissues. (c) The sera contained antibodies for specific components inside the tumor cells, but could not reach these intracellular components and affect them. (d) The sera contained antibodies which did localize in the tissue, but did not produce an observable physiological effect, and, since the results were actually dependent upon a physiological effect of the antiserum, negative results were recorded.

In the atmosphere of 1946 when I first became interested in the problem of an immunotherapy of cancer using heteroantibodies (and was supported in this endeavor as a Senior Fellow of the American Cancer Society), I realized that it had to be proven that there are antibodies in an antiserum prepared against a tumor which do go to the tumor and that this could be accomplished by the use of radioactive tracers. If an antiserum against the tissue was prepared and the antibodies were tagged by coupling radioactive substances to them or by having radioactive elements incorporated in the antibody molecule, disposition of the antibody could be traced by following the disposition of the radioactivity. Then if it were possible to demonstrate that antibodies did go to the tumor, it should be possible to use them to carry sufficient amounts of radioactivity to be useful therapeutically or diagnostically even though the original antibodies were physiologically ineffective by themselves (70).

We were able to show that antibodies prepared in rabbits against certain animal tumors contained antibodies which do get to the tumor (47, 81). This has been confirmed by subsequent experiments and in the laboratory of Bale and Spar (1955) (6). In 1958, Dr. Day, Dr. Blau, and I were able to show that radioiodinated antibodies could be used diagnostically since antibodies localized in a tumor could be determined by scanning (74). That tumor-localizing antibodies could be made to carry a therapeutic dose of radioactivity to the tumor was first demonstrated by Bale, Spar, and Goodland in 1960 (5). Since then several groups of investigators have used radiolabeled antitumor antibodies both diagnostically and therapeutically (vide infra) and indeed Ghose et al. (25) last year reported therapeutic benefits in humans due to the localized radioactivity.

When I started the problem I first had to choose a suitable means of labeling the antibody and then show that the label did not destroy antibody activity. The fact that various substances can be coupled to antibodies without destroying the ability of the latter to combine with antigen had been shown previously. Thus, as early as 1930, Reiner (95) showed that arsanilic acid can be diazotized and coupled to antibodies without destroying antibody specificity. Eagle et al. showed similar effects in 1936 (19). It is not too surprising that this is possible, since the antibody molecule is very large, with a molecular weight of about 160,000 and the antibody specific region is just a small part of the surface of the molecule. Marrack in 1934 (57) was able to couple a red dye to antityphoid serum and showed that the typhoid bacteria, when agglutinated with the antiserum, were colored red. The serum was labeled by coupling "R-salt" to one end of bisdiazotized benzidine and the serum to the other. Later, in 1941 Coons, Creech, and Jones (11) prepared a labeled antipneumococcus type 3 antibody by coupling the protein with β-anthrylisocyanate to give β-anthrylcarbamido groups. Pneumococcus type 3 organisms, when agglutinated with this reagent, showed a blue fluorescence. Then in 1952 Coons, Creech *et al.* (12) coupled fluorescein-4-isocyanate with antibody against type 3 pneumococcus, and the pneumococci, agglutinated, showed a green fluorescence. They were able to show the presence of pneumococcus type 3 in tissues by means of this reagent. Their technique was to sacrifice an animal heavily infected with pneumococcus type 3, prepare slides of the various tissues and stain the slides with the fluorescein labeled antibody. The regions of the tissue which showed the green fluorescence were considered to be those containing either the pneumococci or the specific polysaccharide. In all the labelings so far described, there has been a known definite chemical bond formed between the antibody and the material coupled. For instance, the diazotized compound coupled with the tyrosine and with the histidine to form an azo linkage and the isocyanates coupled with free amino groups of the protein to form carbamido linkages. McClintock and Friedman in 1945 (61) reported that they "combined" "metallic" uranium and malachite green with antibodies against pneumococcus polysaccharide and claimed localization of the label in regions which had been heavily infiltrated with the pneumococcus polysaccharide. From the relative quantities of label and antibody and from the methods used it would appear that any observed effect was not due to labeled antibody.

For my work, I decided on the use of radioiodine-131 as a tracer. It has the advantages that iodine will directly iodinate the tyrosine and, probably, the histidine of a protein molecule, and this forms a definite chemical bond with the protein molecule. It is easily obtained, easily counted, and has a convenient half-life. Iodine has the disadvantage that it goes to the thyroid, but it is known that this can be controlled by feeding non-radioactive potassium iodide.

The first iodine I used was the short-lived, 25-minute half-life, [128]I made by the Szilard-Chalmers nuclear excitation reaction by bombardment of ordinary [127]I ethyl iodide with neutrons from the Van de Graaff machine at Caltech (courtesy of Dr. Charles C. Lauritsen). The [131]I I first used came from the nuclear facility at Oakridge, Tenn., as the neutron irradiated tellurium target from which I had to isolate the [131]I. Using the short-life [128]I, I was able to determine the conditions for coupling iodine to globulin and show that antibodies could be made radioactive by iodination. Subsequently, with ^{131}I, I was able to show the iodination did not destroy antibody activity. Antiovalbumin antibody iodinated with radiolabeled iodine was shown to be still specifically precipitable (79).

For the next step we studied radiolabeled antibodies to rat kidney. Since Masugi (58) and later Smadel (102) had shown that antisera raised in rabbits against rat kidney were nephrotoxic and produced physiological changes in the structure of the rat kidney when administered intravenously into the rat, it seemed logical that such a serum contained antibody which goes to the kidney. Then, if the antibody were labeled, it should be possible to follow it to the kidney. We reported this experiment in 1948 by preparing such an antiserum against kidney tissue, separating out the globulin fraction by alcohol precipitation and then iodinating with iodine containing tracer concentrations of ^{131}I (79). We injected several rats with this radioiodinated globulin fraction of antikidney serum and others with a similarly prepared radioiodinated globulin fraction of antiovalbumin serum as a control, waited for 4 days and then sacrificed the animals. On analyzing the various tissues, we found evidence for specific localization. With the antikidney preparation there was appreciable accumulation of radioactivity in the kidney, whereas with the antiovalbumin there was practically no accumulation in the kidney. This showed definitely that there were antibodies in the antikidney serum which localized in the kidney. The localization was not due to a general property of globulin molecules since there was no localization for the antiovalbumin preparation.

There was an accumulation of radioactivity by other organs when radioiodinated antikidney antibody was administered, but to a lower extent than was observed with the kidney. This cross-reaction was due to the presence of common types of tissue in the various organs, such as blood vessels, etc. The cross-reacting antibodies could be removed by suitable absorption with preparations from other organs.

Subsequently we showed that the actual localization was in the glomerular tuft by making radioautographs of sections of the kidney. Kidneys from animals receiving normal rabbit globulin labeled with iodine showed no such localization (76, 78).

The rate of removal of antikidney antibodies from the circulation was determined and it was found that they were essentially completely removed from the blood as it passed through the kidney (76, 77), and it took a tremendous amount of antibody to saturate the kidney (75).

Antibody remained fixed in kidney for months, being removed with a half-life of 20 days in the case of the rat (70).

Antibodies with specificities for other tissues and organs have been found by radioiodine methods; for example, antibodies favoring localization in adrenal, liver, lung, placenta have been studied (35, 46, 82, 103, 108, 109).

That antibodies prepared against a tumor and injected into the tumor-bearing animal can be fixed in the tumor was first shown in our laboratory in 1953 in the case of the Wagner osteogenic sarcoma of mice (81), and then in 1954 in the case of the Murphy lymphosarcoma of rats (47).

By the use of the paired label methods (vide infra) fixation of iodine labeled antitumor antibodies raised in rabbits has been found with the

2-acetaminofluorene induced hepatoma of rats (15), the L1210 lymphoma of mice (45) and the MOPC 104E plasmacytoma of mice (90). Iodine labeled antibodies raised in the same species were found by the Bale group to localize in a transplantable methyl cholanthrene induced tumor of rats (1, 42).

All of the tumors mentioned above were transplantable tumors except for the 2-acetaminofluorene induced hepatoma. In the latter case each animal used bore autochthonous tumors. Extensive studies have been carried out with them (39, 40, 41). Radioiodinated antihepatoma antibodies, after purification in vivo from induced hepatomas in rats, localized in the total hepatic region (liver with hepatoma) of hepatoma-bearing rats to an extent as high as 60% of the injected dose (39). The localized antibodies were shared almost equally by hepatoma and non-neoplastic portions. When the purified antibodies were passively transferred through normal rats, cross-localizing antibodies were absorbed from the circulation. Antibodies that remained in the serum, when assayed in hepatoma-bearing rats, preferentially localized in discrete hepatomas and localized to as high as 40 percent of the injected dose in the total hepatic region. When assayed in normal rats, the same preparation localized at the 4 percent level in liver. Antihepatoma antibodies, when purified in vivo from normal liver of normal rats and assayed in hepatoma-bearing rats, preferentially localized in the non-neoplastic portions of the hepatic region.

A more precise evaluation of just where the tumor localization took place in the acetamino-induced hepatoma was made by Kyogoku et al. (48). The localization of antibodies to the hepatoma and to normal liver were compared by radioautography and fluorescent antibody techniques and their localizations in hepatoma and liver were different showing tumor specificity following suitable absorption techniques.

The amount of radioactivity which can be incorporated into antibody molecules certainly is sufficient to be useful therapeutically or diagnostically. The main problem is to have a sufficient proportion located in the tumor. That sufficiently large amounts of radioactivity can be incorporated and reach the tumor has been shown by the fact that therapy has been reported to be achieved with radioiodinated antibody injected into the tumor-bearing host in the case of tumors in rats (105), in mice (23), and in humans (25).

That the radiation from radioiodinated antibodies can kill tumor cells in vitro has been shown by Ghose et al. (21).

That radioiodinated antibodies can be used diagnostically in radioscanning for tumor has been shown to be possible in animals (22, 23, 25, 28, 74) and in humans (25, 36, 52, 53, 54, 60, 69, 94).

Calculations have been published on the amounts which can be fixed in tissues and the effective dose required (3, 62, 76, 110, 111).

Paired Label

A complication in the determination of localization of antibody in a tumor became evident in the early experiments. Tumors pick up globulins (and other macromolecules) nonspecifically and there are large variations in the size and uniformity of the tumor which affect the apparent specific localization.

Although it is possible to determine the localization of the antikidney antibody by injecting one group of rats with antikidney antibody and another group with radiolabeled control protein such as antiovalbumin antibody and show that there was greater localization of antibody in the kidney, this procedure is not nearly as satisfactory in the case of tumor. Even if rats are all implanted with the same size pieces of tumor, the tumors grow at different rates and achieve different sizes and different parts of the tumor are of different quality; one part may be avascular, another part may be necrotic and another part may be very vascular. The different parts will pick up control protein and antibody protein to different extents. Also, tumors frequently show a relatively high nonspecific pickup of macromolecules such as globulin as first reported by Duran-Reynolds in 1939 (18). Because of these complications in the case of tumor, the paired radioiodine label technique was developed in which the antitumor antibodies are labeled with one radioactive isotope of iodine, for example, ^{125}I, and normal control globulins are labeled with another, e.g., ^{131}I. The two preparations are mixed and injected into tumor-bearing animals. It is possible then to cut the tumor into small pieces and determine how much antibody and how much control protein is present in each piece. In this manner, a small differential pickup of antibody can be determined even though the pickup is not uniform throughout the tumor mass (73).

The paired label technique has been extended to the triad label technique in which the localization of three protein preparations, i.e., antitumor antibody, antinormal tissue antibody, and control globulin, can be determined simultaneously using three different isotopes of iodine, a different one to label each protein (16). In order to handle the computations involved in the paired and triad label techniques computer programs have been developed (83, 84).

Mechanism of Localization

Most rapid localization of antibodies takes place when the antigen involved is in the lumen of the blood vessel exposed to the circulation. This is the situation in the glomerular tuft in the kidney. The blood is cleared of the antibody as it passes through the kidney (7). The cleared blood is returned to the intravascular pool of blood and rapidly mixed with it diluting the remaining labeled antibody. It would take an infinite time for all of the antibody molecules to pass through the kidney. Indeed, although the kidneys receive one-third of the cardiac output and clear the blood of antibody as it passes through, it still requires 15 minutes to remove 90 percent of the antibody from the circulation. The rapid localization was also observed for antibodies showing preferential localization in the lung (108, 109), liver (7) and in adrenal (35). These specificities are an indication that the vascular beds of these organs are different and this must be due to exposure of tissue specific antigen to the blood (72).

In the case of tumors, for the radiolabeled antibody to localize on the tumor cell, it must react with an antigen in the cell surface. If this antigen and the corresponding portion of cell surface are part of the lumen of the blood vessel, then localization is most rapid, although still probably slow because of the small fraction of the cardiac output received by the tumor. If the tumor cells are not exposed directly to the blood then we must depend on the extravascular fluid to carry the antibody to the cell. This greatly slows down the rate of localization and limits the fraction of specific antibody present which can be fixed on the cell before the antibody is metabolized (3). The situation can be helped, in a practical way, in these problems of distribution, by keeping the antibody in the vicinity of the tumor cell by the use of either a circulation isolation technique which permits continued circulation in a limited portion of the body without involving the main blood volume of the individual or perfusion of the involved region of the body by bringing the labeled antibody by catheter into juxtaposition with the tumor as described by Order (69).

If the antibody localizes on the surface of cells capable of capping it can be interiorized as shown by Lewis, Pegram, and Evans (50) and by Robert et al. (96, 97) and thus expose internal cell components to agents coupled to the tumor which are cytotoxic to interior components.

If the antibody is not directed to a cell surface constituent but is directed to an interior component and depends on pinocytosis for delivery inside the cell, there would not be any difference from delivery of normal globulin to the inside of the cell and the uptake would be much too slow for effective diagnostic or therapeutic use.

Weissman et al. (111) have measured the fixation of radiolabeled tumor localizing antibodies by determining the reduction of tumor reactive radioactivity remaining in the circulation at various times. They found that Moloney lymphoma bearing mice, regardless of whether the tumor had been implanted intravenously, subcutaneously or intraperitoneally, showed appreciable loss of in vivo filtered rat anti-tumor antibodies from the circulation apparently indicating good contact of circulating antibody with tumor substances. However they did not determine whether or not the localization was on tumor tissue or as fixation of antigen-antibody complexes in various tissues.

Preparation of Specific Antibody Reagents

During the course of these investigations it became apparent we had to develop methods for purifying antibodies, i.e., isolating antibodies which localized specifically in the tumor. We made use of specific absorbents to concentrate antibodies capable of localizing in the tumor and made use of other specific absorbents to remove cross-localizing antibodies which can and do localize elsewhere than in the tumor. We also put effort into the preparation of more specific antibodies in the first place either by using a purer tumor antigen preparation for raising antibodies or by rendering animals tolerant to normal tissue antigens so that they would produce antibodies only to the tumor specific antigens. Originally we used the insoluble portions of tissues, normal or tumor, and subsequently the microsome fraction as absorbents on the basis that specific localization would be limited to the cell membranes and the insoluble microsome fraction represents cell membrane. Indeed in experiments involving the fractionation of tumor tissue by differential centrifugation of the homogenate following injection of iodine labeled antibody to the MOPC 104E plasmacytoma into mice bearing the tumor, the principle localization was observed on the microsome fraction (90).

In some earlier investigations, some antibodies were purified by injecting the radioiodinated antibody into tumor-bearing animals and the antibodies fixed in the tumor (or normal tissue of interest) were eluted and then used for assay in a second animal with increased localizing activity (4, 87).

In other cases the original preparation of radiolabeled antibody or antibody purified in vivo as above was injected into normal rats to remove antibodies capable of reacting with normal tissue constituents and then the animals were bled and the radiolabeled globulin remaining in the circulation assayed for localizing activity. They showed a particularly high specific localization in the tumor in the case of the acetaminofluorene induced hepatoma of rats (15, 17).

A great step forward is the use of a purified antigen so that when it is used for raising antibody, a large part of the antibody which is produced will be capable of reacting with the tumor specific antigen and so that it is more effective when used for purifying the antibodies. Thus the isolation of pure CEA antigen from human colonic cancers has given a very fruitful means of producing and purifying anti-CEA antibodies and determining their localization in human colonic tumors carried by nude mice or hamsters and still producing CEA (9, 10, 27, 28, 36, 51, 92, 93).

Also the availability of a highly specific Hodgkin's ferritin has permitted the preparation of sufficiently pure and specific radioiodinated antibody to permit visualization of the tumor when the antibody was infused directly in the tumor region (69).

In order to reduce nonspecific binding of radiolabeled antibody to normal cells it has been suggested that Fab fragments made by papain digestion of the antibody molecule be used in place of the intact molecule. This would reduce the nonspecific binding to Fc receptors on cells giving a more specific reaction. However there may be a problem of avidity of binding of Fab to tumor. We made a study of localization of Fab fragments in the rat kidney from rabbit anti-rat kidney serum and found that there was very transitory localization since the Fab fragment was removed after being fixed very much faster than the intact antibody (107). Apparently the univalent nature of the Fab fragment greatly reduces its apparent binding constant with antigen similar to that observed with the difference in precipitating activity of IgG and IgM antibodies (see Ref. 44). Nevertheless, Coates et al. (10) have reported localization of radioiodinated Fab fragments of anti-CEA antibodies in transplanted human colonic tumors in hamsters.

Another possible problem is the possible presence of antigen in the circulation which would bind to antibody rendering it non-localizing or excess antibody in the circulation which might compete successfully for sites on the cell. If antigen or antibody in circulation becomes a problem, it might be removed by the thoracic fistula method of Rose (99) in which humoral factors in the circulation are removed along with the cellular constituents as lymph from the thoracic duct. The cellular components are returned and the humoral components removed. Plasma is used to replace the removed lymph fluid.

Another problem is sensitization by the heteroantiserum. The latter might well be overcome when it becomes a problem by desensitization by sequentially using antibody prepared in various species by using chemical alteration to the antibody to alter its antigenicity or by using immunosuppressive agents.

The Iodination Procedure

Oxidized iodine in the form of hypoiodous acid, HOI, reacts with the tyrosines and histidines of the antibody molecule. In the initial studies the triiodide ion was used to produce HOI (79). However this method has the limitation that theroretically only one-third of the radioactive label at most can be incorporated in the antibody. Usually a much smaller fraction is incorporated. Then oxidation of iodide to HOI by nitrous acid became popular. Both of these methods depend on exchange of the radiolabel with the iodide added. Any radioactivity present as iodate does not exchange and thus reduces the yield on radioactivity incorporation. For cases where it is necessary to know precisely the number of iodines incorporated, the HOI was generated by the use of iodine monochloride (86). It is still used for qantitative work. It has the advantage that theoretically 100% of the radioactivity can be incorporated in the protein and yields of 70% are not uncommon.

Subsequently the chloramine T method (29) has replaced the first two methods since chloramine T will oxidize iodide to HOI and will continue to do so for any reduced iodine until all the iodine is incorporated. The chloramine T itself exerts some oxidizing power which usually does not seem to be very important in connection with antibody activity if its concentration is kept low but is very deleterious for certain other biologically active proteins. Weissman, Nord, and Baird (110) have shown that particularly at higher levels of chloramine T, there is marked inactivation of the antibody molecule, even when less than 1 atom of iodine is present per antibody molecule.

A fifth method of iodination involves the use of peroxidase and hydrogen peroxide (56, 65). Iodide in the presence of this system is oxidized and attached, in the oxidized state, to the active site of the peroxidase which then transfers it to a tyrosine. This is a very mild reaction and is used to iodinate surface proteins on cells on the basis that only the surface is accessible to the large peroxidase molecule. It even is considered to offer the advantage of iodinating only the surface of the immunoglobulin avoiding the specificity determining cleft on steric grounds. This would avoid loss of antibody activity during iodination (see below).

The number of iodines incorporated per molecule of antibody is not the same for all molecules present except where the average number of iodines per molecule is appreciably less than 1 (88). Then only a small proportion of the molecules are iodinated and these bear only 1 iodine each. When the average number approaches 1 or more there is a distribution of iodine such that various molecules of antibody have different numbers of iodine on a probability basis. Molecules with the same number of iodines may well differ from each other since they would have the iodines distributed over different tyrosines.

The effect of extent of iodination on antibody activity was first studied by us in an antihapten system where we showed that antibenzoate and anti-benzenearsonate antibodies lose their ability to precipitate when iodinated extensively (25 iodines per antibody molecule) and this loss can be prevented by the presence of the specific hapten protecting the site during iodination (88). Subsequently, Johnson, Day and I (43) studied the effect in the following systems: (a) The localizing activity of antikidney antibody, (b) the specific precipitation of antiovalbumin and of antibovine serum albumin, (c) the binding activity of antierythrocyte antibody. In each system the antibody activity decreased with iodination. However over 30 iodine atoms per antibody molecule were required to destroy activity. The destruction is interpreted as being due to iodination of a particular group, probably tyrosine, in the antibody specific site which may be more reactive or less reactive than other tyrosines in the molecule. Iodination below 2 atoms/molecule does not affect antibody activity of antibodies requiring only one site for activity, i.e., localizing, binding, or hemolytic antibodies.

It appears that low levels of iodination which can carry therapeutic levels of radioactivity have little effect on localization at least for normal organs. Thus with anti-rat kidney antibodies, the localizing activity was still 30% of the original localizing activity in the kidney when 19 atoms of iodine were present per molecule of globulin. The liver localizing activity was 50% of the original activity at the level of 19 atoms of iodine.

The effect on the precipitin reaction is interesting in that low levels of iodination of antihapten antibody with protection results in a greater precipitability of antibody than was observed with the original globulin fraction. It would appear that the hydrophobic nature of the iodines is probably necessary for increased interaction between the lightly iodinated molecules giving rise to a precipitation of antibodies which normally were not incorporated in the precipitate (85).

The effect of the extent of the iodination has been studied in many antihapten systems where iodination inactivates the antibody on extensive iodination by iodinating the tyrosine in the antigen combining site. The loss of activity increases with increasing iodination. However, appreciable binding activity is present even at levels of 30 iodines/molecule or greater (30). The activity can be protected during iodination by the presence of the specific hapten which protects tyrosines in the site against the iodination reaction. Indeed this type of experiment has permitted the determination of the sequences of the antibody molecule which form the antihapten binding site (86). The extent of loss of activity depends on the individual systems studied and the particular antibody produced since the various antibody molecules raised by the same hapten antigen have different degrees of inactivation by iodination (98).

Weissman and his colleagues (66, 67, 68, 110, 111) have made a very extensive study of the effect of iodination and the effect of the radioiodination on antibody activity. They have particularly studied the effect on the nonspecific pick up of the iodinated molecules in vivo since, if they are removed from circulation, they can no longer fix to tumor cells.

Other Labels Used

Methods other than iodination have been used for labeling antibodies with iodine although they offer little or no advantage for therapeutic or diagnostic purposes. Thus p-iodobenzoyl groups have been used (8). Although direct iodination seems to have very little effect on the localizing activity of the antibody particularly at low levels of iodination since increasing the amount of iodine per molecule has very little effect on the distribution of the radiolabeled antibody in the animal while there is evidence that some labels can affect localization nonspecifically. For example, fluorescein coupled to kidney localizing antibodies cause them to locate in the liver nonspecifically (91). Other labels can be used of course. ^{35}S labeled benzene sulfonic acid has been used as a label (77). Carbon and tritium of course can be used and these along with labels like sulfur require assay methods which will permit the determination of low energy beta particles emitted.

Hughes in 1957 suggested the possible use of astatine (just below iodine in the periodic table) as a label for antibody particularly in connection with immunotherapy (37). It reacts with protein as iodine does. Since the astatine emits an alpha particle in its decomposition, a very large amount of destructive energy is available right close to the localized antibody molecule.

Antifibrin Antibody Localization

In the course of our investigations, we made the observation that antibody to fibrin or fibrinogen will localize in fast growing tumors such as the Murphy lymphosarcoma of rats, or wherever fibrin is being deposited (13, 14). Almost simultaneously Spar, Goodland and Bale (106) reported the localization of anti-rat fibrin antibodies in the Murphy lymphosarcoma of rats. Following our original observation that antibodies made against the insoluble portion of the Murphy lymphosarcoma in rats would localize in the homologous tumor, we converted the tumor to the ascites form in hopes of getting a better antitumor antibody preparation by using tumor cells to raise antibody. These antibodies showed good localization in the Murphy lymphosarcoma. However, they showed good localization in several mouse tumors and it was subsequently found that fibrin was present in the preparation of ascites cells used as antigen and raised antibodies to fibrin which, when labeled and injected, were deposited in locations where fibrin clots were forming or had been formed. Thus a rapidly growing tumor induces fibrin deposition and will cause localization of the antifibrin antibodies. Since antifibrin was found to be fixed by several rapidly growing animal tumors, it indicated that fibrin might be a common tumor-associated antigen. It is interesting that the antifibrin localizes since it must form complexes with the fibrinogen in the circulation and either the antibody is more tightly bound to the fibrin clot and thus removed from the fibrinogen antibody complex or is deposited along with the fibrinogen as a fibrinogen is converted to fibrin on the clot. The use of the antifibrin antibody to locate animal and human tumors has been investigated by Spar, Bale and their colleagues (105) and McCardle et al. (60). The general use of the radiolabeled antifibrin antibodies in locating blood clots has also been investigated by these investigators.

Isolation of Localizing Activity from Normal Globulin

In carrying out controlled experiments for localization assays, there are two aspects to consider. The first is the comparison of the localizing properties of the purified antibody preparation with the properties of normal globulin. The second is the comparison with the properties of the product obtained when normal globulin is passed through the same specific purification procedure used for purifying antitumor antibodies, which includes absorption with a specific solid absorbent and subsequent elution. These isolates from the normal globulin substances act like localizing antibody. This is because normal globulin is a mixture of globulins, some of which may be able to bind with the antigens on the absorbent. These are retained in the purification process and act similar to the antibody isolated by the same absorbents. This was first shown by isolating globulins from normal globulin capable of localizing in different organs when components in these organs had been used as specific absorbents (80). Subsequently the same situation was shown by Winkler et al. to hold when normal globulin is treated with absorbents containing simple haptens (112). Globulins remarkably like raised antibodies in ability to bind the hapten are isolated.

It might be well to use a myeloma protein as the control globulin since a myeloma protein will be homogeneous having only one particular species of globulin and thus give a better base of reference than the complex and variable mixture termed normal globulin usually used. Perhaps the in vivo filtered globulin used by Bale et al. (1) is a good base line.

Antibodies as Carriers
for Cytotoxic Agents

Radiolabeling can play an important role in the recent efforts aimed at using cytotoxic agents coupled to antitumor antibodies to kill tumor cells selectively (20, 24, 25, 38, 49, 59, 63, 64, 100, 101). Although good results can be obtained in vitro where the antibody-cytotoxic agent conjugate is tested on a suspension of cells and contact with the cells is assured, there is still the problem of how effectively can the antibody get to the tumor in vivo. This is the same problem the radiolabeled antibody studies have been trying to overcome, i.e., means of increasing the fraction of injected material localized.

Tests should be carried out to determine whether the conjugated antibodies are still localizing on the tumor and this can be done by the use of radiolabeled techniques. The distribution of conjugated antibodies in vivo may well be affected by the substance coupled. The iodination seems to have relatively little effect on the localization whereas some of the other substances exert appreciable effects. We have found that when fluorescein isocyanate is coupled to antibodies it has the tendency to fix the antibody molecule or immunoglobulin in general in the liver. Thus antikidney antibodies labeled with fluorescein show a decreased localization in kidney and an increased localization in liver due to the nonspecific effect of the label (91).

Similar effects were observed when ^{35}S-labeled azobenzenesulfonate groups were coupled to immunoglobulin (77). Gitlin (26) reported that casein coupled with various diazonium salts accumulate differently in various tissues depending on the attached azo group.

Many of the cytotoxic substances being studied may be ineffective for the same reason: they fix the antibody to their preferred localization site rather than vice versa. In addition to the problem of localization, the molecules bearing most cytotoxic agents would depend on being interiorized in order for the toxic agent to be effective. As pointed out above, this interiorization can take place by capping for those cells which can cap.

In connection with antibodies carrying toxic substances to the tumor, a variation has been to use antibodies to carry boron derivatives to a tumor on the basis that subsequent neutron irradiation of the individual would result in high-dose radiation to the tumor through the decomposition of the boron-10 to helium and lithium residues on neutron absorption (31).

REFERENCES

1. Bale, W. F., Contreras, M. A., Izzo, M. J., Della Penta, D., and Buchsbaum, D. J. 1974. Preferential *in vivo* localization of ^{125}I-labeled antibody in a carcinogen-induced syngeneic rat tumor, *in* V. Richards (ed.), *Immunology of Cancer Progress in Experimental Tumor Research*, Vol. 19, pp. 270–283. S. Karger, Basel.

2. Bale, W. F., and Spar, I. L. 1954. *In vivo* localization of rat organ antibodies in ovaries, adrenals, and other tissues. *J. Immunol.* 73: 125–133.

3. Bale, W. F., and Spar, I. L. 1957. Studies directed toward the use of antibodies as carriers of radioactivity for therapy, *in* J. H. Lawrence and C. A. Tobias (eds.), *Advances in Biological and Medical Physics*, Vol. 5, pp. 285–356. Academic Press, New York.

4. Bale, W. F., Spar, I. L., and Goodland, R. L. 1958. *In vivo* purification of ^{131}I labeled localizing antirat lymphosarcoma antibody. *J. Immunol.* 80: 482–494.

5. Bale, W. F., Spar, I. L., and Goodland, R. L. 1960. Experimental radiation therapy of tumors with I[131]-carrying antibodies to fibrin. *Cancer Res.* 20: 1488–1494.

6. Bale, W. F., Spar, I. L., Goodland, R. L., and Wolfe, D. E. 1955. *In vivo* and *in vitro* studies of labeled antibodies against rat kidney and Walker carcinoma. *Proc. Soc. Exp. Biol. Med.* 89: 564–568.

7. Blau, M., Day, E. D., and Pressman, D. 1957. The rate of localization of anti-rat kidney antibodies. *J. Immunol.* 79: 330–333.

8. Blau, M., Johnson, A. C., and Pressman, D. 1958. p-iodobenzoyl groups as a paired label for *in vivo* protein distribution studies: specific localization of anti-tissue antibodies. *Int. J. Applied Rad. Isotopes* 3: 217–225.

9. Chao, H.-F., Peiper, S. C., Philpott, G. W., Parker, C. W., and Aach, R. D. 1974. Selective uptake of specifically purified antibodies to carcinoembryonic antigen of human adenocarcinoma. *Chem. Pathol. Pharmacol.* 9: 749–761.

10. Coates, J. E., Koch, M., Beaver, P. F., McPherson, T. A., and Noujaim, A. A. 1975. Radioiodinated antibody to carcinoembryonic antigen: Binding to normal and cancerous human colon *in vitro*. *J. Natl. Cancer Inst.* 55: 25–27.

11. Coons, A. H., Creech, H. J., and Jones, R. N. 1941. Immunological properties of an antibody containing a fluorescent group. *Proc. Soc. Exp. Biol. Med.* 47: 200–202.

12. Coons, A. H., Creech, H. J., Jones, R. N., and Berliner, E. 1942. The demonstration of pneumococcal antigen in tissues by the use of fluorescent antibody. *J. Immunol.* 45: 159–170.

13. Day, E. D., Planinsek, J. A., and Pressman, D. 1959. Localization *in vivo* of radioiodinated anti-rat-fibrin antibodies and radioiodinated rat fibrinogen in the Murphy rat lymphosarcoma and in other transplantable rat tumors. *J. Natl. Cancer Inst.* 22: 413–426.

14. Day, E. D., Planinsek, J. A., and Pressman, D. 1959. Localization of radioiodinated rat fibrinogen in transplanted rat tumors. *J. Natl. Cancer Inst.* 23: 799–812.

15. Day, E. D., Planinsek, J. A., and Pressman, D. 1960. Localization of

radioiodinated antibodies in rats bearing tumors induced by N-2-fluorenylacetamide. *J. Natl. Cancer Inst.* 25: 787–802.

16. Day, E. D., Planinsek, J. A., and Pressman, D. 1961. Triadic labeling with I^{130}, I^{131}, and I^{133} for controlled determinations of tumor-localizing antibodies. *J. Natl. Cancer Inst.* 26: 1321–1333.

17. Day, E. D., Planinsek, J. A., and Pressman, D. 1961. Specific localization *in vivo* of antihepatoma antibodies in autochthonous rat hepatomas. *J. Natl. Cancer Inst.* 27: 1107–1114.

18. Duran-Reynolds, F. 1939. Studies on the localization of dye and foreign proteins in normal and malignant tissues. *Amer. J. Cancer* 35: 98.

19. Eagle, H., Smith, D., and Vickers, P. 1936. The effect of combination with diazo compounds on the immunological reactivity of antibodies. *J. Exp. Med.* 63: 617–643.

20. Flechner, I. 1973. The cure and concomitant immunization of mice bearing Ehrlich ascites tumors by treatment with an antibody-alkylating agent complex. *Eur. J. Cancer* 9: 741–745.

21. Ghose, T., Cerini, M., Carter, M., and Nairn, R. C. 1967. Immunoradioactive agent against cancer. *Brit. Med. J.* 1: 90–93.

22. Ghose, T., and Guclu, A. 1974. Cure of a mouse lymphoma with radioiodinated antibody. *Eur. J. Cancer* 10:787–792.

23. Ghose, T., Guclu, A., Tai, J., MacDonald, A. S., Norvell, S. T., and Aquino, J. 1975. Antibody as carrier of ^{131}I in cancer diagnosis and treatment. *Cancer* 36: 1646–1657.

24. Ghose, T., Norvell, S. T., Guclu, A., Cameron, D., Bodurtha, A., and MacDonald, A. S. 1972. Immunochemotherapy of cancer with chlorambucil-carrying antibody. *Brit. Med. J.* 3: 495–499.

25. Ghose, T., Tai, J., Guclu, A., Norvell, S. T., Bodurtha, A., Aquino, J., and MacDonald, A. S. 1976. Antibodies as carriers of radionuclides and cytotoxic drugs in the treatment and diagnosis of cancer. *Ann. N.Y. Acad. Sci.* 277: 671–689.

26. Gitlin, D. 1950. Distribution of azoproteins in the tissues of the normal mouse. *Proc. Soc. Exp. Biol. Med.* 74: 138–142.

27. Goldenberg, D. M., and Hansen, H. J. 1972. Carcinoembryonic antigen present in human colonic neoplasms serially propagated in hamsters. *Science* 175: 1117–1118.

28. Goldenberg, D. M., Preston, D. F., Primus, F. J., and Hansen, H. J. 1974. Photoscan localization of GW-39 tumors in hamsters using radiolabeled anticarcinoembryonic antigen immunoglobulin G. *Cancer Res.* 34: 1–9.

29. Greenwood, F. C., Hunter, W. M., and Glover, J. S. 1963. The preparation of ^{131}I-labeled human growth hormone of high specific radioactivity. *Biochem. J.* 89: 114–123.

30. Grossberg, A. L., Radzimski, G., and Pressman, D. 1962. Effect of iodination on the active site of several antihapten antibodies. *Biochemistry* 1: 391–401.

31. Hawthorne, M. F., Wiersema, R. J., and Takasugi, M. 1972. Preparation of tumor-specific boron compounds. I. *In vitro* studies using boron-labeled antibodies and elemental boron as neutron targets. *J. Med. Chem.* 15: 449–452.

32. Hericourt, J., and Richet, C. 1888. De la transfusion peritoneal et de l'immunité qu'elle confère. *C.R. Acad. Sci.* 107: 748–750.

33. Hericourt, J., and Richet, C. 1895. Traitement d'un cas de sarcome par la serotherapie. *C.R. Acad. Sci.* 120: 948–950.

34. Hericourt, J., and Richet, C. 1895. De la serotherapie dans le traitment du cancer. *C.R. Acad. Sci.* 121: 567–569.

35. Hiramoto, R., Yagi, Y., and Pressman, D. 1958. *In vivo* fixation of antibodies in the adrenal. *Proc. Soc. Exp. Biol. Med.* 98: 870–874.

36. Hoffer, P. B., Lathrop, K., Bekerman, C., Fang, V. S., and Refetoff, S. 1974. Use of ^{131}I-CEA antibody as a tumor scanning agent. *J. Nucl. Med.* 15: 323–327.

37. Hughes, W. L. 1957. The chemistry of iodination. *Ann. N.Y. Acad. Sci.* 70: 3–18.

38. Isliker, H., Cerottini, J. C., Jaton, J. C., and Magnenat, G. 1964. Specific and nonspecific fixation of plasma proteins in tumors, in P. A. Plattner (ed.), *Chemotherapy of Cancer*, Proceedings of International Symposium, Lugano, Switzerland, p. 278. Elsevier, Amsterdam.

39. Isojima, S., Bernecky, J., Planinsek, J., Yagi, Y., Pressman, D. 1965. Differences between antibodies against the dense sediment and microsome fractions of the N-2-fluorenylacetamide-induced rat hepatoma. *Cancer Res.* 25: 968–975.

40. Isojima, S., Planinsek, J., Yagi, Y., and Pressman, D. 1966. Differences between the microsomes of normal rat liver and of N-2-fluorenylacetamide-induced rat hepatoma as determined by the paired label antibody technic. *Cancer Res.* 26: 1527–1533.

41. Isojima, S., Yagi, Y., Planinsek, J., and Pressman, D. 1965. Purification of localizing antibodies formed against microsomes of the N-2-fluorenylacetamide-induced rat hepatoma. *Cancer Res.* 25: 962–967.

42. Izzo, J. J., Buchsbaum, D. J., and Bale, W. F. 1972. Localization of an ^{125}I-labeled rat transplantation antibody in tumors carrying the corresponding antigens. *Proc. Soc. Exp. Biol. Med.* 139: 1185–1188.

43. Johnson, A., Day, E. D., and Pressman, D. 1960. The effect of iodination on antibody activity. *J. Immunol.* 84: 213–220.

44. Karush, F. 1976. Multivalent binding and functional affinity, in H. N. Eisen and R. A. Reisfeld (eds.), *Contemporary Topics in Molecular Immunology*, Vol. 5, pp. 217–228. Plenum Press, New York.

45. Kitano, M., Mihich, E., and Pressman, D. 1972. Antigenic differences between leukemia L1210 and a subline resistant to methylglyoxal-bis(guanylhydrazone). *Cancer Res.* 32: 181–186.

46. Korngold, L., and Pressman, D. 1953. The *in vitro* purification of tissue localizing antibodies. *J. Immunol.* 71: 1–5.

47. Korngold, L., and Pressman, D. 1954. The localization of antilymphosarcoma antibodies in the Murphy lymphosarcoma of the rat. *Cancer Res.* 14: 96–99.

48. Kyogoku, M., Yagi, Y., Planinsek, J., Bernecky, J., and Pressman, D. 1964. Localizing properties of anti-rat hepatoma antibodies *in vivo*. *Cancer Res.* 24: 268–279.

49. Levy, R., Hurwitz, E., Maron, R., Arnon, R., and Sela, M. 1975. The specific cytotoxic effects of daunomycin conjugated to antitumor antibodies. *Cancer Res.* 35: 1182–1186.

50. Lewis, C. M., Pegrum, G. D., and Evans, C. A. 1974. Intracellular location of specific antibodies reacting with human lymphocytes. *Nature* 247: 463–465.

51. Mach, J.-P. Carrel, S., Merenda, C., Sordat, B., and Ceroltini, J.-C. 1974. *In vivo* localization of radiolabeled antibodies to carcinoembryonic antigen in human colon carcinoma grafted into nude mice. *Nature* 248: 704–706.

52. Mahaley, M. S., Jr. 1968. Immunological consideration of the malignant glioma problem. *Clin. Neurosurg.* 15: 175–189.

53. Mahaley, M. S., Jr., Day, E. D., and Bigner, D. 1969. Problems inherent to the *in vivo* localization of anti-brain tumor antibodies. *Ann. N.Y. Acad. Sci.* 159: 451.

54. Mahaley, M. S., Jr., Mahaley, J. L., and Day, E. D. 1965. The localization of radioantibodies in human brain tumors. II. Radioautography. *Cancer Res.* 25: 779–793.

55. Mallinger, A. G., Jozwiak, E. L., Jr., and Carter, J. C. 1972. Preparation of boron-containing bovine γ-globulin as a model compound for a new approach to slow neutron therapy of tumors. *Cancer Res.* 32: 1947–1950.

56. Marchalonis, J. J. 1969. An enzymatic method for the trace iodination of immunoglobulins and other proteins. *Biochem. J.* 113: 299–305.

57. Marrack, J. 1934. Nature of antibodies. *Nature* 133: 292–293.

58. Masugi, M. 1933. Über das weden der spezifischen veränderungen der niere und der leber durch das nephrotoxin bzw. das hepatotoxin. *Beitr. Pathol.* 91: 82.

59. Mathe, G. 1958. Effet sur la leucemie 1210 de la souris d'une combinaison par diazotation d'A-methopterine et de γ-globulines de hamsters porteurs de catte leucemie par heterogreffe. *C.R. Acad. Sci.* pp. 1626–1628.

60. McCardle, R. J., Harper, P. V., Spar, I. L., Bale, W. F., Andros, G., and Jiminez, F. 1966. Studies with iodine-131-labeled antibody to human fibrinogen for diagnosis and therapy of tumors. *J. Nucl. Med.* 7: 837–847.

61. McClintock, L. A., and Friedman, M. M. 1945. Utilization of antibody for the localization of metals and dyes in the tissues. *Amer. J. Roentgenol. Radium Ther.* 54: 704–706.

62. McGaughey, C. 1974. Feasibility of tumor immunoradiotherapy using radioiodinated antibodies to tumor-specific cell membrane antigens with emphasis on leukemias and early metastases. *Oncology* 29: 302–319.

63. Moolten, F. L., and Cooperband, S. R. 1970. Selective destruction of target cells by diphtheria toxin conjugated to antibody directed against antigens on the cells. *Science* 169: 68–70.

64. Moolten, F., Zajdel, S., and Cooperband, S. 1976. Immunotherapy of experimental animal tumors with antitumor antibodies conjugated to diphtheria toxin or ricin. *Ann. N.Y. Acad. Sci.* 277: 690–699.

65. Morrison, M., Bayse, G. S., and Webster, R. G. 1971. Use of lactoperoxidase catalyzed iodination in immunochemical studies. *Immunochemistry* 8: 289–297.

66. Nord, S., and Weissman, I. L. 1974. Radiolabeled antitumor antibodies. I. Antibody-specific and immunoglobulin-specific binding sites on Moloney lymphoma cells (LSTRA). *J. Natl. Cancer Inst.* 53: 117–124.

67. Nord, S., and Weissman, I. L. 1974. Radiolabeled antitumor antibodies. II.

Quantitative analysis of Moloney tumor antigens on Moloney lymphoma cells (LSTRA). *J. Natl. Cancer Inst.* 53: 125–130.

68. Nord, S., and Weissman, I. L. 1974. Radiolabeled antitumor antibodies. III. Highly iodinated and highly radioiodinated antibodies. *J. Natl. Cancer Inst.* 53: 959–965.

69. Order, S. E. 1976. The history and progress of serologic immunotherapy and radiodiagnosis. *Radiology* 118: 219–223.

70. Pressman, D. 1949. The zone of localization of antibodies. IV. The *in vivo* disposition of anti-mouse-kidney serum and anti-mouse-plasma serum as determined by radioactive tracers. *J. Immunol.* 63: 375–388.

71. Pressman, D. 1949. The zone of activity of antibodies as determined by the use of radioactive tracers. *Ann. N.Y. Acad. Sci.* 11: 203–206.

72. Pressman, D. 1957. Current status of the tissue localization of ^{131}I-labeled antitissue antibodies. *Ann. N.Y. Acad. Sci.* 70: 72–81.

73. Pressman, D., Day, E. D., and Blau, M. 1957. The use of paired labeling in the determination of tumor-localizing antibodies. *Cancer Res.* 17: 845–850.

74. Pressman, D., Day, E. D., and Blau, M. 1958. Radioactive anti-tumor antibodies. *Proc. 2nd UN Intl. Conference on Peaceful Uses of Atomic Energy,* Geneva, 24: 236.

75. Pressman, D., and Eisen, H. N. 1950. The zone of localization of antibodies. V. An attempt to saturate antibody-binding sites in mouse kidney. *J. Immunol.* 64: 273–279.

76. Pressman, D., Eisen, H. N., and Fitzgerald, P. J. 1950. The zone of localization of antibodies. VI. The rate of localization of anti-mouse-kidney serum. *J. Immunol.* 64: 281–287.

77. Pressman, D., Eisen, H. N., Siegel, M., Fitzgerald, P. J., Sherman, B., and Silverstein, A. 1950. The zone of localization of antibodies. X. The use of radioactive sulfur 35 as a label for anti-kidney serum. *J. Immunol.* 65: 559–569.

78. Pressman, D., Hill, R. F., and Foote, F. W. 1949. The zone of localization of anti-mouse-kidney serum as determined by radioautographs. *Science* 109: 65–66.

79. Pressman, D., and Keighley, G. 1948. The zone of activity of antibodies as determined by the use of radioactive tracers; the zone of activity of nephritoxic antikidney serum. *J. Immunol.* 59: 141–146.

80. Pressman, D., and Korngold, L. 1952. Experimental hypersensitivity. *Science* 116: 443.

81. Pressman, D., and Korngold, L. 1953. The *in vivo* localization of anti-Wagner osteogenic sarcoma antibodies. *Cancer* 6: 619–623.

82. Pressman, D., and Korngold, L. 1957. Localizing properties of anti-placenta serum. *J. Immunol.* 78: 75–78.

83. Pressman, D., and Pressman, R. 1965. Computer programs for paired and triad radioiodine label techniques in radioimmunochemistry. *Int. J. Appl. Rad. Isotopes* 16: 617–622.

84. Pressman, D., and Pressman, R. 1965. Computer programmes for multiple labelling techniques involving two or more radioiodines, *in Radioisotope Sample Measurement Techniques in Medicine and Biology,* pp. 223–234. Intl. Atomic Energy Agency, Vienna, Austria.

85. Pressman, D., and Radzimski, G. 1962. Increased precipitability of antibody as a result of iodination. *J. Immunol.* 89: 367–376.

86. Pressman, D., and Roholt, O. 1961. Isolation of peptides from an antibody site. *Proc. Natl. Acad. Sci.* 47: 1606–1610.

87. Pressman, D., and Sherman, B. 1951. The zone of localization of antibodies. XI. The in vivo purification of kidney-localizing anti-kidney antibody. *J. Immunol.* 67: 15–20.

88. Pressman, D., and Sternberger, L. A. 1950. The relative rates of iodination of serum components and the effect of iodination on antibody activity. *J. Amer. Chem. Soc.* 72: 2226–2233.

89. Pressman, D., and Sternberger, L. A. 1951. The nature of the combining sites of antibodies. The specific protection of the combining site by hapten during iodination. *J. Immunol.* 66: 609–620.

90. Pressman, D., and Watanabe, T. 1975. Tumor localization of radiolabeled antibodies raised by a mouse plasma cell tumor. *Immunochemistry* 12: 581–584.

91. Pressman, D., Yagi, Y., and Hiramoto, R. 1958. A comparison of fluorescein and I^{131} as labels for determining the in vivo localization of anti-tissue antibodies. *Intl. Arch. Allergy* 12: 125–136.

92. Primus, F. J., Wang, R. H., Cohen, E., Hansen, H. J., and Goldenberg, D. M. 1976. Antibody to carcinoembryonic antigen in hamsters bearing GW-39 human tumors. *Cancer Res.* 36: 2176–2181.

93. Primus, F. J., Wang, R. H., Goldenberg, D. M., and Hansen, H. J. 1973. Localization of human GW-39 tumors in hamsters by radiolabeled heterospecific antibody to carcinoembryonic antigen. *Cancer Res.* 33: 2977–2983.

94. Quinones, J., Mizejewski, G., and Beierwaltes, W. H. 1971. Choriocarcinoma scanning using radiolabeled antibody to chorionic gonadotrophin. *J. Nuclear Med.* 12: 69–75.

95. Reiner, L. 1930. On the chemical alteration of purified antibody-proteins. *Science* 72: 483–484.

96. Robert, M., and Revillard, J. P. 1976. Fate of antibodies bound to lymphocyte surface. I. Study with complement-dependent cytotoxicity, indirect immunofluorescence and radiolabeled antibodies. *Ann. Immunol.* 127: 129–144.

97. Robert, M., Vincent, C., Arnaud, P., and Revillard, J. P. 1976. Fate of antibodies bound to lymphocyte surface. II. Degradation and release of immune complexes. *Ann. Immunol.* 127: 145–161.

98. Roholt, O. A., and Pressman, D. 1968. Structural differences between antibodies produced against the same hapten by individual rabbits. *Immunochemistry* 5: 265–275.

99. Rose, S. 1973. Augmentation of immune activity by elimination of antibody and its implications in cancer. *J. Surg. Oncol.* 5: 137–166.

100. Rubens, R. D. 1974. Antibodies as carriers of anticancer agents. *Lancet* (7856) 1 (Pt. 1): 498–499.

101. Rubens, R. D., and Dulbecco, R. 1974. Augmentation of cytotoxic drug action by antibodies at cell surface. *Nature* 248: 81–82.

102. Smadel, J. E. 1936. Experimental nephritis in rats induced by injection of anti-kidney serum. *J. Exp. Med.* 64: 921.

103. Spar, I. L., and Bale, W. F. 1954. In vivo localization of labeled rat

adrenal antibodies. *J. Immunol.* 73: 134–137.

104. Spar, I. L., Bale, W. F., and Goodland, R. L. 1959. *In vivo* localization studies of ^{131}I-labeled anti-Murphy-Sturm lymphosarcoma antibodies. *Extrait de Acta Union Internationale Contre le Cancer* 15: 980.

105. Spar, I. L., Bale, W. F., Goodland, R. L., Casarette, G. W., and Michaelson, S. M. 1960. Distribution of injected ^{131}I-labeled antibody to dog fibrin in tumor-bearing dogs. *Cancer Res.* 20: 1501–1504.

106. Spar, I. L., Goodland, R. L., and Bale, W. F. 1959. Localization of I[131] labeled antibody to rat fibrin in a transplantable rat lymphosarcoma. *Univ. Rochester Atomic Energy Report* UR-536, pp. 1–11, 1958. *Proc. Soc. Exp. Biol. Med.* 100: 259–262.

107. Stelos, P., Yagi, Y., and Pressman, D. 1961. Localization properties of radioiodinated fragments of antirat kidney antibody. *J. Immunol.* 87: 106–109.

108. Tamanoi, I., Yagi, Y., Hiramoto, R., and Pressman, D. 1961. Lung localizing antibodies in anti-lung and anti-kidney serum. *Proc. Soc. Exp. Biol. Med.* 106: 661–663.

109. Tamanoi, I., Yagi, Y., and Pressman, D. 1961. Rate of localization of anti-rat lung antibody. *Proc. Soc. Exp. Biol. Med.* 106: 769–772.

110. Weissman, I., Nord, S., and Baird, S. 1972. Immunotherapy and immunodiagnosis of metastatic neoplasms. *Front. Rad. Ther. Onc.* 7: 161–178.

111. Weissman, I. L., Nord, S., and Ellis, R. 1974. Radiolabeled antibodies: Their potential as quantitative tools for *in vitro* and *in vivo* tumor diagnosis, in Interaction of Radiation and Host Immune Defense Mechanisms in Malignancy, pp. 379–398. Brookhaven National Laboratory, Associated Universities, Inc., under contract No. AT(30-1)-16 with the United States Atomic Energy Commission.

112. Winkler, M. H., Adetugbo, K., and Lehrey, G. M. 1972. Specific hapten binding activity in normal sera. *Immunol. Commun.* 1: 51–68.

CHAPTER 3

THE ROLE OF MACROPHAGES IN CANCER RESISTANCE AND THERAPY

J. Brice Weinberg
John B. Hibbs, Jr.

Division of Hematology-Oncology and
Division of Infectious Diseases
Veterans Administration Hospital and
University of Utah
College of Medicine
Salt Lake City, Utah

Macrophages from animals with enhanced resistance to cancer induced by chronic infection with agents like BCG or *Toxoplasma gondii* can kill tumor cells *in vivo*. Normal macrophages can be activated by a lymphokine (possibly MIF) which is secreted by lymphocytes responding to mitogens or specific antigens. The activated macrophages can kill tumor cells nonspecifically. The killing requires close contact between activated macrophage and tumor target cell and apparently involves the macrophage's vacuolar system. The activated macrophage, with its potent tumoricidal capacity and powers to discriminate between normal and neoplastic cells, probably plays an important role in surveillance against cancer, and represents an important source to tap for more effective treatment of established tumors.

I. Introduction

Macrophages (mononuclear phagocytes) originate in the bone marrow from pluripotent stem cells and enter the blood as monocytes. After a short residence as circulating blood monocytes, they take up long-term residence in various tissues where they undergo further differentiation. The majority reside in the liver (von Kuppfer cells), lung (alveolar macrophages), spleen and lymph nodes, serous cavities (pleural and peritoneal macrophages), and the nervous system (microglial cells). There is also evidence that tissue macrophages can proliferate in situ when exposed to severe physiologic stress and in this manner supplement the recruitment of marrow-derived blood monocytes.

Phylogenetically, macrophages are primitive cells functioning in invertebrates in the absence of lymphocytes and plasma cells. Vertebrate macrophages play a central role in immunologic responses modulating B lymphocyte activities (proliferation and antibody production) and T lymphocyte activities (proliferation, lymphokine production, mixed lymphocyte reactions, and lymphocyte killing). In addition, macrophages participate as effector cells in the mediation of cellular resistance to viral and bacterial infection. More recent studies have shown that macrophages are also proficient killers of neoplastic cells.

Host resistance to tumor growth is complex, involving interactions of lymphocytes, antibodies, macrophages, tumor cells, and possibly other factors. We will discuss the macrophage and its role in mediating specific and nonspecific tumor cell destruction. Attention will be given to studies which suggest that nonspecific resistance to intracellular pathogens and tumor development are related and that the activated macrophage is a common effector cell for expression of this resistance. We will review evidence that activated macrophages can discriminate between normal and neoplastic cells by nonimmunological means. The importance of intimate contact between activated macrophages and their neoplastic target cells will be emphasized. Investigations into possible mechanisms involved in the killing process will be discussed.

II. Role of Immune Macrophages in the Specific Destruction of Tumor Cells

The participation of macrophages as effector cells in the immunologic destruction of tumor cells was first suggested by Gorer. He studied histologically the regression of two allogeneic ascites sarcomas growing subcutaneously in mice and described the invasion of macrophages from the periphery into the tumor. He remarked that macrophages surrounded the malignant cells and apparently destroyed them (52). Subsequently, a similar macrophage response was described to the DBA/2 lymphoma L1210 and the C57BL lymphoma E.L.4 growing in the ascites for m in histoincompatible C3H mice. Intact lymphoma cells were phagocytized by host macrophages and were noted to undergo degenerative changes inside phagocytic vacuoles (7, 73). Baker and her associates examined, sequentially, the changes in cellular composition of ascites fluid during the rejection of sarcoma I cells in allogeneic C57BL/6K mice (13). They found that the macrophage was the only host cell that showed a marked increase in concentration in the ascites fluid prior to the onset of tumor destruction. They noted that most of the larger macrophages were in contact with tumor cells and that no other host cell seemed to display such affinity for the tumor cells. The destruction of sarcoma I cells by macrophages was described as a contact phenomenon requiring many minutes or hours for completion. Phagocytosis did not appear to play a major role in tumor cell destruction by macrophages. Strong circumstantial evidence suggesting that immune macrophages are capable of acting as effector cells in the in vivo destruction of allogeneic tumor cells was supplied by Bennett (19). He demonstrated that purified suspensions of peritoneal macrophages from mice immunized with allogeneic tumor inhibited tumor growth in irradiated recipients.

Granger and Weiser demonstrated that specifically immune mouse peritoneal macrophages were cytotoxic to allogeneic target cells in vitro by a nonphagocytic mechanism (53). Until this report, lymphocytes were the only cells which had been shown to cause the immunologic destruction of target cells by a nonphagocytic mechanism (123). Subsequent experiments showed that the nonphagocytic macrophage cytotoxic reaction was divided into two steps. First, there was passive specific adherence of immune macrophages to target cells, which was thought to be due to a specific hemagglutinin which could be eluted from well washed immune macrophages by heat treatment. The second step occurred subsequent to adherence and resulted in the mutual destruction of both immune macrophage and target cells. Its nature was not defined, but it apparently required the biosynthetic activities of the immune macrophages because it could be blocked by inhibitors of RNA and protein synthesis (54). It was later suggested that inhibitors of RNA and protein synthesis may block specific macrophage cytotoxic activity by interfering with surface membrane function of immune macrophages (91). Later work by Lohmann-Matthes et al. also provided evidence that immune macrophages, in the apparent absence of lymphocytes, were potent specifically cytotoxic effector cells (84).

Evans and Alexander conducted a series of studies designed to establish the mechanism of acquisition of specific cytotoxic activity by macrophages. They observed that after a single immunization, syngeneic DBA/2 mice became resistant to challenge with irradiated L5178Y lymphoma cells. This resistance could be transferred to normal mice by spleen and lymph node cells from immune mice. However, in vitro, spleen cells from the immune mice were not cytotoxic to L5178Y cells. Thus, immune syngeneic spleen cells could transfer activity in vivo but were inactive by themselves in vitro suggesting that in the syngeneic system the immune lymphoid cells must act in cooperation with macrophages to destroy the lymphoma cells. In addition, they demonstrated that syngeneic peritoneal macrophages from mice immunized with L5178Y cells were specifically cytotoxic to lymphoma cells in vitro and that syngeneic macrophages from unimmunized mice were rendered cytotoxic following incubation with immune spleen cells. The lymphoma cells were killed by a nonphagocytic mechanism which required intimate contact with immune macrophages (44). A T-lymphocyte-derived factor induced specific killing of lymphoma cells by macrophages.

The nature of the "specific macrophage activating factor" (SMAF) is still in question. It has properties of cytophilic antibody in that it specifically adsorbs to the macrophages or the tumor cells used for immunization, but it has no characteristics of any known immunoglobulins. Chromatographic separation of SMAF reveals activity in the > 300,000 MW and in the 40,000 MW range (possible subunit?), and speculation is that it is an immunoglobulin-like T cell product (46). The relationship of SMAF to migration inhibition factor (MIF) is unknown, but it is certainly functionally distinct since MIF induces nonspecific killing (to be discussed in more detail below).

III. Nonspecific Stimulation of Host Resistance to Neoplasia

Host resistance to microorganism or tumor cell growth is complex and multifactorial. It can be stimulated nonspecifically by agents which are able to enhance the ability of the host to respond more effectively than a normal untreated control to a pathogenic microorganism or to tumor growth. This resistance is said to be nonspecific when there is no immunologic cross reactivity between the stimulating agent and the microorganism or tumor cell being eliminated from the host.

Infection with intracellular agents can stimulate increased resistance to tumor growth. Included are infections with the facultative intracellular bacteria Bacillus Calmette-Guérin (BCG) (81, 90, 100, 103, 104, 157) and

Salmonella enteriditis (56), the lactic dehydrogenase elevating virus (121), the M-P virus (98), filterable hemolytic anemia virus (127), and protozoa (63, 86). In addition, resistance to tumor growth has been conferred by a variety of nonliving agents. Included are the polyanions poly I:C (83) and pyran copolymer (99, 119); dead organisms [*Corynebacterium parvum* (152), *Bordetella pertussis* (139), and *Mycobacterium butyricum* (64, 119)]; and the products of microorganisms [zymosan (21), methanol insoluble fraction of BCG (149), other mycobacterial cell wall extracts (120), and endotoxin (136)].

It is evident that a great variety of agents are capable, under certain experimental conditions, of stimulating nonspecific host resistance to allogeneic or syngeneic tumor growth. However, each of these agents stimulates multiple resistance factors of the host and their actual mechanism of action in increasing tumor resistance has not been defined with certainty. It has been generally believed that treatment of animals with these agents induces an augmented response to unrelated antigens subsequently administered. Indeed, enhanced development of an immune response to challenge with a non-cross-reacting antigen appears to contribute to increased resistance in animals treated with many of these agents (154). However, caution should be exercised in attributing the increased resistance to tumor growth stimulated by these agents, in all circumstances, to an enhanced immune response to antigenic stimulation. In a series of experiments we observed that mice chronically infected with the obligate intracellular protozoan parasite *Toxoplasma gondii* had nonspecific resistance to tumor development (63). We believe this increased resistance to tumor development may be due to persistent activation of macrophages by the chronic toxoplasma infection because peritoneal macrophages from these mice are nonspecifically cytotoxic to tumor cells *in vitro* (65). Peritoneal lymphocytes from these mice did not kill tumor cells *in vitro* even at effector target:cell ratios of 66:1 (65). Normal mice did not have increased resistance to tumor development and their peritoneal macrophages were not cytotoxic to tumor cells *in vitro*.

Furthermore, there is evidence of a generalized immunosuppression in animals with increased resistance to neoplasia induced by chronic protozoal infection. Thus, in mice with chronic toxoplasma infection, we have noted a marked impairment of primary skin allograft rejections (Table 1) and primary antibody responses to the T-cell-dependent antigens tetanus toxoid (Table 2) and sheep red blood cells (Table 3) (67, and Hibbs, Lambert, and Remington, manuscript in preparation). All secondary responses were normal. This paradoxical lymphoid immunosuppression in animals with enhanced nonspecific resistance to tumor development further emphasizes the importance of macrophages as effector cells in mediating this resistance.

Table 1. Effect of chronic toxoplasma infection on the rejection of allografts on normal skin[a]

Experimental Groups[b,c]	Average Weight	Graft	Number	Day of Rejection	Mean Survival Time (days)
SWR/J female control (H-2[b])	26 gm	primary	10	(1×10) (3×11) (6×12)	11.5 ± 1.5
SWR/J female chronic toxoplasma infection	25.8 gm	primary	11	(1×14) (1×15) (1×17) (1×18) (2×19) (1×20) (1×21) (2×22) (1×23)	19.1 ± 5.0
C3H/He female control (H-2[k])	25.1 gm	primary	10	(2×10) (6×11) (2×12)	11.0±1.0
C3H/He female chronic toxoplasma infection	24.5 gm	primary	10	(1×13) (2 × 14) (1×16) (1×18) (1×19) (2×21) (2×22)	18.0 ± 5.0
SWR/J female control	—	secondary	6	(2×7) (1×8) (3×9)	8.2 ± 1.2
SWR/J female chronic toxoplasma infection	—	secondary	7	(2×5) (3×6) (1×12) (1×13)	7.6 ± 5.6

a. From Hibbs, Lambert, Remington; unpublished data.

b. Mice were infected with the C_{56} strain of toxoplasma as previously described (63) seven weeks prior to primary skin grafting. Two weeks before primary skin grafting the toxoplasma-infected mice were boosted with 5×10^3 trophozoites IP of the RH strain of toxoplasma.

c. Second-set grafts were applied approximately three weeks after rejection of primary grafts.

Table 2. Comparison of antitoxin response in mice with and without chronic *Toxoplasma gondii* infection[a]

| Dose of Toxoid/ Mouse[c] | No. of Mice | Day of Death After Inoculation | | | | | | Survivors | | Mean Score |
		2	3	4	5	6	7	With Tetanus	Without Tetanus	
A. Primary Immunization of Uninfected Mice E.D.$_{.50}$ = 0.0053 ml/mouse of tetanus toxoid 22Lf/ml[b]										
0.1000	3								3	6
0.0500	3								3	6
0.0250	3								3	6
0.0125	3								3	6
0.0064	3	1							2	4
0.0032	3	2		1						1.3
0.0016	3	3								0
no toxoid	3	3								0
Score:		0	2	2	3	3	3	4	6	
B. Primary Immunization of Mice with Chronic Toxoplasma Infection[d] E.D.$_{.50}$ = >0.1 ml/mouse of tetanus toxoid 22 Lf/ml[b]										
0.1000	3	1						2		3
0.0500	3		2					1		2.0
0.0250	3	1	1					1		1.7
0.0125	3	2				1				1.3
0.0064	3	3								0
0.0032	3	3								0
0.0016	3	3								0
no toxoid	3	3								0
Score:		0	2	2	3	3	3	4	6	

a. From Hibbs, Lambert, Remington; unpublished data.

b. The bioassay for tetanus antitoxin is a modification of the method described in Ipsen (71).

c. Tetanus toxoid was obtained through the courtesy of Dr. Leo Levine, Department of Public Health, Boston, Mass. The tetanus toxoid was diluted to give the appropriate dose for each group of mice and was administered SC in the right flank. Challenge with 15 MLD of tetanus toxin (also kindly supplied by Dr. Levine) was 14 days after immunization with tetanus toxoid.

d. Mice were infected with the C$_{56}$ strain of toxoplasma as previously described (63) 8 weeks prior to primary immunization with tetanus toxoid. Two weeks before primary immunization the mice were boosted with 5 × 10^3 trophozoites of the RH strain of toxoplasma.

Table 3. Effect of chronic protozoan infection on hemagglutinin response to sheep red blood cells

Group[a]	No. of	Primary Response[c]		Secondary Response[d]	
		IP	IV	IP	IV
Normal controls	12	9(9–10)	8(7–10)	12(12–13)	11(10–12)
Chronic toxoplasma infection[e]	12	7(4–8)	6(4–9)	12(11–13)	11(10–12)
Chronic besnoitia infection[e]	12	6(3–8)	5(4–7)	12(11–13)	12(11–13)

Hemagglutinin Titers[b]

a. All groups were immunized with 0.2 ml of a 10% suspension of SRBC.

b. Log_2 of reciprocal of highest serum dilution showing complete agglutination median (range).

c. Mice bled 7 days after primary injection of SRBC.

d. Mice received a second 0.2-ml injection of 10% SRBC 12 days after the primary immunization and bled 3 days after.

e. Infection with toxoplasma or besnoitia was initiated 8 weeks before primary immunization with SRBC as previously described. Two weeks prior to SRBC immunization the mice were boosted with the appropriate protozoan as described.

Others have also documented the lymphoid immunosuppression in animals treated with "immunostimulants" known to produce nonspecific resistance to neoplasia. Scott noted that certain T cell functions (responsiveness to phytohemagglutinin or allogeneic lymphocytes *in vitro* and graft versus host reactivity) were decreased in spleen cells from *C. parvum*-infected mice. The responses were returned to normal when macrophages were removed from the preparations (132, 133). Others have confirmed these findings (75) and noted similar defects in animals injected with BCG (97). In addition, impaired responses to sheep red blood cells (141) and poliovirus vaccine (70) have been noted in mice with chronic toxoplasma infections. The mechanism of this immunosuppression is complex but probably relates to certain macrophage-derived soluble factors (see Section VIII and Ref. 101). Most important for this discussion, however, is the fact that enhanced nonspecific resistance to neoplasia occurs in the setting of immunosuppression.

The fact that macrophages can be recruited and activated by an immunological reaction, but as participant cells in that reaction utilize nonimmunologic mechanisms of response was first elucidated by Mackaness in studies of resistance to intracellular bacteria in mice (87, 88). He demonstrated that expression of acquired resistance to intracellular bacteria depends on three factors: (1) recognition residing in specifically immune lymphocytes, (2) the presence in tissue of bacteria which can act as specific antigenic stimuli for the immune lymphocytes, and (3) the production of activated macrophages with increased microbicidal activity which are the effector cells in the expression of this nonspecific resistance. For the appearance of a local and/or systemic population of activated macrophages in the host, the first two factors must coexist in the tissues. As the bacteria, which are the specific stimuli for the sensitized lymphocytes, are cleared from the tissue by the activated macrophages, the production of the macrophage activating factor(s) by the sensitized lymphocytes wanes, and macrophage function gradually reverts to normal. Mackaness also showed that, although the induction of acquired resistance to intracellular bacteria was highly specific (lymphocytes sensitized to specific microbial antigens), its expression was nonspecific (population of activated macrophages). Using mice chronically infected with the protozoa *Toxoplasma gondii,* Ruskin and Remington (124) showed an increased resistance to *Listeria monocytogenes* challenge. This demonstrated that increased nonspecific resistance to microbial agents crosses phylogenetic lines.

Subsequently, Zbar *et al.* showed that rejection of syngeneic tumor grafts in guinea pigs also required several steps (157, 158). Recognition, the first step, resided in sensitized lymphocytes, but tumor cell destruction, the second step, was nonspecific. These workers demonstrated that close contact between sensitized cells, sensitizing antigen, and the antigenically unrelated tumor cells was required to nonspecifically suppress growth of the antigenically unrelated tumor cells.

In a series of studies, we provided strong circumstantial evidence that the nonspecific component in mediating tumor resistance in mice is due to a population of activated macrophages. Our results suggest that the mechanisms of host resistance to intracellular pathogens and neoplasia are related and that the activated macrophage is a common effector arm for expression of this resistance. *In vivo* experiments showed that mice chronically infected with intracellular protozoa had increased resistance to autochthonous and transplanted tumors (Fig. 1) (63). In this experimental model the protozoal antigens persist in the tissues for an extended period but the mice remain healthy. This provides the necessary context, coexistence of specific antigen and sensitized lymphocytes, for the expression of acquired as well as nonspecific resistance to intracellular bacteria and tumors.

We observed an impressive delay in time to death due to spontaneous leukemia in protozoal-infected AKR mice. In one group of mice infected with *Besnoitia jellisoni,* deaths due to leukemia did not occur until ten

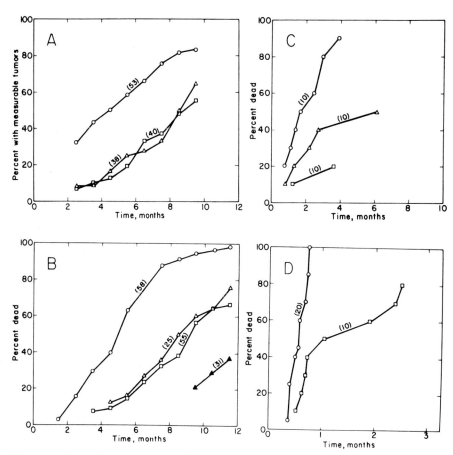

Fig. 1. Effect of chronic intracellular protozoal infection on autochthonous and transplanted tumors in mice. *A*—Incidence of spontaneous mammary tumor in C3H/He mice. *B*—Incidence of death due to spontaneous leukemia in AKR mice. The difference between subgroup (△) and subgroup (▲) was the interval between infection and treatment sulfadiazine, 48 hours in (△) and 96 hours in (▲). *C*—Incidence of death due to Friend leukemia in Swiss-Webster mice. *D*—Incidence of death due to sarcoma 180 in ascites form in Swiss-Webster mice. In *A* and *B*, time 0 = date of infection. In *C* and *D*, time 0 = date of tumor transplant. Figures in parentheses = number of mice. (0) = controls; (□) = chronically infected with C56 strain of *Toxoplasma gondii*; (△) = chronically infected with *Besnoitia jellisoni*. (Reprinted from Ref. 63 with permission of the publisher.)

months after chronic infection was established. By that time 97% of control mice had died of leukemia (63).

Challenge with *Listeria monocytogenes* was used to determine whether mice infected with protozoa had resistance to a phylogenetically unrelated intracellular pathogen. Mice from the same groups tested for nonspecific resistance to neoplasia had increased resistance to listeria challenge (Table 4) (63). Therefore, in addition to stimulating nonspecific resistance to phylogenetically unrelated intracellular pathogens, chronic infection with intracellular protozoa also stimulates nonspecific resistance to both autochthonous and transplanted tumors.

A more recent investigation has further defined the requirements for the in vivo expression of nonspecific resistance and has provided further evidence that the nonspecific effector cell in the expression of this resis-

Table 4.   Challenge of experimental groups with L. monocytogenes[a]

Tumor Evaluated	Strain of Mice[b]	Experimental Group[c]	Percent Survival	Time to Death (Days After Challenge)[d]						
				2	3	4	5	6	7	8
Mammary carcinoma	C3H/He	Control	0	1	7	2				
		T. gondii	60			1	1	1	1	
		B. jellisoni	80			1			1	
AKR leukemia	AKR	Control	0	10						
		T. gondii	60			2	1	1		
		B. jellisoni	80					1		1
Friend leukemia	SW	Control	10	1	5	3				
		T. gondii	90				1			
		B. jellisoni	70				1	1	1	
S-180	SW	Control	10	3	2	3	1			
		T. gondii	90				1			
L1210	DBA/2	Control	0	2	8					
		T. gondii	80				1			1
	DBA/2	Control	10		8	1				
		B. jellisoni	40					2	3	1

a. Reprinted from Ref. 63 with permission of the publisher.
b. All were females except for the *B. jellisoni* infected DBA/2 group and their controls.
c. Control = mice inoculated with saline or HBSS; TG = mice chronically infected with *T. gondii*; BJ = mice chronically infected with *B. Jellisoni*.
d. Numbers in columns show number of mice that died on each day.

tance is the tumoricidal activated macrophage (61, 62). We found that there is a requirement for local persistence of inducing antigen for the continued presence of a population of tumoricidal activated macrophages in an anatomical compartment, e.g., in mice high levels of BCG tend to remain localized in the anatomical compartment(s) into which they were administered. Likewise, the presence of tumoricidal activated macrophages in the tissue tends to be a local phenomenon, also confined to the anatomical compartment(s) that contain high levels of inducing antigen (62). (See Table 5.)

In nonspecific tumor cell destruction the activated macrophages induced by a heterologous antigen, e.g., BCG or toxoplasma, were present in the tissues before grafting the tumor cells and could be detected after the tumor cells had been rejected (62). This continuing presence may be due to the fact that the specific antigen (BCG or toxoplasma) which induced the production of cytotoxic activated macrophages remains in the tissues and provides a continuing stimulus for elaboration of a chemical signal that maintains macrophage activation.

Table 5.   Correlation of BCG in peritoneal lymph nodes with *in vitro* cytotoxic effect of peritoneal macrophages and resistance to i.p. grafts of S180[a]

Group	Route of Administration of BCG[b]	Colonies of BCG Cultured from Peritoneal Lymph Nodes[c]	Cytotoxic Effect of Peritoneal Macrophages for 3T12 Target Cells[d]	Result of i.p. Graft of 4 × 10^5 S180 Cells: No. of Mice Dead of Tumor Growth/ No. of Mice Tested
A	Control	0	0	20/20
B	BCG i.p.	3 to 4+	4+	9/20($P < 0.001$)
C	BCG i.v.	0 to 1+	0	20/20
D	BCG i.m.R	0 to 1+	0	19/20

a. Reprinted from Ref. 62 with permission of the publisher.

b. Intraperitoneal (i.p.), intravenous (i.v.), and right gastrocnemius muscle (i.m.R).

c. Quantitation of BCG growth: 0, no growth; 1+, 1–5 colonies per petri dish; 2+, 6–20 colonies per petri dish; 3+, 21–50 colonies per petri dish; 4+, 51–100 colonies per petri dish.

d. Cytotoxic effect of macrophages for 3T12 cells: 0, multilayer of 3T12 cells among macrophages (no cytotoxic or cytostatic effect); 1+, patchy areas of confluent 3T12 growth among macrophages (slight cytostatic effect); 2+, 10–20 3T12 cells per 430X field among macrophages (cytostatic effect); 3+, 3–9 cells per 430X field among macrophages (cytotoxic effect); 4+, 2 or fewer 3T12 cells per 430X field among macrophages (marked cytotoxic effect). The results are given as the range obtained from three separately performed experiments.

In contrast to our results with the induction of nonspecific resistance with BCG, the specific rejection of lymphoma L1210 cells was not restricted anatomically. CBA mice immunized with L1210 cells i.m.R rejected secondary L1210 grafts (2×10^7 cells) i.p., as can be seen in Table 6.

We noted that the specific rejection of secondary grafts of the allogeneic L1210 lymphoma in immunized CBA mice (inducing antigens are present on the lymphoma cell surface) produces activated macrophages with tumoricidal effect for antigenetically unrelated SV40 transformed WI-38 cells. However, we found that the tumoricidal activated macrophages rapidly revert to normal when the antigen that induced their mobilization (allogeneic L1210 cells) is cleared from the tissues and that they are not cytotoxic for tumorigenic 3T12 cells which share common $H-2^d$ antigens. It is important to note that the population of tumoricidal activated macrophages was confined to the anatomical compartment containing the inducing antigen (the tumor allograft). When the secondary graft of L1210 cells was administered i.m.R, cytotoxic activated macrophages did not appear in the peritoneal cavity. (See Table 6.)

It is interesting that activated macrophages with nonspecific cytotoxic effect for tumor cells comprise 70 to 85 percent of the peritoneal

Table 6. Correlation of presence of viable L1210 cells in peritoneal cavity of CBA mice with cytotoxic effect of peritoneal macrophages *in vitro*[a]

Group	Site of Primary L1210 Graft	Site of Secondary L1210 Graft	Time Interval Between Secondary L1210 Graft and Collection of Peritoneal Cells for Cytotoxicity Test (hr)	Cytotoxic Effect[b] 3T12	Cytotoxic Effect[b] VA-13
A	i.m.R	i.p.	24	4+	4+
B	i.m.R	i.p.	48	4+	4+
C	i.m.R	i.p.	72	2 to 3+	2 to 3+
D	i.m.R	i.p.	96	0	0
E	i.m.R	i.m.R	24	0	0
F	i.m.R	i.m.R	48	0	0
G	i.m.R	i.m.R	72	0	0
H	i.m.R	—	—	0	0
I	L1210 i.p.[c]	—	—	0	0
J	—	—	—	0	0

a. Reprinted from Ref. 62 with permission of the publisher.
b. See footnotes to Table 4 for interpretation of symbols used.
c. The primary immunizing dose of L1210 cells was 2×10^6.

exudate cells in CBA mice 48–72 hours after a secondary graft of L1210 cells (Hibbs, unpublished data). These results clearly show that activated macrophages with nonspecific cytotoxic effect for tumorigenic cells are produced in large numbers at the site of specific rejection of allogeneic lymphoma cells in mice. Whether or not cytotoxic activated macrophages are significant effector cells in clearing allogeneic L1210 cells from the tissues was not determined in this study. Other effector mechanisms are certainly not excluded and it is probable that they have a major role in the destruction of L1210 cells in immunized allogeneic mice.

IV. Mechanisms of Acquisition of Nonspecific Tumoricidal Capacity by Macrophages

Normal mouse peritoneal macrophages are not tumoricidal under usual or unstressed physiologic conditions as determined by their interaction with tumor cells in vitro (65). But activated peritoneal cells, as reviewed above, are tumoricidal when tested in vitro. In the mouse, merely inducing a sterile inflammatory peritoneal exudate with agents such as starch, mineral oil, thioglycollate, or peptone is not sufficient stimulus to convert macrophages into tumoricidal cells (30, 65).

This suggests that specific chemical stimuli induced by host reaction to infection mediates the acquisition of tumoricidal capacity by macrophages. Piessens et al. have provided evidence of a source of the chemical signal (110). They demonstrated that normal guinea pig macrophages become cytotoxic to syngeneic tumor cells after they have been activated in vitro by mediator-rich supernatants prepared from sensitized lymphocytes responding to the sensitizing antigen which is unrelated to the tumor cells. The mediator was distinct from lymphotoxin. A chromatographically fractionated supernatant component was effective in activating the macrophages to kill nonspecifically even in the absence of the stimulating antigen (27), thus differentiating it from SMAF (discussed above). The exact lymphokine responsible for this activation is unknown, but its activity appears in the same fraction as migration inhibition factor (MIF) activity. Injection of MIF-containing supernatants into sites of guinea pig tumor transplants suppresses the growth of the syngeneic tumor graft (20).

The polyanions endotoxin, double-stranded RNA, poly I:C, and pyran copolymer are also capable of rendering normal macrophages cytotoxic to tumor cells (3, 74). Endotoxin, dsRNA, and poly I:C effectively activate macrophages in vitro and in vivo, whereas pyran copolymer is effective only in vivo. All will protect animals from tumor growth (99, 108). Endotoxin has some coagulative and vascular effects which contribute to resolution of established tumors (108). The mechanisms of activation of macrophages is not totally clear. Pyran copolymer can induce tumor regression and a population of cytotoxic activated macrophages in thymectomized, irradiated, bone-marrow-reconstituted mice (74). Endotoxin and pyran copolymer are both B cell mitogens (8, 12), suggesting the possibility that the activating factor is derived from stimulated B cells. B lymphocytes, like T lymphocytes, can secrete MIF when stimulated with B cell mitogens. Thus, B cell mitogens cause MIF production by B lymphocytes (26, 155). Wilton *et al.* (151) found that activation of guinea pig macrophages (as monitored by glucosamine uptake) by endotoxin required the presence of B cells. The report that BCG administration to athymic nude mice induces regression of tumor xenografts (111) also suggests the possible participation of B cell factors in the *in vivo* activation induced by chronic infection. Previous claims that endotoxin directly activates macrophages (3, 59) will now have to be reexamined realizing that con-

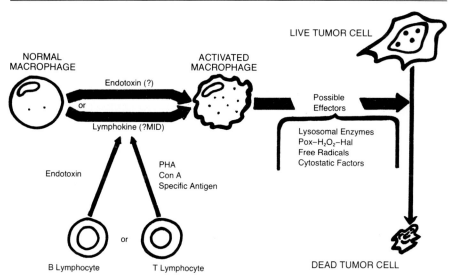

Fig. 2. Proposed mechanisms of macrophage activation and nonspecific tumor killing. Normal macrophages can be activated by a lymphokine(s) (possibly MIF) which is secreted by stimulated B or T lymphocytes. Endotoxin possibly acts directly on normal macrophages without the involvement of lymphocytes. Activated macrophages kill tumor cells by incompletely understood, contact-dependent mechanisms. Possible effectors of this killing include lysosomal enzymes, the peroxidase–H_2O_2–halide (Pox–H_2O_2–Hal) system, free radicals, cytostatic factors, and/or other factors.

taminating B lymphocytes can represent a source of MIF when they are stimulated by endotoxin. (See Fig. 2.)

Macrophages made specifically cytotoxic by SMAF (Section II) become nonspecifically cytotoxic when exposed to the antigen used for original immunization (46). Thus, macrophages from mice immunized with a specific tumor are capable of killing only that tumor. However, if these specifically activated macrophages are incubated with the specific tumor, they then become nonspecifically activated, acquiring the capacity to kill other tumor lines (45). Similarly, tumoricidal macrophages from mice immunized against BCG or sheep red blood cells are made nonspecifically tumoricidal when exposed to PPD or red blood cells (47). Furthermore, specifically tumoricidal macrophages are converted to nonspecifically tumoricidal effector cells when exposed to rabbit anti-mouse gamma globulin (43). As Evans has stated, this suggests that an immune complex, either antigen-antibody or antigen-SMAF, is instrumental in rendering macrophages nonspecifically cytocidal to tumor cells.

V. Selectivity of Macrophage-Mediated Cytotoxicity

In our initial studies we made the observation that the cytotoxic effect of activated macrophages was selective (65). Activated peritoneal macrophages from mice with chronic toxoplasma, besnoitia, listeria, or BCG infection did not destroy contact-inhibited allogeneic fibroblast or kidney cell strains that have surfaces of high immunogenic potential, but were markedly cytotoxic to both syngeneic and allogeneic tumorigenic cell lines. These experiments suggest that normal cells may acquire a property in parallel with neoplastic transformation that elicits nonimmunologic recognition and makes them more susceptible to destruction by activated macrophages.

To test this hypothesis, we studied the cytotoxic activity of activated mouse macrophages against mouse embryo fibroblasts before and after spontaneous transformation of the fibroblasts in vitro (66). We found that activated C3H/HeJ macrophages did not destroy two allogeneic fibroblast cell strains differing from them at a strongly antigenic H-2 locus. In contrast, these macrophages were markedly cytotoxic for the same allogeneic fibroblasts (and also for syngeneic fibroblasts) after the fibroblasts had spontaneously developed abnormal growth properties that included loss of contact inhibition of cell division. Because H-2 antigens are more immunogenic than tumor specific transplantation antigens or fetal antigens expressed on tumor cells, this study strongly suggests that a change associated with the acquisition of abnormal growth properties by target cells, rather than a change in antigens, is responsible for the increased susceptibility of tumor cells to destruction by activated macrophages.

To show the importance of cell-surface factors in the nonimmunologic cytotoxic reaction between activated macrophages and target cells, the following cell lines were evaluated: BALB/3T3 fibroblasts (a contact-inhibited, nontumorigenic cell line), BALB/3T12 fibroblasts (a non-contact-inhibited, tumorigenic cell line from the same original pool of mouse cells as the BALB/3T3 line), and BALB/SV-3T3 fibroblasts (a non-contact-inhibited, tumorigenic cell line). The results show that under the conditions of the experiment, BALB/3T3 fibroblasts were not destroyed whereas BALB/3T12 and BALB/SV-3T3 fibroblasts were destroyed by syngeneic and allogeneic activated macrophages (59). This suggests that surface alterations related to loss of contact inhibition, a property of the BALB/3T12 and BALB/SV-3T3 lines, are important factors in target cell recognition and destruction. Abnormal characteristics of the BALB/3T3 fibroblast line seeming not to be factors in nonimmunologic recognition and destruction by activated macrophages include (1) loss of normal cell morphology, (2) hypotetraploid karyotype, (3) maximum growth *in vitro* to confluency from a low inoculum, and (4) continuous multiplication *in vitro*.

These results indicate that surface modification of non-contact-inhibited cells may be so extensive that it can evoke nonimmunologic recognition and response by activated macrophages even without specific sensitization to the target cell.

The cell surface is extensively modified after loss of contact inhibition (102, 114, 129, 137, 153). Others working with the BALB/3T3, BALB/3T12, and BALB/SV-3T3 series of mouse fibroblasts showed that tumorigenicity (1) and cell agglutination after plant lectin binding (114) correlate with loss of contact inhibition. Likewise, we demonstrated that nonimmunologic destruction by activated macrophages is also associated with loss of contact inhibition by these target cells. All these findings may be related to extensive biochemical and topographic differences (or both) in the surface membrane of non-contact-inhibited (BALB/SV-3T3) fibroblasts.

The observation of selective cytotoxic effect of activated macrophages for neoplastic target cells has been confirmed by several laboratories (14, 30, 68, 74, 95, 96, 110). In addition, using a mixture of neoplastic and nonneoplastic cell lines prelabeled with ^{3}H-thymidine, Meltzer *et al.* demonstrated that BCG-activated macrophages selectively destroyed neoplastic cells. The nonneoplastic cells were not affected as "innocent bystanders" (95).

It should be noted that although the discriminatory capacity between normal and malignant cells is reproducible and of impressive magnitude, it is not absolute. Thus, some killing of nonmalignant cells can be achieved by increasing macrophage/target cell ratios (Hibbs, unpublished data), but neoplastic cells are uniformly much more susceptible to the cytotoxic effects of activated macrophages. This could relate to the fact that certain membrane properties of malignant cells present throughout the cell cycle [for example, increased membrane fluidity (85) and increased clustering of lectin binding sites (117)] are also usual properties of normal cells in mitosis (117).

VI. Importance of Macrophage-Tumor Cell Contact in Macrophage-Mediated Cytotoxicity

Several investigators have demonstrated the apparent dependence for intimate contact between cytotoxic macrophages and tumor cells for destruction of those tumor cells (30, 60, 65, 68, 74). However, other workers have successfully demonstrated soluble factors produced by macrophages that have cytolytic or cytostatic effects on target cells in the absence of intact macrophages. We have not been able to identify a soluble cytotoxic mediator (SCM) elaborated by cytotoxic activated macrophages. No cytopathic effect was noted when supernatant media, taken from cultures in which activated macrophages had mediated target cell destruction, was added to target cell monolayers growing alone (65). Further studies were done to determine if evidence for an SCM could be implicated in the destruction of target cells by cytotoxic activated macrophages (60).

Figure 3 shows petri dishes stained with giemsa at the end of a 60 hour cytotoxicity assay. BALB/3T12 cells completely overgrow normal macrophages. On the other hand, wherever BALB/3T12 cells come into contact with BCG-activated macrophages there is a marked cytotoxic effect with absence of tumor cells. This holds true even when narrow strips of adherent macrophages are removed with a rubber policeman prior to BALB/3T12 cell challenge. Macrophage-free substrate is always overgrown with tumor cells, even though it is surrounded by fully viable tumoricidal activated macrophages. Microscopically, the BALB/3T12 cells grow to the edge of the macrophage-free areas. Comparable results occur when activated macrophages are seeded onto established BALB/3T12 monolayers. This is evidence that the cytotoxic mechanism does not involve an SCM. To further test for a possible SCM elaborated by activated macrophages, we removed culture medium every three hours and each time replaced it with fresh medium warmed to 36.5°C. The cytotoxic

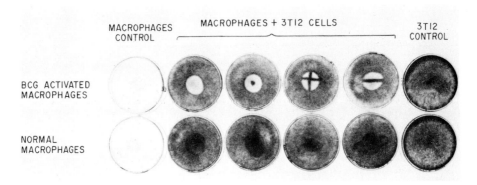

Fig. 3. Photo of petri dishes demonstrating the importance of activated macrophage-tumor target cell contact in macrophage mediated cytotoxicity. Peritoneal cells (5×10^5) from BCG-infected or normal Balb/c mice in 0.1 ml media were added to the center of 35 mm petri dishes and incubated at 37°C in 5% CO_2/air for 60 minutes to allow macrophages to adhere. Nonadherent cells were then removed by washing. The residual central monolayer of macrophages covered an area the size of a 0.1-ml drop. A rubber policeman was then used to remove narrow strips or a dot from the centrally located monolayer. Then Balb/3T12 target cells (1×10^5) were added in 2 ml of media to cover the entire dish. The dishes were stained with giemsa after 60 hours.

effect was identical to that of control cultures (where the medium was not changed), suggesting that destruction was independent of an SCM whose effect could be diminished by dilution. To promote the thorough distribution of an SCM, we mixed the culture medium with a sterile Pasteur pipette every 60 minutes during the 72-hour incubation period. This did not interfere with BALB/3T12 cell destruction among activated macrophages, nor did it produce inhibition of BALB/3T12 cell growth on the periphery of the cover slip which was free of activated macrophages. It was also possible that an SCM was present but active only in cooperation with macrophages. To test this we removed the supernatant medium after 24, 48, and 72 hours of incubation from monolayers of activated macrophages or from activated macrophages that had been challenged with BALB/3T12 cells. Both types of activated-macrophage-conditioned medium were added to normal macrophages that had been challenged with BALB/3T12 cells one hour earlier, and the cultures were evaluated for cytotoxic effect after a 72-hour incubation period. Activated-macrophage-conditioned medium did not render normal macrophages cytotoxic.

VII. Role of the Macrophage Vacuolar System in Macrophage-Mediated Cytotoxicity

Nonenzymatic agents that accumulate and are stored in the vacuolar system of macrophages were used to study the nonphagocytic contact-dependent mechanism or mechanisms of target cell destruction. Normal and activated macrophages readily take up dextran sulfate which is concentrated in secondary lysosomes (51). Dextran sulfate is indigestible and nontoxic, and it stains metachromatically with toluidine blue 0 (51). Tumorigenic BALB/3T12 cells that had been in contact with labeled activated macrophages contained metachromatic cytoplasmic vacuoles whereas those tumor cells at the periphery of the coverslip not in contact with activated macrophages did not contain the metachromatic granules (Fig. 4). Moreover, tumor cells in contact with dextran sulfate-labeled normal macrophages and nontransformed mouse embryo fibroblasts in contact with labeled activated macrophages did not contain metachromatic granules.

These results suggest that activated macrophages directly transfer the contents of secondary lysosomes into susceptible target cells. Such a process of exocytosis involves membrane fusion which should be partially inhibited by membrane stabilization (115). Hydrocortisone, a known membrane stabilizing agent (150), was added to normal and activated macrophages for 6 to 24 hours before the target cells were challenged (60). Preliminary treatment of activated macrophages with hydrocortisone inhibited their cytotoxic effect. Maximum inhibitory effect was seen with doses as low as 2.8×10^{-7} M if maintained in the culture medium throughout the 72-hour incubation period. Hydrocortisone also inhibited the transfer of dextran sulfate to BALB/3T12 cells from labeled activated macrophages.

These results provide evidence that transfer of the contents of activated macrophage lysosomes is associated with target cell destruction. Experiments were done to determine whether lysosomal enzymes of activated macrophages could be the effectors of target cell heterolysis. Trypan blue, an inhibitor of lysosomal hydrolases (17) is readily taken up by macrophages, is nontoxic, and is stored in secondary lysosomes (16). Normal and activated macrophages were vitally stained in vitro by incubation with 4.2×10^{-4} M trypan blue in culture medium for 18 hours prior to challenge with target cells. Peritoneal macrophages were also labeled in vivo by inoculation of 4 mg of trypan blue intraperitoneally 48 hours before the mice were used as a source of macrophages for the cytotoxicity test. The cytotoxic effect of BCG- and toxoplasma-activated macrophages containing trypan blue in their vacuolar system was inhibited. However, there was transfer of trypan blue from activated macrophages to BALB/3T12 cells. These results suggest that lysosomal enzymes of activated

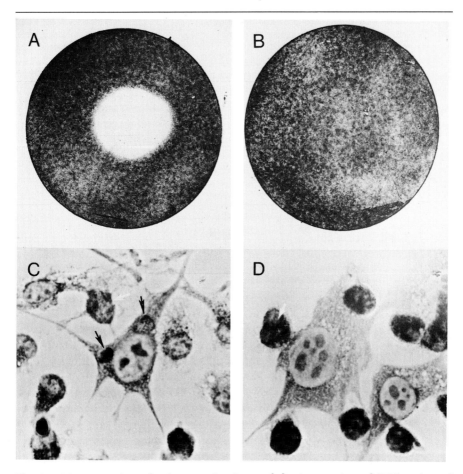

Fig. 4. Macroscopic and microscopic views of the interaction of BCG-activated and normal Balb/c macrophages with 3T12 target cells. The cytotoxicity test is described briefly in the caption to Figure 2. *A* and *B* were stained with giemsa 72 hours after 3T12 cell challenge. In *C* and *D*, macrophages were first labeled with dextran sulfate, challenged with 3T12 cells, and 24 hours later were stained with toluidine blue 0. *Macrophages are marked with white arrows.* (A) A thick multilayer of 3T12 cells grows to the immediate edge of a central monolayer of activated macrophages, which have destroyed the 3T12 cells (0-4 3T12 cells per field at × 400) with which they were in initial contact. (B) The central monolayer of normal macrophages has been completely overgrown by a thick multilayer of 3T12 cells. (C) A 3T12 cell in contact with activated macrophages is undergoing degenerative changes which include clumping of nuclear chromatin, vacuolation, and partial retraction of cytoplasm. The vacuoles (*black arrows*) of the 3T12 cell contain large dark dextran sulfate particles, which were strongly metachromatic when viewed with bright-field microscopy. (D) Healthy 3T12 cells, which are in contact with normal macrophages, contained no metachromatic granules when viewed with bright-field microscopy. Darker staining normal macrophages were strongly metachromatic [(A) and (B), × 2; (C) and (D), × 790].

macrophage origin may be the final molecular effectors of target cell destruction in this cytotoxicity system.

The inhibitory effect of trypan blue is not shared by the other tested nonenzymatic agents stored in secondary lysosomes. Dextran sulfate had no inhibitory effect on the cytotoxic reaction, and similar results were found with sucrose and Ficoll (average molecular weight, 400,000)—carbohydrates not digested by macrophages—that are taken up by macrophages and stored in secondary lysosomes (31). Normal macrophages with large secondary lysosomes containing sucrose or Ficoll were not cytotoxic for BALB/3T12 cells. Activated macrophages containing sucrose and Ficoll were cytotoxic for BALB/3T12 cells.

The interaction of macrophages and target cells in Sykes-Moore chambers maintained at 37°C was observed by phase-contrast microscopy (60). Initial contact between macrophages and target cells began as the target cells were spreading on the coverslip among the macrophages. Long thin extensions of macrophage cytoplasm (pseudopods) made contact with the target cell surface (Fig. 4). Activated macrophages were more active in extending pseudopods than were normal macrophages. Phase-dense granules could be seen to move from the macrophage perinuclear region to the pseudopod which they entered and slowly traversed centrifugally toward the target cell. Phase-dense granules were observed to be transferred from activated macrophages into the cytoplasm of BALB/3T12 cells. Activated macrophages vitally stained with neutral red or trypan blue were observed to transfer secondary lysosomes containing dye to BALB/3T12 cells. The cytoplasmic bridges between activated macrophages and target cells were always temporary, lasting several minutes to many hours. Activated macrophages were only rarely seen to transfer phase-dense granules or vitally stained secondary lysosomes to normal target cells. Normal macrophages were not observed to transfer phase-dense granules or vitally stained secondary lysosomes to either normal or tumorigenic target cells.

The findings suggest that the critical modification underlying the destruction of tumorigenic cells by activated macrophages may be local or general membrane destabilization in both cells, which favors focal and temporary membrane fusion (85, 115). The apparent universal susceptibility of tumorigenic cells to destruction by activated macrophages suggests that decreased membrane stability (increased membrane fluidity) may be fundamental to expression of the neoplastic phenotype. In addition to morphologic (89) and biochemical modifications (143), the results suggest that destabilization of macrophage membranes may occur in parallel with activation. Therefore, normal macrophages may not be cytotoxic because their stable membranes do not participate in the fusion reactions required for target cell heterolysis. Likewise, activated macrophages may have little or no cytotoxic effect for normal target cells because the stability of the latter's membranes does not favor the temporary cell fusion reaction required for heterolysis. Bucana et al. have confirmed the transfer of lysosomal material from activated guinea pig macrophages into syngeneic tumor target cells (22). Using a combination of cinemicrophotography, immunofluorescence, and electron microscopy, they demonstrated the lysosomal transfer from activated (but not normal) macrophages into the line 10 hepatoma cells. When viewed at the ultrastructural level, fusion between activated macrophages and tumor target cells was not seen in this study. It is possible that the transfer of lysosomal material occurred via exocytosis-endocytosis coupling, but the exact mechanism was not defined.

Trypan blue administered to mice suppresses the rejection of tumor allografts and reverses toxoplasma- or BCG-induced nonspecific resistance to tumor growth (61). It also inhibits the effects of pyran copolymer on tumor regression (99). Furthermore, it inhibits the rejection of allogeneic tumors mediated by immunologically specific mechanisms (61). Trypan blue does not alter the antibody response to the T cell-dependent antigen sheep red blood cells and does not alter the in vitro mitogenic response of lymph node cells to Concanavalin A, even though in mice receiving comparable regimens of trypan blue, rejection of allogeneic skin grafts is delayed (Kripke, Gruys, Hibbs, unpublished data). Trypan blue is not ingested by lymphocytes, basophils, eosinophils, or neutrophils (106). These results, although not conclusive, imply that the in vivo and in vitro effects of trypan blue in decreasing tumor cell killing and tumor regression are reflections of relatively specific alterations of macrophage killing function by inhibition of lysosomal enzymes.

VIII. Contribution of Macrophage-Soluble Factors to Macrophage-Mediated Cytotoxicity

Despite our and others' inability to demonstrate soluble cytotoxic mediators produced by macrophages, some have shown that macrophage cultures supernatants can lyse susceptible target cells in immune (80, 113) and nonimmune systems (34, 58, 94, 112, 118, 134). In general, the demonstration of the cytolytic factors has required various manipulations, e.g., use of reducing agents and especially sensitive assays (94, 118). The factors have differed widely in physical characteristics. The relevance of macrophage mediated destruction of red blood cells to tumor cell killing is not clear (94). The discriminatory capacity of a cell-free macrophage cytolytic factor between normal and tumor cells has been shown in one study (34). (See Table 7.)

Table 7. Macrophage-elaborated soluble cytotoxic factors

Investigator	Target Cell	Source of Factor	Effect	Molecular Weight	System Immune for Target Cell	Specificity for Neoplastic Cells
Pincus (112)	L cells	Isolated macrophages	Lysis	30–40K	No	None
Heise (58)	L cells	Isolated macrophages	Lysis	250K	No	Not tested
Kramer (80)	L cells, HeLa, fetal fibroblast	Macrophage with specific target cell	Lysis	47K, 50K	Yes	None
Piper (113)	Specific target cell	Macrophage with specific target cell	Lysis		Yes	None
Melsom (94)	RBC	Isolated macrophages	Lysis	"Low"	No	Not tested
Reed (118)	L cells	Isolated macrophages	Lysis	45K	No	None
Sethi (134)	Various normal and counterpart transformed cells	Isolated macrophages	Lysis		No	Some
Currie (34)	Sarcoma cells, normal rat kidney cells	Isolated macrophages	Lysis		No	Yes
Waldman (148)	Lymphoid cells	Isolated macrophages	Stasis	"Low"	No	Not tested
Nelson (101)	Lymphoid cells	Isolated macrophages	Stasis		No	Not tested
Calderon (24, 25)	Lymphoid cells, leukemic cells, mastocytoma cells	Isolated macrophages	Stasis	1.4K	No	None

Adapted from Ref. 118 with permission of the authors and publisher.

Other workers have demonstrated soluble factors elaborated by macrophages that have cytostatic but not cytolytic properties (24, 25, 101, 148). These substances inhibit DNA synthesis and proliferation of various cells including nonlymphoid tumor cells. The possibility of assay system artifacts (69, 105) has been eliminated by actual cell counting and determination of mitotic indices (24). They are elaborated by normal and activated macrophages in comparable amounts, and normal as well as neoplastic cells are affected. Evans and Alexander have noted that the killing in their system involves a combination of both cytostatic and cytolytic features (46). Some classes of activated macrophages were rapidly cytolytic in vitro, whereas others had cytostatic effects on the target cells with later target cell disintegration.

In our hands, supernatants from cultures of peritoneal macrophages activated in vivo by chronic BCG infection or in vitro by endotoxin are not able to cause release of tritiated thymidine from labeled tumor cells. However, supernatants from either activated or normal macrophages suppress tumor cell proliferation and DNA synthesis (Weinberg and Hibbs, unpublished data). The role of macrophage soluble cytolytic and cytostatic agents in production of cell death in macrophage mediated cytotoxicity continues to be not well understood. Table 7 summarizes various reports of macrophage-elaborated soluble factors affecting target cells and serves to emphasize the heterogeneity of the methods of production, methods of assay, and physical characteristics of the factors. The apparent requirement for activated macrophage-target cell contact in the in vitro cytotoxicity systems used by us and others implies that if soluble factors are important, they act only locally and are either rapidly deactivated in media or diffuse poorly in media.

IX. Ultimate Mechanisms of Killing

In comparison to the knowledge of mechanisms of microbial killing, little is known about the ultimate process of tumor killing by macrophages. The best characterized cellular microbicidal mechanism is the peroxidase-H_2O_2-halide (Pox-H_2O_2-Hal) system (79). This potent antimicrobial system is effective against bacteria (76), viruses (18), fungi (82), and mycoplasma (72). After polymorphonuclear leukocytes (PMN) phagocytize the microorganisms, peroxidase is released into the phagosome as fusion of the primary lysosome and phagosome occurs, and H_2O_2 is produced via the NADPH oxidase reaction set into action by the phagocytosis (109, 144). Peroxidase and H_2O_2 act in conjunction with chloride or iodide ions in the phagolysosome. In addition, peroxidase and H_2O_2 can be released extracellularly with phagocytosis (9, 10). Mammalian tumor cells can be destroyed when exposed to the components of the Pox-H_2O_2-Hal system *in vitro* (29) and PMN in the presence of phagocytosable particles and a halide cofactor can kill tumor cells without internalizing them (28).

Promonocytes and peripheral blood monocytes contain peroxidase in their lysosomes, but as they mature into macrophages, this activity is lost (36). Whereas noninduced mouse peritoneal macrophages have no detectable lysosomal peroxidase, peritoneal macrophages induced with sterile, inflammatory stimulants like casein or peptone have appreciable amounts of lysosomal peroxidase (138). Activated, noninduced peritoneal macrophages have no more peroxidase than do normal, noninduced peritoneal macrophages, but they are cytotoxic to tumor cells (59). Macrophages do contain catalase (50) which in the low pH environment of the lysosome also functions as a peroxidase (77).

Highly reactive free radicals are other potential macrophage weapons for tumor killing. Superoxide anion (O_2^-) is formed by the univalent reduction of oxygen (48). It is produced by phagocytizing PMN and macrophages (39) and contributes to bactericidal activity (78, 156). Superoxide dismutase, a metalloenzyme present in many cells including macrophages (38, 48) converts O_2^- to H_2O_2. H_2O_2 and O_2^- will react to form the highly destructive hydroxyl radical ($\cdot OH$) (55), the proposed effector in cell death induced by ionizing irradiation. In addition, singlet oxygen, another free radical with cidal capacity (4, 122) is generated by phagocytizing PMN or macrophages as evidenced by the chemiluminescence generated in the process (128).

The inhibition of macrophage mediated tumor cell killing by the lysosomal enzyme inhibitor trypan blue suggests a role for lysosomal enzymes in the killing process. The peroxidatic activity (be it peroxidase or catalase) present in macrophages could function in the Pox-H_2O_2-Hal system. Singlet oxygen or O_2^-, being generated in the vacuolar system as intermediates or by-products in the production of H_2O_2 by NADPH oxidase, could act as destructive effector molecules. The hydroxyl radical, generated by O_2^- and H_2O_2 interaction, also represents a potent killer molecule. Thus, although the exact molecular mechanism of neoplastic cell killing by activated macrophages is unknown, the killing may involve lysosomal enzymes, the Pox-H_2O_2-Hal system, and/or free radicals.

X. Macrophages in Established Tumors

The mass of a tumor is comprised of the neoplastic cells, supporting stroma and musculature, and inflammatory cells including PMN, lymphocytes, and macrophages. Evans demonstrated that macrophages comprise up to 60 percent of the cellular content of some tumors (42). The tumors with the highest content of macrophages were in general those considered most immunogenic. In addition, there was a relationship between the tumor macrophage content and the incidence of metastases— the more tumor infiltration with macrophages, the less the incidence of metastases (40). These relationships held true in experimentally induced animal tumors and in human breast carcinomas and melanomas (2). Currie (32, 35) has shown that serum lysozyme levels indirectly reflect the tumor macrophage content and the extent of disease. Russel et al. (125) demonstrated that spontaneously regressing Moloney sarcomas had more macrophages per gram of tumor than did advancing tumors. In addition, infiltration of macrophages into the tumor was associated with a decrease in the mitotic activity of the tumor cells. Macrophages removed from tumors have been shown to inhibit the growth of or kill tumor cells *in vitro* without additional activating manipulation (43, 57, 140).

XI. Macrophages in Immune Surveillance

The concept of immune surveillance against neoplasia as formulated by Thomas (145) and Burnet (23) has been coming under increasing scrutiny. Experimental evidence is accumulating that makes one question the full validity of the original concept that specific immunity against tumor neoantigens reduces the occurrence of clinically detectable cancer. The following points seem most relevant: (1) Although patients with severe congenital or acquired immunodeficiency have a greatly increased incidence of malignant neoplasms, the cancers are almost all of lymphoid origin with a slight increase in the incidences of skin, lip, and cervix cancers (93). These malignancies are all of suspected viral origin making one suspect defective surveillance against oncogenic viruses rather than defective surveillance against tumor neoantigens as the cause of increased tumor incidence. Patients with some diseases associated with pronounced immunosuppression (e.g., leprosy and sarcoidosis) do not have increased incidences of cancer (93). (2) Congenitally athymic, nude mice do not develop spontaneous tumors (126), but they are quite susceptible to experimental induction of tumors by oncogenic viruses (5). (3) If tumor development were the result of release from a surveillance mechanism, one would expect multiple and polyclonal tumor development. However, tumors usually arise at one site and are almost exclusively monoclonal in origin (49). Despite these discrepancies, we would not discard the concept of surveillance against cancer. Rather, we suggest that surveillance against neoplasia can involve both immune and nonimmune mechanisms. Immune responses would require lymphocytes, and nonimmune responses would involve macrophages functioning without the need for lymphocytes.

Phylogenetically, macrophages are primitive cells, functioning in invertebrates in the absence of lymphocytes and antibody (142). Invertebrates can recognize foreign tissue grafts and bacteria and eliminate them. The cockroach (131) and earthworm (11) reject foreign grafts. This rejection is apparently mediated by the amoeboid phagocytic haemocyte, a cell which morphologically and functionally is comparable to the vertebrate's macrophage. In the freshwater crayfish, the haemocytes, in cooperation with soluble, nonimmunoglobulin opsonins, phagocytize and kill bacteria. Crayfish that have received bacterial endotoxin have enhanced resistance to bacteria (92, 146). Furthermore, haemocytes from crayfish can kill mammalian tumor cells by nonphagocytic, nonspecific means. Sensitization of the crayfish to the tumor cells does not enhance the killing (147). Ontogenetically, macrophages may participate in certain types of tissue remodeling involving cell death during normal vertebrate embryogenesis before the onset of lymphopoeisis (130).

In summary, surveillance against cancer should probably be perceived as involving macrophages as well as lymphocytes and as having both nonimmune as well as immune components. Immune responses to tumors would involve lymphocyte recognition of neoantigens with subsequent responses like specific antibody production, killer lymphocyte generation, and the mobilization, activation, and focusing of macrophages in areas of tumor growth via lymphokine production. In the latter case, the cooperation of sensitized lymphocytes and activated macrophages in an immune response to tumor growth could involve both specific (sensitized lymphocytes) and nonspecific (activated macrophages) components.

In addition, nonimmune surveillance responses not involving lymphocytes could also utilize macrophage tumoricidal mechanisms. Macrophages activated directly by substances like endotoxin introduced via mouth or gut flora could recognize and destroy neoplastic cells by nonimmunologic mechanisms (see Section V). The failure of nonimmune macrophage surveillance against small numbers of neoplastic cells would then require a vigorous host response if the exponential proliferation of larger numbers of tumor cells were to be contained. At that point the amplification and focusing capability of a specific immune response to tumor specific antigenic stimulation would seem to offer the only means for mobilization of sufficient numbers of macrophages within areas of tumor growth for successful containment. However, the major unanswered question remains. Why do these surveillance mechanisms in the usual clinical setting fail?

XII. Tumor Defense Mechanisms

It would be naive to consider the tumor cell as a passive participant in the macrophage–target cell interaction. The shedding of tumor
specific transplantation antigen (TSTA) or histocompatibility antigens
may be a factor in the evading cytotoxic effects of macrophages. This
"decoy" mechanism is supported by studies showing that aggressive,
metastastizing tumors shed more TSTA (33), or have a higher surface
turnover rate of H-2 antigens (37) than do less aggressive tumors. Tumor
cells are very active metabolically. They synthesize and secrete certain
enzymes like plasminogen activator (116) which could conceivably interfere with macrophage effector mechanisms. The hypoxia created in the
tumor environment *in vivo* (135) could interfere locally with certain
oxygen-dependent killing systems, e.g., the Pox-H_2O_2-Hal system discussed above.

XIII. Conclusions

Over the past five to ten years, the importance of macrophages in
resistance to cancer has become more apparent. Not only can macrophages function in immunologically specific ways to eliminate tumors,
but they can also kill tumor cells by nonimmune means after being activated by lymphokines or agents like endotoxin. Treatment of animals
with agents like BCG or *C. parvum* reduces the incidences of spontaneously occurring or experimentally induced cancers. Activated macrophages have the unique capacity to selectively kill neoplastic cells
while not affecting normal cells. With increased awareness and more
clever techniques of examining tumors, we now appreciate that tumors
contain many macrophages and that these macrophages are capable of
killing those tumor cells.

Clinically, nonspecific immunotherapy is becoming more and more
popular. Unfortunately, the only consistent beneficial results have occurred in the treatment of cutaneous tumors by intralesional injection
(15). Treatment of other forms of cancer or of other "minimal residual
disease" states show promise, but as yet, the results show only marginal
or questionable benefit (41, 128a). A preliminary trial using macrophage-
activating lymphoid supernatants for injection into cutaneous metastases
(146) represents a logical attempt for immunotherapy using concepts derived from more basic research. But, clearly, clinical immunotherapy as
practiced today, leaves much to be desired.

The real challenge remains. We must more clearly understand the basic mechanisms of carcinogenesis and the body's pathophysiologic responses to cancer. The evasive defensive maneuvers of tumors must be understood and means of overriding these developed. Safe, effective means of manipulating and enhancing the body's inherent defense mechanisms against cancer will then be more easily developed. The macrophage, with its capability of being nonspecifically activated, its potent tumoricidal capacity and its selectivity of tumor destruction, is undoubtedly an important effector in surveillance against cancer and represents a potent source to tap for eventually developing more rational therapy of established tumors.

ACKNOWLEDGMENTS

This work was supported by the Veterans Administration, Washington, D.C., and by National Institutes of Health Grants CA 14045 and CA 15811.

NOTES

Recent in vitro studies have further characterized the modulation of macrophage tumor cell killing capability (25a, 67a). Various factors can influence the differentiation of macrophages to the tumoricidal state. Macrophages activated in vivo in BCG-infected ainmals are not tumoricidal in in vitro assays done in endotoxin-free cultures with endotoxin-free adult sera. But the isolated 40,000-90,000 dalton factor of normal serum, factor(s) in endotoxin-free fetal bovine serum, or picogram-nanogram amounts of endotoxin can make these nontumoricidal activated macrophages kill tumor cells. Similarly, macrophages isolated from progressing murine tumors are nontumoricidal in vitro, but they are "activated" since picogram-nanogram quantities of endotoxin make them tumoricidal (125a). Low density lipoprotein from normal serum or cholesterol-containing liposomes can inhibit the tumoricidal capability of activated macrophages, suggesting that macrophage membrane lipid composition may influence the modulation of the macrophage tumor cell killing (25a).

By using lymphocyte-free cloned macrophages, we have shown that endotoxin can act directly on macrophages to induce tumor cell killing without the need for the small numbers of B lymphocytes that commonly contaminate peritoneal exudate cell monolayers. This endotoxin effect was shown to be related to the lipid moiety of the molecule (148b, and Weinberg, J. B., Chapman, H. A., Jr., and Hibbs, J. B., Jr., Unpublished Results).

Although the exact mechanism of killing remains unknown, our further studies have shown that endocytosis of red blood cells, hemoglobin, or iron by activated macrophages inhibits their tumoricidal effect, thus further emphasizing the importance of the macrophage vacuolar system in the killing process (148a). Furthermore, in this study we showed that endotoxin-free catalase or superoxide dismutase had no effect on killing, thus decreasing the likelihood that the superoxide anion or the peroxidase-H_2O_2-halide system is instrumental in the killing.

REFERENCES

1. Aaronson, S. A., and Todaro, G. 1968. Basis for the acquisition of malignant potential by mouse cells cultivated in vitro. Science 162: 1024–1026.

2. Alexander, P., Eccles, S. A., and Gauci, C. L. L. 1976. The significance of macrophages in human and experimental tumors. Ann. N. Y. Acad. Sci. 276: 124–133.

3. Alexander, P., and Evans, R. 1971. Endotoxin and double stranded RNA render macrophages cytotoxic. Nature New Biol. 232: 76–78.

4. Allen, R. C., Stjernholm, R. L., and Steele, R. H. 1972. Evidence for the generation of an electronic excitation state(s) in human polymorphonuclear leukocytes and its participation in bactericidal activity. Biochem. Biophys. Res. Commun. 47: 679–684.

5. Allison, A. C., Monga, J. N., and Hammond, V. 1974. Increased susceptibility to virus oncogenesis of congenitally thymus-deprived nude mice. Nature 252: 746–747.

6. Allison, A. C., and Young, M. R. 1964. Uptake of dyes and drugs by living cells in culture. Life Science 3: 1407–1414.

7. Amos, D. B. 1960. Possible relationship between the cytotoxic effects of isoantibody and host cell function. Ann. N. Y. Acad. Sci. 87: 273–290.

8. Andersson, J., Möller, G., and Sjöberg, O. 1972. Selective induction of DNA synthesis in T and B lymphocytes. Cell. Immunol. 4: 381–393.

9. Baehner, R. L., Karnovsky, M. J., and Karnovsky, M. L. 1969. Degranulation of leukocytes in chronic granulomatous disease. J. Clin. Invest. 48: 187–192.

10. Baehner, R. L., Nathan, D. G., and Castle, W. B. 1971. Oxidant injury of caucasian glucose-6-phosphate dehydrogenase-deficient red blood cells by phagocytosing leukocytes during infection. J. Clin. Invest. 50: 2466–2473.

11. Bailey, S., Miller, B. J., and Cooper, E. L. 1971. Transplantation immunity in annelids. II. Adoptive transfer of the xenograft reaction. Immunology 21: 81–86.

12. Baird, L. G., and Kaplan, A. M. 1975. Immunoadjuvant activity of pyran copolymer: I. Evidence for direct stimulation of T-lymphocytes and macrophages. Cell. Immunol. 20: 167–176.

13. Baker, P., Weiser, R. S., Jutila, J., Evans, C. A., and Blandau, R. J. 1962. Mechanisms of tumor homograft rejection: The behavior of sarcoma I ascites tumor in the A JAX and C57BL/6K mouse. Ann. N. Y. Acad. Sci. 101: 46–62.

14. Basic, I., Milas, L., Grdina, D. J., and Withers, H. R. 1974. Destruction of hamster ovarian cell cultures by peritoneal macrophages from mice treated with Corynebacterium granulosum. J. Natl. Cancer Inst. 52: 1839–1841.

15. Bast, R. C., Jr., Zbar, B., Borsos, T., and Rapp, R. J. 1974. BCG and Cancer. N. Eng. J. Med. 290: 1413–1420 and 1458–1469.

16. Beck, F., and Lloyd, J. B. 1969. Histochemistry and electron microscopy of lysosomes, Ch. 21, in Lysosomes in Biology and Pathology, pp. 567–599. North-Holland Publishing, Amsterdam.

17. Beck, F., Lloyd, J. B., and Griffiths, A. 1967. Lysosomal enzyme inhibition by trypan blue: a theory of teratogenesis. *Science* 157: 1180–1182.

18. Belding, M. E., Klebanoff, S. J., and Ray, C. G. 1970. Peroxidase-mediated virucidal systems. *Science* 167: 195–196.

19. Bennett, B. 1965. Specific suppression of tumor growth by isolated peritoneal macrophages from immunized mice. *J. Immunol.* 95: 656–664.

20. Bernstein, I. D., Thor, D. E., Zbar, B., and Rapp, H. J. 1971. Tumor immunity: Tumor suppression *in vivo* initiated by soluble products of specifically stimulated lymphocytes. *Science* 172: 729–731.

21. Bradner, W. T., Clarke, D. A., and Stock, C. C. 1958. Stimulation of host defense against experimental cancer I. Zymosan and sarcoma 180 in mice. *Cancer Res.* 18: 347–351.

22. Bucana, C., Hoyer, L. C., Hobbs, B., Breesman, S., McDaniels, M., and Hanna, M. G., Jr. 1976. Morphologic evidence for the translocation of lysosomal organelles from cytotoxic macrophages into the cytoplasm of tumor target cells. *Cancer Res.* 36: 4444–4458.

23. Burnet, F. M. 1970. The concept of immunological surveillance. *Prog. Exp. Tumor Res.* 13: 1–28.

24. Calderon, J., and Unanue, E. R. 1975. Two biological activities regulating cell proliferation found in cultures of peritoneal exudate cells. *Nature* 253: 359–361.

25. Calderon, J., Williams, J. T., and Unanue, E. R. 1974. An inhibitor of cell proliferation released by cultures of macrophages. *Proc. Natl. Acad. Sci. U.S.A.* 71: 4273–4277.

25a. Chapman, H. A., Jr., and Hibbs, J. B., Jr. 1977. Modulation of macrophage tumoricidal capability by components of normal serum: a central role for lipid. *Science* 197: 282–285.

26. Chess, L., MacDermott, P. M., Sondel, P. M., and Schlossman, S. F. 1974. Isolation and characterization of cells involved in human cellular hypersensitivity. *Progress in Immunology* II, 3: 125–132.

27. Churchill, W. H., Jr., Piessens, W. F., Sulis, C. A., and David, J. R. 1975. Macrophages activated as suspension cultures with lymphocyte mediators devoid of antigen become cytotoxic for tumor cells. *J. Immunol.* 115: 781–786.

28. Clark, R. A., and Klebanoff, S. J. 1975. Neutrophil-mediated tumor cell cytotoxicity: Role of the peroxidase system. *J. Exp. Med.* 141: 1442–1447.

29. Clark, R. A., Klebanoff, S. J., Einstein, A. B., and Fefer, A. 1975. Peroxidase-H_2O_2-halide system: Cytotoxic effect on mammalian tumor cells. *Blood* 45: 161–170.

30. Cleveland, R. P., Meltzer, M. S., and Zbar, B. 1974. Tumor cytotoxicity *in vitro* by macrophages from mice infected with *Mycobacterium bovis* strain BCG. *J. Natl. Cancer Inst.* 52: 1887–1894.

31. Cohn, Z. A., and Ehrenreich, B. A. 1969. The uptake, storage and intracellular hydrolysis of carbohydrates by macrophages. *J. Exp. Med.* 129: 201–225.

32. Currie, G. A. 1976. Serum lysozyme as a marker of host resistance. II. Patients with malignant melanoma, hypernephroma, or breast carcinoma. *Brit. J. Cancer* 33: 593–599.

33. Currie, G. A., and Alexander, P. 1974. Spontaneous shedding of TSTA by

viable sarcoma cells: its possible role in facilitating metastatic spread. *Brit. J. Cancer* 29: 72–75.

34. Currie, G. A., and Basham, C. 1975. Activated macrophages release a factor which lyses malignant cells but not normal cells. *J. Exp. Med.* 142: 1600–1605.

35. Currie, G. A., and Eccles, S. A. 1976. Serum lysozyme as a marker of host resistance. I. Production by macrophages resident in rat sarcomata. *Brit. J. Cancer* 33: 51 59.

36. Daems, W. T., Wisse, E., Brederoo, P., and Emeis, J. J. 1975. Peroxidatic activity in monocytes and macrophages, in R. van Furth (ed.), *Mononuclear Phagocytes in Immunity, Infection, and Pathology*, pp. 57–82. Blackwell Scientific Publications, Oxford.

37. Davey, G. C., Currie, G. A., and Alexander, P. 1976. Spontaneous shedding and antibody induced modulation of histocompatibility antigens on murine lymphomata: correlation with metastatic capacity. *Brit. J. Cancer* 33: 9–14.

38. DeChatelet, L. R., McCall, C. E., McPhail, L. C., and Johnson, R. B., Jr. 1974. Superoxide dismutase activity in leukocytes. *J. Clin. Invest.* 53: 1197–1201.

39. Drath, D. B., Karnovsky, M. L. 1975. Superoxide production by phagocytic leukocytes. *J. Exp. Med.* 141: 257–262.

40. Eccles, S. A., Alexander, P. 1974. Macrophage content of tumours in relation to metastatic spread and host immune reaction. *Nature* 250: 667–669.

41. Eilber, F. R., Morton, D. L., Holmes, E. C., Sparks, F. C., and Ramming, K. P. 1976. Adjuvant immunotherapy with BCG in treatment of regional-lymph-node metastases from malignant melanoma. *N. Engl. J. Med.* 294: 237–240.

42. Evans, R. 1972. Macrophages in syngeneic animal tumors. *Transplantation* 14: 468–473.

43. Evans, R. 1975. Macrophage-mediated cytotoxicity: its possible role in rheumatoid arthritis. *Ann. N. Y. Acad. Sci.* 256: 275–287.

44. Evans, R., and Alexander, P. 1970. Cooperation of immune lymphoid cells with macrophages in tumour immunity. *Nature* 228: 620–622.

45. Evans, R., and Alexander, P. 1972. Mechanism of immunologically specific killing of tumour cells by macrophages. *Nature* 236: 168–170.

46. Evans, R., and Alexander, P. 1976. Mechanisms of extracellular killing of nucleated mammalian cells by macrophages, in D. S. Nelson (ed.), *Immunobiology of the Macrophage*, pp. 536–573. Academic Press, London.

47. Evans, R., Cox, H., and Alexander, P. 1973. Immunologically specific activation of macrophages armed with the specific macrophage arming factor (SMAF). *Proc. Soc. Exp. Biol. Med.* 143: 256–259.

48. Fridovich, I. 1972. Superoxide radical and superoxide dismutase. *Accounts of Chemical Research* 5: 321–326.

49. Friedman, J. M., and Fialkow, P. J. 1976. Cell marker studies on human tumorigenesis. *Transplant. Rev.* 28: 17–33.

50. Gee, J. B. L., Vassallo, C. L., Bell, P., Kaskin, J., Basford, R. E., and Field, J. B. 1970. Catalase-dependent peroxidative metabolism in the alveolar macrophage during phagocytosis. *J. Clin. Invest.* 49: 1280–1287.

51. Gordon, S., and Cohn, Z. 1970. Macrophage-melanocyte heterokaryons. I. Preparation and properties. *J. Exp. Med.* 131: 981–1003.

52. Gorer, P. A. 1956. Some recent work on tumor immunity. *Adv. Cancer Res.* 4: 149–186.

53. Granger, G. A., and Weiser, R. S. 1964. Homograft target cells: Specific destruction in vitro by contact interaction with immune macrophages. *Science* 145: 1427–1429.

54. Granger, G. A., and Weiser, R. S. 1966. Homograft target cells: Contact destruction in vitro by immune macrophages. *Science* 151: 97–99.

55. Haber, F., and Weiss, J. 1934. The catalytic decomposition of hydrogen peroxide by iron salts. *Proc. Roy. Soc.,* Ser. A 147: 332–351.

56. Hardy, D., and Kotlarski, I. 1971. Resistance of mice to Ehrlich ascites tumour after immunization with live *Salmonella enteritidis* 11RS. *Aust. J. Exp. Biol. Med. Sci.* 49: 271–279.

57. Haskill, J. S., Proctor, J. W., and Yamamura, Y. 1975. Host responses within solid tumors. I. Monocytic effector cells within rat sarcomas. *J. Natl. Cancer Inst.* 54: 387–393.

58. Heise, E. R., and Weiser, R. S. 1969. Factors in delayed sensitivity: lymphocyte and macrophage cytotoxins in the tuberculin reaction. *J. Immunol.* 103: 570–576.

59. Hibbs, J. B., Jr. 1973. Macrophage nonimmunologic recognition: target cell factors related to contact inhibition. *Science* 180: 868–870.

60. Hibbs, J. B., Jr. 1974. Heterocytolysis by macrophages activated by Bacillus Calmette-Guérin: lysosome exocytosis into tumor cells. *Science* 184: 468–471.

61. Hibbs, J. B., Jr. 1975. Activated macrophages as cytotoxic effector cells. I. Inhibition of specific and nonspecific tumor resistance by trypan blue. *Transplantation* 19: 77–81.

62. Hibbs, J. B., Jr. 1975. Activated macrophages as cytotoxic effector cells. II. Requirement for local persistence of inducing antigen. *Transplantation* 19: 81–87.

63. Hibbs, J. B., Jr., Lambert, L. H., Jr., and Remington, J. S. 1971. Resistance to murine tumors conferred by chronic infection with intracellular protozoa, *Toxoplasma gondii,* and *Besnoitia jellisoni. J. Infect. Dis.* 124: 587–592.

64. Hibbs, J. B., Jr., Lambert, L. H., Jr., and Remington, J. S. 1972. Adjuvant induced resistance to tumor development in mice. *Proc. Soc. Exp. Biol. Med.* 139: 1053–1056.

65. Hibbs, J. B., Jr., Lambert, L. H., Jr., and Remington, J. S. 1972. Possible role of macrophage mediated nonspecific cytoxicity in tumor resistance. *Nature New Biol.* 235: 48–50.

66. Hibbs, J. B., Jr., Lambert, L. H., Jr., and Remington, J. S. 1972. Control of carcinogenesis: a possible role for the activated macrophage. *Science* 177: 998–1000.

67. Hibbs, J. B., Jr., Lambert, L. H., Jr., and Remington, J. S. 1973. Activated macrophage mediated nonspecific tumor resistance associated with immunosuppression. *J. Reticuloendothel. Soc.* 13: 368.

67a. Hibbs, J. B., Jr., Taintor, R. R., Chapman, H. A., Jr., and Weinberg, J. B. 1977. Macrophage tumor killing: influence of the local environment. *Science* 197: 279–282.

68. Holtermann, O. A., Klein, E., and Casale, G. P. 1973. Selective cytotoxicity of peritoneal leucocytes for neoplastic cells. *Cell. Immunol.* 9: 339–352.

69. Houck, J. C. 1973. General introduction to the chalone concept. *Natl. Cancer Inst. Monogr.* 38: 1–4.

70. Huldt, G., Gard, S., and Olovson, S. G. 1973. Effect of *Toxoplasma gondii* on the thymus. *Nature* 244: 301–303.

71. Ipsen, J. 1959. Differences in primary and secondary immunizability of inbred mice strains. *J. Immunol.* 83: 448–457.

72. Jacobs, A. A., Low, I. E., Paul, B. B., Strauss, R. R., and Sbarra, A. J. 1972. Mycoplasmacidal activity of peroxidase H_2O_2 halide system. *Infect. Immunity* 5: 127–131.

73. Journey, L. J., and Amos, D. B. 1962. An electron microscope study of histiocyte response to ascites tumor homografts. *Cancer Res.* 22: 998–1001.

74. Kaplan, A. M., Morahan, P. S., and Regelson, W. 1974. Induction of macrophage-mediated tumor-cell cytotoxicity by pyran copolymer. *J. Nat. Cancer Inst.* 52: 1919–1921.

75. Kirchner, H., Holden, H. T., and Herberman, R. B. 1975. Splenic suppressor macrophages induced in mice by injection of *Corynebacterium parvum*. *J. Immunol.* 115: 1212–1216.

76. Klebanoff, S. J. 1967. Iodination of bacteria: a bactericidal mechanism. *J. Exp. Med.* 126: 1063–1079.

77. Klebanoff, S. J. 1969. Antimicrobial activity of catalase at acid pH. *Proc. Soc. Exp. Biol. Med.* 132: 571–574.

78. Klebanoff, S. J. 1974. Role of the superoxide anion in the myeloperoxidase-mediated antimicrobial system. *J. Biol. Chem.* 249: 3724–3728.

79. Klebanoff, S. J. 1975. Antimicrobial mechanisms in neutrophilic polymorphonuclear leukocytes. *Semin. Hematol.* 12: 117–142.

80. Kramer, J. J., and Granger, G. A. 1972. The *in vitro* induction and release of a cell toxin by immune C57Bl6 mouse peritoneal macrophages. *Cell Immunol.* 3: 88–100.

80a. Kriske, M. L., Norbury, K. C., Gruys, E., and Hibbs, G. B., Jr. 1977. Effects of trypan blue treatment on the immune responses of mice. *Infect. Immun.* 72: 121–129.

81. Larson, C. L., Ushijima, R. N., Florey, M. J., Baker, R. E., and Baker, M. B. 1971. Effect of BCG on Friend disease virus in mice. *Nature New Biol.* 229: 243–244.

82. Lehrer, R. I. 1969. Antifungal effects of peroxidase systems. *J. Bacteriol.* 99: 361–365.

83. Levy, H. B., Law, L. W., and Rabson, A. S. 1969. Inhibition of tumor growth by polyinosinic-polycytidylic acid. *Proc. Natl. Acad. Sci. U.S.A.* 62: 357–361.

84. Lohmann-Matthes, M. L., Schipper, H., and Fischer, H. 1972. Macrophage mediated cytotoxicity against allogeneic target cells *in vitro*. *Eur. J. Immunol.* 2: 45–49.

85. Lucy, J. A. 1970. The fusion of biological membranes. *Nature* 227: 815–817.

86. Lunde, M. N., and Gelderman, A. H. 1971. Resistance of AKR mice to lymphoid leukemia associated with a chronic protozoan infection, *Besnoitia jellisoni*. *J. Natl. Cancer Inst.* 47: 485–488.

87. Mackaness, G. B. 1962. Cellular resistance to infection. *J. Exp. Med.* 116: 381–406.

88. Mackaness, G. B. 1969. The influence of immunologically committed lymphoid cells on macrophage activity *in vivo. J. Exp. Med.* 129: 973–992.

89. Mackaness, G. B. 1970. The monocyte in cellular immunity. *Seminars in Hematology* 7: 172–184.

90. Mathé, G., Pouillart, P., and Lapeyraque, F. 1969. Active immunotherapy to L1210 leukemia applied after the graft of tumour cells. *Brit. J. Cancer* 23: 814–824.

91. McIvor, K. L., and Weiser, R. S. 1971. Mechanisms of target cell destruction by alloimmune peritoneal macrophages. I. The effect of treatment with sodium fluoride. *Immunology* 20: 307–313.

92. McKay, D., Jenkin, C. R., and Tyson, C. J. 1973. Effect of endotoxin on resistance of the freshwater crayfish (*Parachaeraps bicarinatus*) to infection. *J. Infect. Dis.* 128: 157–161.

93. Melief, C. M., and Schwartz, R. S. 1975. Immunocompetence and malignancy. (Cited in Möller, G. and Möller, E. 1976. The concept of immunological surveillance against neoplasia. *Transplant. Rev.* 28: 3–12, 1976).

94. Melsom, H., Kearn, Y. G., Gruca, S., and Seljelid, R. 1974. Evidence for a cytolytic factor released by macrophages. *J. Exp. Med.* 140: 1085–1096.

95. Meltzer, M. S., Tucker, R. W., Sanford, K. K., and Leonard, E. J. 1975. Interaction of BCG-activated macrophages with neoplastic and nonneoplastic cell lines *in vitro*: quantitation of the cytotoxic reaction by release of tritiated thymidine from prelabeled target cells. *J. Natl. Cancer Inst.* 54: 1177–1184.

96. Meltzer, M. S., Tucker, R. W., and Breuer, A. C. Interaction of BCG-activated macrophages with neoplastic and nonneoplastic cell lines *in vitro*: cinemicrographic analysis. *Cell. Immunol.* 17: 30–42.

97. Mitchell, M. S., Kirkpatrick, D., Mokyr, M. B., and Gery, I. 1973. On the mode of action of BCG. *Nature New Biol.* 243: 216–218.

98. Molomut, N., and Padnos, M. 1965. Inhibition of transplantable and spontaneous murine tumours by the M-P virus. *Nature* 208: 948–950.

99. Morahan, P. S., Kaplan, A. M. 1976. Macrophage activation and antitumor activity of biologic and synthetic agents. *Int. J. Cancer* 17: 82–89.

100. Morton, D. L., Eilber, F. R., Malmgren, R. A., and Wood, W. C. 1970. Immunological factors which influence response to immunotherapy in malignant melanoma. *Surgery* 68: 158–164.

101. Nelson, D. S. 1973. Production by stimulated macrophages of factors depressing lymphocyte transformation. *Nature* 246: 306–307.

102. Nicolson, G. L. 1971. Difference in topology of normal and tumour cell membranes shown by different surface distributions of ferritin-conjugated concanavalin A. *Nature New Biol.* 233: 244–246.

103. Old, L. J., Benacerraf, B., Clark, D. A., Carswell, E. A., and Stockert, E. 1961. The role of the reticuloendothelial system in the host reaction to neoplasia. *Cancer Res.* 21: 1281–1300.

104. Old, L. J., Clarke, D. A., and Benacerraf, B. 1959. Effect of Bacillus Calmette-Guérin infection on transplanted tumours in the mouse. *Nature* 184: 291–292.

105. Opitz, H., Niethammer, D., Jackson, R. C., Lemke, H., Huget, R., and Flad, H. 1975. Biochemical characterization of a factor released by macrophages. *Cell. Immunol.* 18: 70–75.

106. Padawer, J. 1973. The peritoneal cavity as a site for studying cell-cell and cell-virus interactions. *J. Reticuloendothel. Soc.* 14: 462–512.

107. Papermaster, B. W., Holterman, O. A., Klein, E., Djerassi, I., Rosner, D., Dao, T., and Costanzi, J. J. 1976. Preliminary observations on tumor regressions induced by local administration of a lymphoid cell culture supernatant fraction in patients with cutaneous metastatic lesions. *Clin. Immunol. Immunopath.* 5: 31–47.

108. Parr, I., Wheeler, E., and Alexander, P. 1973. Similarities of the antitumor actions of endotoxin, lipid A, and double-stranded RNA. *Brit. J. Cancer* 27: 370–389.

109. Patriarca, P., Cramer, R., Moncalvo, S., Rossi, F., and Romeo, D. 1971. Enzymatic basis of metabolic stimulation in leukocytes during phagocytosis: The role of activated NADPH oxidase. *Arch. Biochem. Biophys.* 145: 255–262.

110. Piessens, W. F., Churchill, W. H., Jr., and David, J. R. 1975. Macrophages activated *in vitro* with lymphocyte mediators kill neoplastic but not normal cells. *J. Immunol.* 114: 293–299.

111. Pimm, M. V., and Baldwin, R. W. 1975. BCG immunotherapy of rat tumours in athymic nude mice. *Nature* 254: 77–78.

112. Pincus, W. B. 1967. Formation of cytotoxic factor by macrophages from normal guinea pigs. *J. Reticuloendothel. Soc.* 4: 122–139.

113. Piper, C. E., McIvor, K. L. 1975. Alloimmune peritoneal macrophages as specific effector cells: characterization of specific macrophage cytotoxin. *Cell. Immunol.* 17: 423–430.

114. Pollack, R. E., and Burger, M. M. 1969. Surface-specific characteristic of a contact-inhibited cell line containing the SV_{40} viral genome. *Proc. Natl. Acad. Sci. USA* 62: 1074–1076.

115. Poste, G., and Allison, A. C. 1971. Membrane fusion reaction: a theory. *J. Theoret. Biol.* 32: 165–184.

116. Quigley, J. P., Ossowski, L., Reich, E. 1974. Plasminogen, the serum proenzyme activated by factors from cells transformed by oncogenic viruses. *J. Biol. Chem.* 249: 4306–4311.

117. Rapin, A. M., Burger, M. M. 1974. Tumor cell surfaces: general alterations detected by agglutinins. *Adv. Cancer Res.* 20: 1–91.

118. Reed, W. P., Lucas, Z. J. 1975. Cytotoxic activity of lymphocytes. V. Role of soluble toxin in macrophage inhibited cultures of tumor cells. *J. Immunol.* 115: 395–404.

119. Regelson, W., and Munson, A. E. 1970. The reticuloendothelial effects of interferon inducers: Polyanionic and nonpolyanionic prophylaxis against microorganisms. *Ann. N. Y. Acad. Sci.* 173: 831–841.

120. Ribi, E. E., Meyer, T. J., Azuma, I., and Zbar, B. 1973. Mycobacterial cell wall components in tumor suppression and regression. *Natl. Cancer Inst. Monogr.* 39: 115–119.

121. Riley, V. 1966. Spontaneous mammary tumors: Decrease in incidence in mice infected with the LDH virus. *Science* 153: 1657–1658.

122. Rosen, H., and Klebanoff, S. J. 1976. Singlet oxygen: A microbicidal product of the myeloperoxidase-mediated antimicrobial system. *Fed. Proc.* 35: 1391.

123. Rosenau, W., and Moon, H. D. 1961. Lysis of homologous cells by sensitized lymphocytes in tissue culture. *J. Natl. Cancer Inst.* 27: 471–483.

124. Ruskin, J., and Remington, J. S. 1968. Immunity and intracellular infection: Resistance to bacteria in mice infected with a protozoan. *Science* 160: 72–74.

125. Russell, S. W., Doe, W. F., and Cochrane, C. G. 1976. Number of macrophages and distribution of mitotic activity in regressing and progressing Moloney sarcomas. *J. Immunol.* 116: 164–166.

125a. Russell, S. W., Doe, W. F., and McIntosh, A. T. 1977. Functional characterization of a stable, noncytolytic stage of macrophage activation in tumors. *J. Exp. Med.* 146: 1511–1520.

126. Rygaard, J., and Povlsen, C. O. 1976. The nude mouse vs. the hypothesis of immunological surveillance. *Transpl. Rev.* 28: 43–61.

127. Sachs, J. H., Clark, R. F., and Egdahl, R. H. 1960. The induction of immunity with a new filterable agent. *Surgery* 48: 244–260.

128. Sagone, A. L., Jr., King, G. W., and Metz, E. N. 1976. A comparison of the metabolic response to phagocytosis in human granulocytes and monocytes. *J. Clin. Invest.* 57: 1352–1358.

128a. Salmon, S. E. 1977. Immunotherapy of cancer; present status of trials in man. *Cancer Res.* 37: 1245–1248.

129. Sanford, K. K. 1965. Malignant transformation of cells *in vitro*. *Int. Rev. Cytol.* 18: 249–311.

130. Saunders, J. W., Jr. 1966. Death in embryonic systems. *Science* 154: 604–612.

131. Scott, M. T. 1971. Recognition of foreignness in invertebrates. Transplantation studies using the American cockroach (*Periplaneta americana*). *Transplantation* 11: 78–86.

132. Scott, M. T. 1972. Biological effects of the adjuvant *Corynebacterium parvum* I. Inhibition of PHA, mixed lymphocyte and GVH reactivity. *Cell. Immunol.* 5: 459–468.

133. Scott, M. T. 1972. Biological effects of the adjuvant *Corynebacterium parvum*. II. Evidence for macrophage-T-cell interaction. *Cell. Immunol.* 5: 469–479.

134. Sethi, K. K., and Brandis, H. 1975. Cytotoxicity mediated by soluble macrophage products. *J. Natl. Cancer Inst.* 55: 393–395.

135. Shapot, V. S. 1972. Some biochemical aspects of the relationship between the tumor and the host. *Adv. Cancer Res.* 15: 253–286.

136. Shear, M. J. 1944. Chemical treatment of tumors. IX. Reactions of mice with primary subcutaneous tumors to injection of a hemorrhage-producing bacterial polysaccharide. *J. Natl. Cancer Inst.* 4: 461–476.

137. Sheinin, R., and Onodera, K. 1972. Studies of the plasma membrane of normal and virus-transformed 3T3 mouse cells. *Biochimica Biophysica Acta* 274: 49–63.

138. Simmons, S. R., and Karnovsky, M. L. 1973. Iodinating ability of various leukocytes and their bactericidal activity. *J. Exp. Med.* 138: 44–63.

139. Sinkovics, J. G., Ahearn, M. J., Shirato, E., and Shullenberger, C. C. 1970. Viral leukemogenesis in immunologically and hematologically altered mice. *J. Reticuloendothel. Soc.* 8: 474–492.

140. Stewart, C. C., Brandt, K., and Adles, C. 1975. Interaction of tumor derived macrophages with autochthonus tumor cells. *J. Reticuloendothel. Soc.* 18: 15b.

141. Strickland, G. T., Pettitt, L. E., and Voller, A. 1973. Immunodepression in mice infected with *Toxoplasma gondii. Amer. J. Trop. Med. Hyg.* 22: 452–455

142. Stuart, A. E. 1970. Phylogeny of mononuclear phagocytes, *in* R. van Furth (ed.), *Mononuclear phagocytes,* pp. 316–334. F. A. Davis, Philadelphia.

143. Stubbs, M., Kuhner, A. V., Glass, E. A., David, J. R., and Karnovsky, M. L. 1973. Metabolic and functional studies on activated mouse macrophages. *J. Exp. Med.* 137: 537–542.

144. Takanaka, K., O'Brien, P. J. 1975. Mechanisms of H_2O_2 formation by leukocytes. Evidence for a plasma membrane location. *Arch. Biochem. Biophys.* 169: 428–435.

145. Thomas, L. 1959. Discussion. P. D. Medawar paper, "Reactions to homologous tissue antigens and relation to hypersensitivity," *in* H. S. Lawrence (ed.), *Cellular and Humoral Aspects of the Hypersensitive States,* pp. 529–532. Hoeber, New York.

146. Tyson, C. J., and Jenkin, C. R. 1974. Phagocytosis of bacteria *in vitro* by haemocytes from the crayfish (*Parachaeraps bicarinatus*) *Aust. J. Exp. Biol. Med.* 52: 341–348.

147. Tyson, C. J., and Jenkin, C. R. 1974. The cytotoxic effect of haemocytes from the crayfish (*Parachaeraps bicarinatus*) on tumour cells of vertebrates. *Aust. J. Exp. Biol. Med.* 52: 915–923.

148. Waldman, S. R., Gottlieb, A. A. 1973. Macrophage regulation of DNA synthesis in lymphoid cells: effects of a soluble factor from macrophages. *Cell. Immunol.* 9: 142–156.

148a. Weinberg, J. B., and Hibbs, J. B., Jr. 1977. Endocytosis of red blood cells or haemoglobin by activated macrophages inhibits their tumoricidal effect. *Nature* 269: 245–247.

148b. Weinberg, J. B., Chapman, H. A., Jr., and Hibbs, J. B., Jr. 1977. Characterization of the effects of endotoxin on macrophage tumor cell killing. *J. Reticuloendothel. Soc.* 22: 23a.

149. Weiss, D. W., Bonhag, R. S., and DeOme, K. B. 1961. Protective activity of fractions of tubercle bacilli against isologous tumours in mice. *Nature* 190: 889–891.

150. Weissmann, G., and Dingle, J. T. 1961. Release of lysosomal protease by ultraviolet irradiation and inhibition by hydrocortisone. *Exp. Cell Res.* 25: 207–210.

151. Wilton, J. M., Rosenstreich, D. L., and Oppenheim, J. J. 1975. Activation of guinea pig macrophages by bacterial lipopolysaccharide requires bone marrow-derived lymphocytes. *J. Immunol.* 114: 388–393.

152. Woodruff, M. F. A., and Boak, J. L. 1966. Inhibitory effect of injection of *Corynebacterium parvum* on the growth of tumor transplants in isogenic hosts. *Brit. J. Cancer* 20: 345–355.

153. Wu, H. C., Meezan, E., Black, P. H., and Robbins, P. W. 1969. Comparative studies on the carbohydrate containing membrane components of normal and virus transformed mouse fibroblasts. I. Glucosamine-labeling patterns in 3T3, and SV-40 transformed 3T3 cells. *Biochemistry* 8: 2509–2517.

154. Yashphe, D. J. 1971. Immunological factors in nonspecific stimulation of host resistance to syngenic tumors. *Israel J. Med. Sci.* 7: 90–107.

155. Yoshida, T., Sonozaki, H., and Cohen, S. 1973. The production of migration inhibition factor by B and T cells of the guinea pig. *J. Exp. Med.* 138: 784–797.

156. Yost, F. J., and Fridovich, I. 1974. Superoxide Radicals and phagocytosis. *Arch. Biochem. Biophys.* 161: 395–401.

157. Zbar, B., Bernstein, I., Tanaka, T., and Rapp, H. J. 1970. Tumor immunity produced by the intradermal inoculation of living tumor cells and living *Mycobacterium bovis* (Strain BCG). *Science* 170: 1217–1218.

158. Zbar, B., Wepsic, H. T., Borsos, T., and Rapp, H. V. 1970. Tumor-graft rejection in syngeneic guinea pigs: Evidence for a two-step mechanism. *J. Natl. Cancer Inst.* 44: 473–481.

CHAPTER 4

BREAST CANCER AND CLINICAL IMMUNOLOGY

Loren J. Humphrey

The University of Missouri
School of Medicine at Kansas City
Kansas City, Missouri 64108

The availability and effectiveness of several modalities for the control of recurrent breast cancer along with a comparative favorable survival rate for treatment of the primary lesion have served to discourage clinical trials of immunotherapy and other clinical immunologic studies that have led to advances in clinical immunology of other cancers. As immunotherapy trials for other cancers continue to show safety and benefit and with the growing realization that even a 70% five-year survival rate for stage I carcinoma of the breast is unacceptable, clinical trials and immunologic studies of breast cancer have increased significantly in number.

While this presentation focuses primarily on the clinical immunology of breast cancer, a few pertinent animal-mammary tumor studies will enhance a grasp of the clinical developments.

I. MAMMARY TUMOR VIRUS

A. Animal-Mammary Tumor Data

The Bittner factor or milk factor is a pertinent starting point. As long ago as 1942, Bittner (5) reported that a factor in the milk of A strain mice was responsible for the development of mammary cancer in offspring. Crucial experiments in which some offspring were used from low mammary tumor strains (CBA) pointed to the existence in the milk of the high mammary tumor strain of a factor responsible for mammary tumors in offspring foster-nursed by low-strain mothers.

The role of the host in mammary carcinogenesis was aided by the work of Foley (26) who used an inbred strain of mice and a sarcoma induced by methylcholanthrene. He ligated the base of transplanted sarcomas when the tumors grew to 1 cm in diameter. The mice were challenged with a second graft at various time intervals and second grafts grew in only 16 of 81 mice rechallenged 2 to 6 days after legation of the first tumor. Interestingly, when a similar experiment was performed using a spontaneous mammary carcinoma, tumors failed to show protection to subsequent tumor challenge.

This seeming lack of antigenicity in spontaneous tissues was confirmed by Prehn and Main (58). When they immunized mice with a methylcholanthrene-induced sarcoma (Mc-Sa), only 20% of the mice developed tumors on rechallenge. In contrast, 71% of controls that received Mc-Sa challenge without prior immunization grew tumors. These investigators found that when a spontaneous sarcoma was studied in a similar fashion, 83% of mice rechallenged with the spontaneous tumor developed "take," whereas tumors grew in 91% of control mice. However, Martinez, Aust, et al. (52) subsequently showed definite immunity in mice transplanted with a mammary tumor. Thus data suggests that the mammary tumors are antigenic but less so when compared to chemically induced tumors.

With the strong growth of virology in the 1960s, work on the antigenticity of mammary tumors was related to the mammary tumor virus (MTV). Simons and Rios (62) demonstrated that Vibrio cholera neuraminidase treatment of mammary tumors increased their antigenicity but this increased antigenicity was unrelated to MTV antigen.

This study brought forth data suggesting that the mammary tumor virus and tumor immunogenicity were not interdependent. Vaage and Medina (67) reported on experiments that support this contention. These workers found that in a mammary tumor virus infected strains of mice (C_0H), 97% of mice developed mammary tumors on an average at 280 days, while in a MTV-free strain (C_3H_f) they found that 69% developed mammary tumors at an average of 708 days. Interestingly, 30% of tumors in the MTV-infected strain had MTV-associated tumor-specific transplantation antigens compared to 6% of tumors in the MTV-free strain.

Further supporting data came from the work of Halpin et al. (32). These workers induced mammary tumors in nonviral and nonantigenic preneoplastic nodules with either methylcholanthrene or dibenzanthracene. Of eight tumors so induced, seven were not antigenic while the eighth tumor gave tumor-specific immunity in BALB/c mice. The authors suggest that carcinogens may not directly induce the appearance of new antigens in the tumor they produce. Conflicting data were brought forth by Ankerst et al. (2) when they reported that lymphocytes from W/Fu rats bearing either a fibroadenoma (adenovirus type 9-induced) or a chemically induced mammary carcinoma not only react with homologous target cells but cross reacted with the unrelated tumor cells. In addition, they reported that sera from these tumor-bearing rats "blocked" the cytotoxicity reaction of the lymphocytes. Unfortunately, the microcytotoxicity test used by these authors has lacked reproducibility in the hands of most investigators. Furthermore, the serum "blocking" experiments as carried out in vitro in a complement-free test system have little correlation to the complement-rich in vivo system.

On the other hand, the positive role of immunity to MTV in mammary tumor development was suggested by the experiments of Goldfeder and Ghosh (28). In these experiments X/Gf mice which are highly resistant to the spontaneous development of mammary tumors were foster nursed by DBA/212 strain mothers who produce mammary tumors in high instance. The X/Gf mice developed mammary tumors after ingestion of MTV from the foster mothers in early generations but by the seventh generation, mammary tumors failed to develop. These data suggest that as the X/Gf mouse develops antibody to MTV, development of mammary tumors is inhibited.

That tumor-specific antigens exist in spontaneous mammary tumors seems beyond doubt as demonstrated by inhibition of macrophage migration tests (68); e.g., tumor antigens from mammary tumors inhibited the migration while antigens from methylcholanthrene-induced sarcomas failed to inhibit. At the same time, as noted above, spontaneous tumors seem less immunogenic than do chemically-induced tumors. From the brief review above, one can conclude that mammary tumors have MTV-associated antigens as well as antigens unrelated (or seemingly so) to MTV. Granted that the strain of mice judged to be MTV-free and mammary tumors found to demonstrate "no" antigenicity may indeed have undetectably low MTV levels and undetectably weak MTV-associated antigens. Also, the crucial question as to the exact role of MTV in mammary tumor development awaits definition. In this respect, the mammary tumor story is not unlike other carcinogenesis models. For example, the work of the Duran-Reynals (19, 20) and of Humphrey (47, 48) also suggests an interaction of chemical carcinogen with oncogenic agents. Thus one can speculate that MTV may accelerate tumor development as the data of Vaage and Medina (67) suggested. The absolute necessity of MTV in tumor development and the necessity of MTV-associated antigens in resistance to development of such tumors remains unanswered due to the lack of precise tools.

Nevertheless, the above review, although much too brief, should serve to alert the reader to the potentials and problems in a consideration of human breast cancer. As depicted in Fig. 1, several factors may be involved in oncogenesis, but when multiple factors interact, perhaps a more aggressive tumor develops.

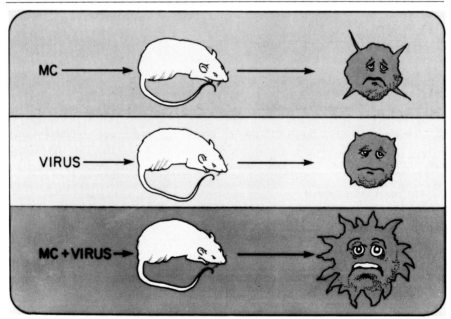

Fig. 1.   Factors operative in oncogenesis. MC = methylcholanthrene; Virus = mammary tumor virus (MTV); MC + Virus = methylcholanthrene (or unknown carcinogens) plus MTV or unknown virus.

B. Clinical Data

The data accumulated on mammary tumors in animals prompts investigation in two areas in human breast cancer: (1) search for a human mammary virus, and (2) search for tumor-specific or tumor-associated antigens in human breast cancer.

Several lines of evidence suggest that a virus may be associated with human breast cancer. In 1964, Lunger et al. (50) reported that milk from breast cancer patients and breast cancer tissue have identical viral particles not found in normal milk. Several reports have described B particles in human milk (18, 22). A fascinating line of evidence is that which points to a relation between murine MTV and human breast cancer. Thus Bowen and co-workers (12) reported that serum antibody from patients with breast cancer reacted with MTV particles. In addition, sera from cancer patients reacted with MTV in tissue sections (39) and had a neutralizing effect on MTV (14). Finally, in another line of evidence, Black et al. (8) showed that milk containing MTV and human breast cancer preparations inhibited human leukocyte migration. Thus, as can be seen, strong evidence exists to implicate a virus in human breast cancer. Nevertheless, the necessity and role of such a virus to the human breast cancer problem awaits proof.

Interestingly, some of the studies in searching for evidence for a virus associated with human breast cancer have produced immunologic data demonstrating an immune response by the patient with breast cancer; e.g., sera from breast cancer patient react with MTV (14, 39) and leukocytes respond in MIF tests to breast cancer preparation (7, 8) and are cytotoxic to breast cancer cells (3). Hickok (37) reported that sera and lymphocytes from breast cancer patients are cytotoxic for breast cancer cells in vitro. Hence data is sufficient to establish that the human host reacts immunologically against antigens in breast cancer tissue. On the other hand, the specificity and significance for the host of these immune responses remains speculative.

II. TUMOR IMMUNITY

A. Role of Regional Lymph Node in Immunologic Defense Against Breast Cancer

The precise role of the regional lymph nodes in defense against breast cancer occupies a central position in recommending treatment of the primary lesion. For years the optimum treatment of breast cancer has encompassed the concept that the regional lymph nodes must be removed with the breast. Knowing that cancer spreads with great proclivity to the axillary lymph nodes led Halsted (33) to recommend the classical radical mastectomy. Thus for half a century, the axillary contents were removed with the breast and pectoral muscles, fulfilling the concept that for solid tumors a procedure should remove the tumor and as much normal surrounding tissue as logically could be included.

Since from 35% (private population) to 65% (non-private patient population) had metastatic disease in the axillary lymph nodes at the time of radical mastectomy, this surgical philosophy was consonant with the principles of good cancer care. While previous authors had recommended an abandonment of procedures that removed the axillary contents, it remained for Crile (15) to evoke immunologic reasons for leaving the axillary contents at the time of mastectomy. This idea, not novel to immunologists, claimed that the axillary lymph nodes served as immunologic memory for the cancer and hence should be left in place for such function until clinically suspicious for cancer. Acceptance of this hypothesis required at least two conditions: (1) proof that the regional nodes were competent and necessary for immunologic memory directed against the cancer, and (2) demonstration that waiting until the axillary lymph nodes were clinically palpable did not represent significant delay.

Thus the role of the regional lymph node in defending against primary breast cancer deserves careful scrutiny. With respect to the first point, what immunologic role does the regional lymph node play? Considerable evidence exists to demonstrate that the regional lymph node responds to the presence of cancer in the host. For example, sinus histocytosis of the regional lymph nodes and lymphocyte infiltration of the tumor have been shown repeatedly to predict a favorable prognosis (1, 6).

1. ANIMAL TUMOR MODELS. Given strong evidence that a host response can be seen in regional lymph nodes, the immunologic function remains to be assessed. Do these lymph nodes act as a railroad station, guiding specifically sensitized lymphocytes and specifically armed macrophages to their proper destination, the primary breast cancer, or do the lymph nodes serve as assembly plants (Fig. 2) putting together the effectors of the immune response and retaining the molds for assembly of these cells? At the same time, one must query if the latter tenet holds. Does the memory remain in the regional nodes or at some point in the natural history of each tumor, does the plant set up memory cells elsewhere—e.g., the spleen?

Several experiments have attempted to answer these questions. Early before inbred animal strains became the sine qua non for separating transplantation immunity from tumor immunity, allogeneic studies using outbred animal strains produced confusing if not meaningless data (15,

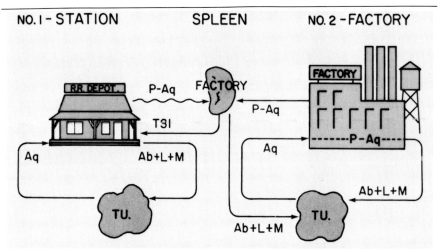

Fig. 2. The regional lymph node: factory or railroad station. *P-Ag* = Processed antigen; *TS1* = tumor-specific immunity; *Ag* = antigen; *TU* = tumor; *AB +L +M* = antibody plus lymphocyte plus macrophage.

23, 70). Interestingly, Mitchison and Duke in 1955 (53) had pointed out the problems encountered in studying tumor immunity in outbred animals.

Using syngeneic animals, Fisher and Hammond (24) showed that spleen cells can inhibit the growth of tumor cells *in vivo* and Humphrey and Goldfarb (45) demonstrated a similar effect using *in vitro* techniques. Further supporting data (34) showed that tumor cells injected in an operative site of mice grew equally as well when the regional lymph nodes were intact as when the nodes were absent. In addition, this report brought forth data concerning the immunologic responsiveness of these mice and showed that the regional lymph nodes were merely one part of the reticuloendothelial response to tumors.

These data showed that immunologic memory is not restricted to the regional lymph nodes. It remained for recent investigations to answer the crucial question, "When does this immunologic memory move beyond the regional lymph nodes?" Hence, when in the natural history of the primary breast lesion should one be concerned about occult metastases in the regional lymph nodes in correlation with movement of immunologic memory beyond these nodes? Solowey *et al.* (63) carried out precise experiments which showed that when the primary tumor is clinically detectable in the mouse, the immunologic memory has moved beyond the regional lymph nodes. This crucial point has been confirmed by others. Furthermore, the work of Friedlander and Baer (27) suggested that under some circumstances, an intact regional lymphatic system may lead to tolerance rather than sensitization.

Evidence in animals strongly suggests that by the time the tumor is clinically palpable, the regional lymph nodes have passed immunologic memory to more central depots.

2. CLINICAL DATA. Unfortunately, the similarity of animal tumor models to the human tumor model is different. The etiology, duration, patterns of dissemination, and other features of the human autochthonous tumor create numerous problems. Thus our scrutiny must be directed to the human model. As noted above (7), sinus histiocytosis is recognized as a predictable sign of a host response to the primary tumor and is correlated with a prognosis much better than for the host whose regional lymph nodes show no sinus histiocytosis. Further data support this, e.g., palpable lymph nodes in the homolateral axilla (17) and lymphocytic infiltration of the primary medullary carcinoma (25) predict a favorable prognosis. Reactive hyperplasia in the ipsilateral apical nodes also indicates a favorable prognosis (4).

Therefore, as in animal studies, data from man point to the regional node as a participant in the host response to a primary carcinoma in the breast. Recent reports have suggested that regardless of the regional nodes as railroad stations and/or assembly plants, very early immunologic memory moves beyond the regional lymph nodes. Thus Hickok (37) has shown that progressive involvement of regional lymph nodes predicts decreased ability of the lymph node cell to respond to soluble tumor antigen. Further data were brought forth by Humphrey et al. (42, 51), who demonstrated that long after radical mastectomy, breast cancer patients retain serum antibody directed against a cancer-associated antigen. Hence immunologic memory moves beyond regional lymph nodes relatively early in the natural history of breast cancer. Continued immune responsiveness of patients following radical mastectomy and the correlation of survival with maintenance of immune response have been detected by hypersensitivity to breast cancer antigen (7) by delayed skin hypersensitivity to breast cancer extracts (38), and by the persistence of serum antibody to breast cancer associated antigens as long as four years after radical mastectomy (43).

Needless to say, the extract role of the regional nodes during carcinogenesis and during the growth of minimal cancers remains a gap in our knowledge of fundamental importance. The observation that women with no evidence of metastatic disease in the regional nodes have serum antibody following radical mastectomy would seem to indicate the immunologic memory has moved centrally (43). Just as important, however, is the observation that 34 women with minimal breast cancer (diameter <

1.0 cm) failed to demonstrate serum antibody either before or after radical mastectomy (43) suggests that not only has the immunologic memory failed to move centrally, but perhaps there is no immune response regionally at this early stage of cancer.

B. Changes in Humoral and Cellular Immunity in the Host with Breast Cancer

1. CELLULAR IMMUNITY. One of the fundamental problems in tumor immunology is the lack of well-established tests that are excellent in vitro correlates of the patient's immune responsiveness. For example, the reproducibility of lymphocyte blastogenesis and microcytotoxicity tests remain in question. Hence the following review must be understood in this context.

While not tumor-specific in the immunologic context, the early reports pointing to a cellular response by the host are nonetheless important. Hence Grace and Kondo (30) showed that patients who made an inflammatory reaction to their tumor were immunologically responsive in that they could reject tumor and skin. In similar fashion, host response in the form of lymphocyte infiltration of tumor and sinus histocytosis of regional lymph nodes (16) indicated a favorable prognosis for that patient.

In some respects, the most reliable test of the patient's cellular immune responsiveness is evaluation of delayed hypersensitivity reactions. Thus Pinsky et al. (57) utilized response to DNCB (2,4-dinitrochlorobenzene) and found that 90% of 21 patients with localized breast cancer and 0 of 3 patients with generalized breast cancer could make a positive skin response. A decrease in skin reactivity was found only in patients terminal with breast cancer (54). These authors also reported a decrease in peripheral lymphocyte response to phtohemagglutinin in terminally ill patients but no decrease in T or B lymphocytes in any stage of disease. They further reported that there was no decrease in total peripheral lymphocyte count in any stage of breast cancer. This latter finding was not supported by the recent work of MacArthur and Humphrey (unpublished data), who noted a decrease in TPLC in patients with disseminated breast cancer but not in patients with localized or "cured" breast cancer. The role of a large tumor burden and its sponge effect on TPLC may well account for this observation.

A significant advance in evaluating the skin test response of breast cancer patients is the determination of response by the patient to preparations of cancer cells; e.g., Stewart (66) has reported extensive experience with cellular extracts of the patient's own malignant tumor. Thus Hollinshead et al. (38) reported that patients react against soluble membrane antigen(s) from breast cancer tissue as well as normal breast tissue. Separation of the antigen preparations by gradient polyacrylamide gel electrophoresis produced two distinct antigens: one was not present in normal breast tissue and the antigen from breast cancer tissues elicited reactivity in patients with localized or disseminated breast cancer.

At this point in time, sufficient clinical evidence exists to indicate that the host makes at least a non-specific immune response to breast cancer and very likely a cell-mediated tumor-specific response as well. The biologic significance of this response and its interrelationship with other aspects of the immune system awaits more reliable in vitro correlates of the host's immunologic responsiveness.

2. HUMORAL IMMUNITY.   Considerable data is available on the humoral response of the host to breast cancer and the availability and facility of reliable serologic tests undoubtedly accounts for this circumstance.

Several forms of serologic data relate a serologic response to breast cancer. For example, Springer and Desai (65) have found that anti-Vicia graminca sera react with human blood group N-like antigen on the cell surface of the TA3 mammary adenocarcinoma. These sera plus complement kill ordinary TA3-S+ cells.

A variety of tumor-associated protein markers and antigens have been reported. Carcinoembryonic antigen, while normal in 9 of 10 patients with localized breast cancer, was abnormal in 15 of 25 with disseminated disease (60). glycoprotein extracts prepared by affinity chromatography with colon and breast cancer tissue showed that primary breast cancers did not contain a CEA that was immunologically identical to CEA glycoprotein present in colon cancers (36). An antigen has been found associated with breast cancer tissue as well as certain benign breast diseases (46) and Zachrau et al. (69) have described protein components of human breast cancer tissues that indicate a favorable prognosis.

Antibody in sera of breast cancer patients was reported by Humphrey et al. (42) in 1971. These sera reacted in immunodiffusion tests with a soluble antigen preparation from breast tissue. Subsequent studies (43) showed this antibody to be present in sera of women with fibrocystic disease and fibroadenoma but rarely in "screenees" of a detection center for breast diseases. In the same year, Edynak et al. (21) reported that antibody was found in sera from 2,500 cancer patients. The antigen used in this was the supernatant (115,000 g) of breast cancer tissue. Sera from 3 of 42 breast cancer patients, 0 of 4 patients with fibrocystic disease, and 0 of 45 blood bank donors were found in immunofluorescence studies to be reactive against breast cancer cells (59). Complement fixation tests were also used (13) in demonstrating that 45% of sera from breast cancer patients, 13% of sera from patients with other breast disease and only 5% sera from controls reacted with a breast cancer cell line (Belev). Further support came from the work of Gorsky and co-workers (29). Using purified radioiodinated antibodies, they found that 52% of sera from breast cancer patients and 16% of sera from patients with other malignancies were more inhibitory in binding of the labeled antibodies to cancer cells than were 95% of the sera from healthy women.

Several authors have shown cross-reactivity of sera from patients with breast cancer against mouse mammary tumor virus antigens (12, 39). However, the work of Newgard et al. (55) seems to indicate that these antibodies may be nonspecific rather than cross-reacting, since the human antibodies reacted not only with MTV but also with mouse lactating mammary gland and dog milk.

Hudson and colleagues (40) found that antibody in the sera of breast cancer patients correlated with sinus histiocytosis of the axillary lymph nodes, lymphocytic infiltration of the tumor, and a favorable prognosis for the patient. Further studies on the antigen preparation to which this antibody is directed have revealed the presence of at least two distinct antigens. One antigen appears to be similar to the Fc fragment of immunoglobulins, and antibody to this antigen is found in sera of patients with breast cancer as well as sera of patients with benign breast diseases and sera of patients with other inflammatory lesions. The other antigen appears to be an altered Fab fragment of immunoglobulin and from the reactivity of sera seems restricted to patients with cancer. In addition, this anti-Fab antibody correlates with a favorable prognosis.

The finding that breast cancer patient's sera contains antibody that reacts with altered immunoglobulin suggests the association of autoimmune phenomena with breast cancer; antibody from the serum of one breast cancer patient cross reacted with heat-altered immunoglobulin. The antibody is found in sera of patients with other cancers but seldom in sera of patients with other diseases: 1 of 89 patients with fibrocystic disease, 0 of 112 patients with fibroadenoma, and only 1 of 916 screenees from a detection center for breast disease (Humphrey—unpublished data). Similarly, Hartman and Lewis (35) have reported that autoimmune phenomena are associated with cancer.

From the above data, one must conclude that the host makes a definite humoral immune response to breast cancer. The specificity of the antigen(s) eliciting this response and the biologic significance of the antibodies needs further elaboration. At this point, some serologic reactions appear strongly cancer associated and some very likely represent autoimmune phenomena. The importance to the host and the interplay of these phenomena is still quite conjectural. However, as depicted in Figure 3, many receptors are on or associated with the cancer cell membrane.

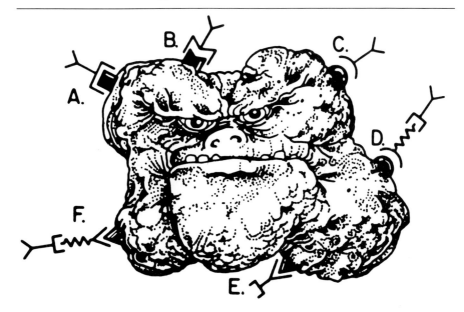

Fig. 3.   Receptors associated with the cancer cell. A = Tissue-specific antigen plus antitissue-specific antibody; B = HLA antigen plus anti-HLA antibody; C = F_c receptor plus immunoglobulin molecule attached by F_c end; D = F_c receptor plus F_c fragment of Igb plus anti-F_c antibody; E = Tumor antigen plus anti-tumor antigen antibody; F = Tumor antigen plus altered Fab fragment of Igb plus anti-Fab antibody.

Hence, of the many antibodies detected, some may be directed against unmasked antigens, against tumor specific markers, tumor viral glycoproteins or even degraded fragments of antibody attached to cell receptors.

III. TRIAL OF IMMUNOTHERAPY

A. Animal Model

Report of a common antigen in MTV-infected tissue from five different mouse strains (9) as well as the numerous reports mentioned above concerning the cross-reactivity of sera from breast cancer patients with MTV suggests that the mouse-MTV model may be similar to the human breast cancer model. The failure to identify MTV in man blunts the enthusiasm for pursuing the immunotherapy studies in animals. Nevertheless, some consideration of the animal model has merit. For example, Simmons *et al.* (63) worked with spontaneous mammary tumors in the C3H/HeJ female mouse. When tumors reached 0.8 cm in diameter, the mice were divided into several groups: (a) inject VCN (neuraminidase) intratumor, (b) inject BCG intratumor, (c) inject sterile medium, (d) inject heat-inactivated VCN and BCG, and (e) inject BCG and VCN. This latter group not only gave most significant regression of these established tumors, but no deaths were noted at 200 days compared to an average time of death in other groups of 88.4 days, 79.5 days, 66.5 days, and 79.5 days respectively. Interestingly, 9 of 13 animals treated with BCG + VCN developed mammary tumors in a second gland during therapy. This curious occurrence suggests that the immunotherapy stimulated immunity to unique antigens in the established tumor but the immunity was not directed to the MTV-related antigen.

In a rat mammary adenocarcinoma model, Bogden *et al.* (11) demonstrated the effectiveness of combination surgery, chemotherapy and immunotherapy. Their data showed that when chemotherapy is used with immunotherapy, optimum results were obtained when used in a short course and at a dose that was not immunosuppressive.

B. Human Model

Due to the effectiveness of several modalities in controlling recurrent and/or disseminated breast cancer, immunotherapy trials have rarely been employed in the patient with breast cancer. In a report of a phase I type study, Humphrey (41) reported that an allogeneic tumor cell vaccine resulted in disappearance of pulmonary lesions in one patient (see Fig. 4) and disappearance of bone lesions in a second patient. Prolongation of life was suggested as well. Other reports, although also involving a small number of patients, suggest that non-specific immunotherapy may be of value for the patient with disseminated breast cancer; both levamisole (61) and transfer factor (66) have given a prolongation of survival.

Recent reports have indicated the value of combination chemotherapy and immunotherapy. Thus Israel and Edelstein (49) used immunotherapy with chemotherapy to demonstrate prolonged survival compared to patients receiving chemotherapy only. This observation was supported by the work of Gutterman *et al.* (31) who used BCG with chemotherapy to demonstrate prolongation of life over controls. Note should be made that prolonged survival is seen in comparison to historical controls. With the voluminous data on results of different chemotherapeutic regimens, historical controls should be adequate for comparison, notwithstanding the fact that a randomized control with the short-term benefit of chemotherapy alone may be contraindicated. Nonetheless, sufficient trials have

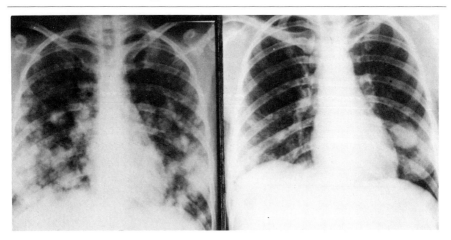

Fig. 4. Response of metastases to immunotherapy: *left*—picture of chest X-ray taken before immunotherapy; *right*—picture of chest X-ray taken 8 weeks after treatment with allogeneic breast cancer vaccine.

been attempted with breast cancer patients to demonstrate their safety and the results have been encouraging enough to stimulate further trials.

CONCLUSIONS

Clinical immunology has much to offer the patient with breast cancer. The work on hormone receptors associated with breast cancer, the studies on serodiagnosis and seroprognosis and the early immunotherapy results support this bold statement. One can only hope that the preliminary and somewhat anecdotal trials of immunotherapy will lead to a very positive role for immunology in controlling breast cancer.

REFERENCES

1. Anastassiades, O. T., and Pryce, D. M. 1966. Immunologic significance of morphologic changes in lymph nodes draining breast. *Cancer* 18: 239–245.
2. Ankerst, J., Steele, G. J., and Sjögren, H. O. 1974. Cross-reacting associated antigen(s) of adenovirus type 9-induced fibroadenomas and a chemically-induced mammary carcinoma in rats. *Cancer Res.* 34: 1794–1800.
3. Avis, F., Mosonov, I., and Haughton, G. 1974. Antigenic cross-reactivity between benign and malignant neoplasma of the human breast. *JNCI* 52: 1041–1049.

4. Berg, J. W., Huvos, A. G., Axtell, L. M., and Robbins, G. F. 1973. A new sign of favorable prognosis in mammary cancer. *Ann. Surg.* 177: 8–12.

5. Bittner, J. J. 1936. Some possible effects of nursing on the mammary gland tumor incidence in mice. *Science* 84: 162.

6. Black, M. M., and Asire, A. J. 1969. Palpable axillary lymph nodes in cancer of the breast. *Cancer* 23: 251–259.

7. Black, M. M., Leis, H. P., Jr., Shore, B., and Zachrau, R. E. 1974. Cellular hypersensitivity to breast cancer: Assessment by a leukocyte migration procedure. *Cancer* 33: 952–958.

8. Black, M. M., Moore, D. H., Shore, B., Zachrau, R. E., and Leis, H. P., Jr. 1974. Effect of murine milk samples and human breast tissues on human leukocyte migration indices. *Cancer Res.* 34: 1054–1060.

9. Blair, P. B. 1965. Immunology of the mouse mammary tumor virus (MTV): A qualitative *in vitro* assay for MTV. *Nature (London)* 203: 165–167.

10. Blair, P. B., and Lane, M. A. 1974. Serum factors in mammary neoplasia: Enhancement and antagonism of spleen cell activity *in vitro* detected by different methods of serum factor assay. *J. Immunol.* 112: 439–443.

11. Bogden, A. E., Esber, H. J., Taylor, D. J., and Gray, J. H. 1974. Comparative study on the effects of surgery, chemotherapy and immunotherapy alone and in combination on metastases of the 13762 mammary adenocarcinoma. *Cancer Res.* 34: 1627–1631.

12. Bowen, J. M., Dmochowski, L., Miller, M. F., Priori, E. S., Seman, G., Dodson, M. L., and Maruyana, K. 1976. Implications of humoral antibody in mice and humans to breast tumor and mouse mammary tumor virus-associated antigens. *Cancer Res.* 36: 759–763.

13. Chan, S. D., Maca, R. D., Levine, P. H., and Ting, R. C. 1971. Immunologic studies of human breast cancer. *JNCI* 47: 511–517.

14. Charney, J., and Moore, D. H. 1971. Neutralization of murine mammary tumor virus by sera of women with breast cancer. *Nature* 229: 627–628.

15. Crile, G. J. 1968. The effect on metastasis of removing or irradiating regional nodes of mice. *Surg. Gyn. Obst.* 126: 1270–1272.

16. Cutler, S. J., Black, M. M., Mork, T., Harvei, S., and Freeman, C. 1969. Further observations on prognostic factors in cancer of the female breast. *Cancer* 24: 653–667.

17. Cutler, S. J., Zippin, C., and Asire, A. J. 1969. The prognostic significance of palpable lymph nodes in cancer of the breast. *Cancer* 23: 243–250.

18. Dmochowski, L., Seman, G., and Gallager, H. S. 1969. Viruses as possible etiologic factors in human breast cancer. *Cancer* 24: 1241–1249.

19. Duran-Reynals, F. 1952. Studies on the combined effects of fowl pox virus and methylcholanthrene in chickens. *Ann. N.Y. Acad. Sci.* 54: 977–991.

20. Duran-Reynals, M. L. 1962. Carcinogenesis in cortisone-treated mice following vaccinia dermal infection and application of methylcholanthrene. *JNCI* 29: 635–647.

21. Edynak, E. M., Lardis, M. P., and Vrana, M. 1971. Antigenic changes in human breast neoplasia. *Cancer* 28: 1457–1461.

22. Feller, W. R., and Chopra, H. C. 1969. Studies of human milk in relation to the possible viral etiology of breast cancer. *Cancer* 24: 1250–1254.

23. Fisher, B., and Fisher, E. R. 1967. Barrier functions of lymph node to tumor cells and erythrocytes. *Cancer* 20: 1907–1913.

24. Fisher, J. C., and Hammond, W. G. 1966. Inhibition of tumor growth by syngeneic spleen cell transfer. *Surg. Forum* 17: 102–104.

25. Flores, L., Arlen, M., Elguezabal, A., Livingston, S. F., and Levowitz, B. S. 1974. Host tumor relationships in medullary carcinoma of the breast. *Surg. Gyn. Obst.* 139: 683–688.

26. Foley, E. J. 1953. Antigenic properties of methylcholanthrene-induced tumors in mice of the strain of origin. *Cancer Res.* 13:835–837.

27. Friedlander, M. H., and Baer, H. 1972. Immunologic tolerance: Role of the regional lymph node. *Science* 176: 312–314.

28. Goldfeder, A., and Ghosh, A. K. 1974. Mammary carcinogenesis in foster nursed X/Gf mice. *Cancer Res.* 34: 2184–2191.

29. Gorsky, Y., Vanky, F., and Sulitzeanu, D. 1976. Isolation from patients with breast cancer of antibodies specific for antigens associated with breast cancer and other malignant diseases. *Proc. Natl. Acad. Sci.* 73: 2101–2105.

30. Grace, J. T., and Kondo, T. 1958. Investigations of host resistance in cancer patients. *Ann. Surg.* 148: 633–641.

31. Gutterman, J. U., Blumenschein, G. R., Hortobagyi, G., Mavligut, G., and Hersh, E. M. 1976. Immunotherapy for breast cancer. *Breast* 2:29.

32. Halpin, Z. T., Vaage, J., and Blair, P. B. 1972. Lack of antigenicity of mammary tumors induced by carcinogens in a non-antigenic preneoplastic lesion. *Cancer Res.* 32: 2197–2200.

33. Halsted, W. S. 1896. The results of operations for the cure of cancer of the breast performed at the Johns Hopkins Hospital from June 1889 to January 1894. *Johns Hopkins Hospital Rep.* 4: 297–328.

34. Hammond, W. G., and Rolley, R. T. 1970. Retained regional lymph nodes: Effect on metastasis and recurrence after tumor removal. *Cancer* 25: 368–372.

35. Hartmann, D., and Lewis, M. G. 1974. Presence and possible role of anti-IgG antibodies in human malignancy. *Lancet* 29: 1318–1319.

36. Harvey, S. R., Girota, R. N., Nemoto, T., Ciani, F., Chu, T. M. 1974. Immunochemical studies on carcinoembryonic antigen-reactive glycoproteins from carcinomas of the colon and breast separated by concanvalin A affinity chromatography. *Cancer Res.* 36: 3486–3494.

37. Hickok, D. F. 1970. The progressive lymph node defect in cancer patients. *Surg. Forum* 21: 114–116.

38. Hollinshead, A. C., Jaffurs, W. T., Alpert, L. K., Harris, J. E., and Herbermann, R. B. 1974. Isolation and identification of soluble skin-reactive membrane antigens of malignant and normal human breast cells. *Cancer Res.* 34: 2961–2968.

39. Hoshino, M., and Dmochowski, L. 1973. Electron microscope study of antigens in cells of mouse mammary tumor cell lines by peroxidase-labeled antibodies in sera of mammary tumor-bearing mice and of patients with breast cancer. *Cancer Res.* 33: 2551–2561.

40. Hudson, M. J. K., Humphrey, L. J., Mantz, F. A., and Morse, P. A., Jr. 1974. Correlation of circulating serum antibody to the histologic findings in breast cancer. *Amer. J. Surg.* 128: 756–762.

41. Humphrey, L. J. 1975. Approaches to immunotherapy in cancer, *in* B. A.

Stoll (ed.), *Host Defense in Breast Cancer*, pp. 191–199. London, England.

42. Humphrey, L. J., Barker, C., Bokesch, G., Fetter, D., Amerson, J. R., and Boehm, O. R. 1971. Immunologic competence of regional lymph nodes in patients with breast cancer. *Ann. Surg.* 174: 383–391.

43. Humphrey, L. J., Estes, N. C., Morse, P. A., Jr., Jewell, W. R., Boudet, R. A., and Hudson, M. J. K. 1974. Serum antibody in patients with mammary disease. *Cancer* 34: 1516–1520.

44. Humphrey, L. J., Estes, N. C., Morse, P. A., Jr., Jowoll, W. R., Boudct, R. A., Hudson, M. J. K., Tsolakidis, P. G., and Mantz, F. A. 1974. Serum antibody in patients with breast disease. *Ann. Surg.* 180: 124–129.

45. Humphrey, L. J., and Goldfarb, P. M. 1966. Immunologic competence of spleen cells from tumor-bearing mice. *Surg. Forum* 17: 262–264.

46. Humphrey, L. J., Jewell, W. R., Mahoney, J. C., and Boehm, O. R. 1972. Kansas breast study. *J. Kans. Med. Soc.* 73: 120–122.

47. Humphrey, L. J., Lincoln, P., Hunter, L., and Jewell, W. R. 1969. Immunologic studies on carcinogenesis. *Curr. Topics in Surg. Res.* 1: 91–103.

48. Humphrey, L. J., and Milgrom, F. 1965. Hermadsorbing factor of malignant tumors. *Surg. Forum* 16: 106–108.

49. Israel, L., Edelstein, R. 1975. Non-specific immunostimulation with C parvum in human cancer, *in Immunologic Aspects of Neoplasia*, pp. 485–493. 26th Annual Symposium, Williams & Wilkins Co., Baltimore.

50. Lunger, P. D., Lucas, J. C., Jr., and Shipley, F. H. 1964. The ultramorpholophy of milk fractions from patients with breast cancer. *Cancer* 17: 549–557.

51. Mahoney, J. C., Boehm, O. R., Boehm, B. J., and Humphrey, L. J. 1972. Studies of serum from patients with breast cancer. *Surg. Forum* 23: 87.

52. Martinez, C., Aust. J. B., Bittner, J. J., and Good, R. A. 1957. Continuous growth of isotransplants of a mammary tumor associated with the development of immunity in mice. *Cancer Res.* 17: 205–207.

53. Mitchison, N. A., and Duke, O. L. 1955. Studies on the immunological response to foreign tumor transplants in the mouse. *J. Exp. Med.* 102: 179–197.

54. Nemoto, T., Han, T., Ninowanda, J., Angkur, V., Chamberlain, A., and Dao, T. L. 1974. Cell-mediated immune status of breast cancer patients. *JNCI* 53: 641–645.

55. Newgard, K. W., Cardiff, R. B., and Blair, P. B. 1976. Human antibodies binding to the mouse mammary tumor virus: A nonspecific reaction. *Cancer Res.* 36: 765–768.

56. Oettgen, H. F., Old, L. J., Farrow, J. H., *et al.* 1974. Effects of dialyzable transfer factor in patients with breast cancer. *Proc. Natl. Acad. Sci.* 71: 2319–2323.

57. Pinsky, C. M., Ep-Domeiri, A. M., Caron, A. S., Knapper, W. H., and Oettgen, H. F. 1974. Delayed hypersensitivity reactions in patients with cancer. *Rec. Results Cancer Res.* 47: 37–41.

58. Prehn, R. T., and Main, J. M. 1957. Immunity to methylcholanthrene-induced sacromas. *JNCI* 18: 769–779.

59. Priori, E. S., Seman, G., Dmochowski, L., Gallager, H. S., and Anderson, D. E. 1971. Immunofluorescence studies on sera of patients with breast carcinoma, *Cancer* 28: 1462–1471.

60. Reynoso, G., Chu, T. M., Holyoke, D., Cohen, C., Nemoto, T., Wang, J-J.,

Chuang, P., Murphy, G. P. 1972. Carcinoembryonic antigen in patients with different cancers. *JAMA* 220: 361–365.

61. Rojas, A. F., Feierstein, J. N., Mickiewicz, E., *et al.* 1976. Levamisole in advanced human breast cancer. *Lancet* 1: 211–215.

62. Simmons, R. L., and Rios, H. 1973. Differential effect of neuraminidase on the immunogenicity of viral associated and private antigens of mammary carcinomas. *J. Immunol.* 111: 1820–1825.

63. Simmons, R. L., Rios, A., and Kersey, J. H. 1972. Regression of spontaneous mammary carcinomas using direct injection of neuraminidase and BCG. *J. Surg. Res.* 12: 57–61.

64. Solowey, M. S., Pendergrast, W. J., and Meyers, G. H., Jr. 1972. Effect of regional lymphadenectomy on development of concomitant immunity. *Surg. Forum* 23: 101–102.

65. Springer, G. F., and Desai, P. R. 1974. Relation of human blood group MN to cancer cell surface antigens and to receptors for oncogenic viruses. *Ann. Clin. Lab. Sci.* 4: 294–298.

66. Stewart, T. H. M. 1969. The presence of delayed hypersensitivity reactions in patients toward cellular extracts of their malignant tumors. *Cancer* 23: 1368–1379.

67. Vaage, J., and Medina, D. 1974. Virus oncogenesis and tumor immunogenicity in the mouse mammary tumor system. *Cancer Res.* 34: 1319–1324.

68. Vaage, J., Jones, R. D., and Brown, B. W. 1972. Tumor-specific resistance in mice detected by inhibition of macrophage migration. *Cancer Res.* 32: 680–687.

69. Zachrau, R. E., Black, M. M., Dion, A. S., Shore, B., Isac, M., Andrade, A. M., and Williams, C. J. 1976. Prognostically significant protein components of human breast cancer tissues. *Cancer Res.* 36: 3143–3146.

70. Zeidman, I., and Buss, J. M. 1954. Experimental studies on the spread of cancer in the lymphatic system. *Cancer Res.* 114: 403–405.

CHAPTER 5

CYCLIC NUCLEOTIDES IN IMMUNE REGULATION AND IMMUNO-POTENTIATOR ACTION

John W. Hadden
and Lilian Delmonte

Laboratory of Immunopharmacology
and Institute Therapy Development
Memorial Sloan-Kettering
Cancer Center
New York, New York 10021

The cyclic nucleotides are implicated as intracellular mediators of diverse hormonal and pharmacologic agents acting on lymphocytes, macrophages, granulocytes, mast cells and platelets. Cyclic GMP is associated with augmentation and cyclic AMP with inhibition of the immunologic functions of each of these cell types. Cyclic AMP is associated with the induction of differentiation in lymphocyte precursors. An analysis of the biological actions and mechanisms of actions of three prototype immunopotentiators (levamisole, poly A:U, and endotoxin) suggest that they act to modify immune responses through changes in cyclic nucleotide levels in these cells. A cyclic-nucleotide-based immunopharmacology appears rational for future drug development.

This chapter will address itself to a discussion of three prototypic, chemically defined immunopotentiators—levamisole, polyadenylic acid:polyuridylic acid (poly A:U), and endotoxin (LPS)—and will discuss the evidence which indicates that the mechanisms of action of these agents involve cyclic 3',5'-adenosine monophosphate (cyclic AMP) and cyclic 3',5'-guanosine monophosphate (cyclic GMP). We will present a background of the roles played by cyclic AMP and cyclic GMP in mediating hormonal influences which modify the functions of lymphocytes, macrophages, granulocytes, basophils and tissue mast cells, and platelets. We will also review the principal *in vivo* and *in vitro* effects of the three immunopotentiators, compare them with those induced by hormonal and hormone-like agents, and discuss experimental data which suggest that these immunopotentiators, like hormonal and hormone-like agents, modify the functions of these cells through cyclic nucleotide mediation. Although Sutherland's criteria for cyclic nucleotide mediation of hormonal action have not been fulfilled for the actions of these immunopotentiators, we feel that our speculation serves two important functions. It offers a theoretical basis for understanding the actions of immunopotentiators by analogy to those of hormonal and hormone-like agents known to act on cells of the immune system. On the basis of observed biological responses, it predicts the mechanisms of action of levamisole, poly A:U and LPS, as well as those of other immunopotentiating agents such as thymosin and thymopoietin, the lymphokines, transfer factor, interferon, BCG, and mixed bacterial vaccines.

The two naturally occurring cyclic nucleotides, cyclic AMP and cyclic GMP, have been extensively evaluated over recent years in a variety of cells and tissues representing almost every phylum, and their roles in mediating events induced by diverse hormones and hormone-like substances have been probed. It is evident that these two cyclic nucleotides represent key intracellular mediators involved in regulating cellular responses which are often opposing in nature (47). Extensive studies of cells involved in the expression of the immune response support the thesis that cyclic nucleotides modulate important intracellular mechanisms by which diverse influences direct and regulate the responses of these cells (see Ref. 52 for review). Similarly, a number of pharmacologic agents and drugs have been found to act on cyclic nucleotides, and their therapeutic effects in a variety of disease states have been attributed to these actions (see Refs. 52 and 138). Intentional development of drugs specifically designed to modify these systems in selected tissues has been suggested as a rational therapeutic approach (138). Before dealing with the application of this approach to immunopotentiating agents, we present the following review of the roles played by the cyclic nucleotides in the regulation of cells involved in immune response.

Cyclic AMP and Lymphocyte Function

The recent development of appropriate culture methods and of agents capable of stimulating proliferation of resting lymphocytes has made possible the detailed study of mechanisms of lymphocyte activation *in vitro*. Studies on the roles played by cyclic nucleotides in lymphocyte functions began in the late 1960s, when a number of laboratories explored the effect of cyclic AMP on the proliferation of lymphocytes. A number of investigators (58, 68, 104, 105, 108, 139) applied cyclic AMP itself, as well as agents acting to increase its intracellular levels through the stimulation of adenylate cyclase (e.g., epinephrine, isoproterenol, and prostaglandin E_1 (PGE_1) or the inhibition of cyclic AMP phosphodiesterase (e.g., aminophylline and theophylline), to both resting lymphocytes and to lymphocytes induced to divide with the mitogenic plant lectin phytohemagglutinin (PHA). It was found that cyclic nucleotides and cyclic nucleotide-stimulating agents had little effect on resting lympho- cytes, blocked the induction of proliferation by PHA, had little effect when presented 6 hours after the initial stimulation by PHA, and aug- mented ongoing DNA synthesis in actively proliferating cells (68–72 hours of culture). These observations conform with those derived from a number of systems employed to study cellular proliferation: cyclic AMP acts to inhibit the induction of proliferation, but plays a complex role to influence the ongoing proliferative process. These studies employed PHA, indicating that the thymus-derived lymphocyte (T cell) is the cell whose functions are being modulated. Extension of these studies to other functions of T cells have indicated that increases of cellular levels of cyclic AMP inhibit antigen-induced secretion of soluble mediators (lym- phokines) (101, 119), rosette formation with sheep erythrocytes (42), and T-lymphocyte-mediated cytotoxicity (67).

Parallel studies on the antibody-producing B lymphocyte support the antiproliferative action of cyclic AMP (152, 153), and suggest further that cyclic AMP may, on the one hand, mediate paralytic (tolerance-inducing) stimuli in the B cell and may, on the other hand, be indirectly involved in the enhancement of antibody formation by B cells through stimulation of T cell helper function (166) or elimination of T cell suppressor function (71).

The concept of an inhibitory role for cyclic AMP in the function of lymphocytes has provided a basis for distinguishing these cells from many other cells for which cyclic AMP represents a positive regulatory influence, and led to the demonstration that the regulation of other cells involved in immune response is similar.

Cyclic AMP and Lymphocyte Differentiation

Recent studies of thymic hormones have yielded data clarifying the process of differentiation of thymocyte precursors into mature thymocytes. A number of studies indicated that in the thymectomized animal, thymic function can be replaced by thymic extracts or by a thymus implanted in a cell-impermeable chamber, suggesting that a hormone-like substance acts to differentiate precursor cells to functional T cells. The efforts of several investigators (see Ref. 75 for review) to purify the active substances from the thymus have yielded several biochemically dissimilar substances which appear to induce differentiation in thymocyte precursors.

The analysis of the action of these thymic agents has been advanced by the development of a variety of in vitro assay systems. The Komuro and Boyse assay (90) has provided a 2-hour assay of the induction of cell surface antigens such as θ, Ly and TL characteristic of intrathymic lymphocytes using mouse spleen- and marrow-derived precursor cells. Prompted by the work of Bach and associates (6), Scheid et al. (132) have presented convincing pharmacologic evidence suggesting that cyclic AMP participates in the mediation of this differentiative process of the T lymphocyte. Hämmerling et al. (66) have developed similar observations for B lymphocyte differentiation. There is no direct evidence demonstrating that the ability of the inducing hormones themselves to increase cyclic AMP levels of the precursor cells correlates directly with their ability to induce the expression of thymocyte surface markers. The pharmacologic observations nevertheless suggest that the antiproliferative role of cyclic AMP in lymphocytes involves the induction of differentiation in lymphocyte precursors and, perhaps, the maintenance of the differentiated state in mature B and T lymphocytes as well. The concept that cyclic AMP acts as an antiproliferative influence favoring differentiated function is consonant with observations in other cell types, made by a number of investigators (see Ref. 17 for review).

The diverse intracellular actions attributable to cyclic AMP in lymphocytes include stimulation of glycogenolysis and gluconeogenesis (55), inhibition of glucose uptake (56) and potassium transport (27), and phosphorylation of non-histone nuclear proteins (82). Each of these intracellular actions is consistent with an antiproliferative action since agents which induce proliferation in lymphocytes have an opposing action on these processes.

Cyclic GMP and Lymphocyte Function

The study of cyclic GMP in lymphocyte function represents a more recent endeavor. We have observed that acetylcholine increases cyclic GMP levels in lymphocytes and augments PHA-induced lymphocyte proliferation through an atropine-sensitive muscarinic receptor mechanism (48, 54, 61). In the absence of PHA, acetylcholine promotes RNA and protein synthesis in lymphocytes. In antigen-stimulated lymphocytes, acetylcholine augments the production of macrophage migration inhibitory factor (54). Strom and coworkers have shown that acetylcholine and related compounds stimulate T-cell-mediated lymphocytotoxicity and the graft-versus-host reaction (143, 144).

Other agents which are known to increase levels of cyclic GMP also appear to augment lymphocyte proliferation and function. Insulin, an agent linked to cyclic GMP in a number of cells (47, 74) including lymphocytes (Hadden and Goldberg, unpublished observation), augments glucose uptake and potassium transport (60), enhances T-cell-mediated cytotoxicity (142), antagonizes the induction by thymic factors of differentiation in thymocyte precursors (132), and augments mitogen-induced lymphocyte proliferation (115). The actions of insulin are not restricted to cyclic GMP, since a direct stimulating effect on lymphocyte membrane ATPases has been observed by us (60).

Cyclic GMP itself has been shown to augment lymphocyte proliferation, cytotoxicity and T-cell-dependent antibody production by mouse lymphocytes (143, 144, 153, 155); however, exogenous cyclic GMP has little or no effect on the human lymphocyte (61). Correspondingly, imidazole, which is both a cyclic AMP phosphodiesterase stimulator and a cyclic GMP phosphodiesterase inhibitor, augments lymphocyte proliferation and cytotoxicity (61, 144).

These observations indicate that each of the mitogen- or antigen-induced functions of lymphocytes which are described as being inhibited by cyclic AMP, are promoted by cyclic GMP.

Cyclic GMP in Mitogen Action

A variety of mitogenic agents have been employed to study the role played by cyclic nucleotides in the induction of both B and T lymphocyte proliferation. While a number of studies have suggested that cyclic AMP might be involved (see Ref. 116 for review), recent studies make it clear that this involvement is related to nonmitogenic, inhibitory aspects of lectin action (57, 59). Cyclic GMP, on the other hand has been extensively linked to mitogen action on both T and B lymphocytes (31, 47, 57, 59, 61, 63, 88, 135, 152, 158). Such diverse mitogenic agents as PHA, Concanavalin A (Con A), succinylated Con A, divalent cation ionophore A23187, periodate, and endotoxin (LPS) have all been demonstrated to increase cyclic GMP levels in lymphocytes. An important difference between the actions of mitogens and those of nonmitogenic hormones or pharmacologic agents which increase lymphocyte levels of cyclic GMP is that only the mitogens have been shown to induce significant calcium influx (61). The requirement of calcium for the induction of proliferation has been extensively documented (see Ref. 7). We have postulated that cyclic GMP and calcium represent the two key components of a mitogen-initiated membrane-to-nucleus signal sequence leading to lymphocyte activation (61, 81). Support for this hypothesis is found in studies demonstrating cyclic GMP binding to nuclear proteins (3, 83, 86) and linking phosphorylation of nuclear acidic proteins (3, 81) to the stimulation of phosphoribosyl pyrophosphate (21) and of DNA-dependent RNA polymerases I and III, and linking cyclic GMP and calcium to RNA synthesis via polymerases I and III in isolated lymphocyte nuclei (85, 86). Each of the effects demonstrated for cyclic GMP and calcium are consonant with those known to occur in the nucleus of the intact mitogen-stimulated lymphocyte.

Cyclic Nucleotides in the Function of Phagocytic Cells

Cyclic nucleotide involvement in the different functions of the polymorphonuclear neutrophil (PMN) and the monocyte or monocyte-derived macrophage has been examined extensively. Both of these cell lines derive from a common precursor cell which requires stimulation by a specific factor (colony stimulating factor, CSF) to proliferate and differentiate. Cyclic AMP and agents which increase its accumulation in the cells (PGE, theophylline) inhibit colony formation induced by CSF, while agents which increase cyclic GMP (imidazole, $PGF_{2\alpha}$, carbachol) augment (92).

The release of lysosomal enzymes, phagocytic activity, motility, chemotactic responses, and adherence of mature PMN also appear to be regulated by cyclic nucleotides (10, 35, 43, 73, 156; see Ref. 72 for review). Cyclic AMP and agents such as catecholamines, PGE_1, PGE_2 and PGA_1, cholera enterotoxin, isoproterenol, histamine, and theophylline tend to inhibit these PMN functions *in vitro* and *in vivo*. Cyclic GMP and agents that increase its intracellular accumulation (cholinergic agents, the divalent cation ionophore, particulate and soluble immune reactants) have the opposite effect. $PGF_{2\alpha}$, which increases cyclic AMP at low doses and cyclic GMP at high doses, appears to have a biphasic effect on PMN functions which parallels its effects on cyclic nucleotide levels. Anti-inflammatory agents such as glucocorticoids appear to inhibit a number of PMN functions, not by increasing intracellular accumulation of cyclic AMP but rather by decreasing intracellular accumulation of cyclic GMP in the PMN during contact with particulate immune reactants. The presence of Ca^{++} appears to be obligatory for lysosomal enzyme release by cyclic GMP-elevating agents. It is postulated that these agents may act by increasing the plasma membrane permeability to Ca^{++}, and that Ca^{++} may activate guanylate cyclase, resulting in biosynthesis and intracellular accumulation of cyclic GMP and subsequent lysosomal enzyme release (72). Elevation of intracellular levels of cyclic AMP may inhibit degranulation of PMN by interfering with microtubule assembly and function, thus limiting translocation of lysosomes to and fusion with the phagosome or the plasma membrane.

The monocyte/macrophage has been less extensively studied than the PMN. Although cyclic nucleotides are involved in the regulation of macrophage functions, their biological roles are less clear. Reports on the effects of cyclic nucleotides and agents which modify their cellular levels on macrophage migration, phagocytosis and enzyme release have been conflicting (see Ref. 118 for review). For example, high concentrations of both cyclic AMP and cyclic GMP inhibit lysosomal enzyme release but not phagocytosis, while low concentrations of both stimulate phagocytosis but not enzyme release. Cyclic AMP-stimulating agents augment phagocytosis in alveolar macrophages but inhibit it in peritoneal macrophages. Cyclic AMP and related agents inhibit macrophage migration yet reverse the inhibition of migration by macrophage inhibitory factor (MIF). A number of variables including drug concentrations, cell heterogeneity, and type of ingestible materials used may account for the fact that the data concerning the modulation of mobility, phagocytosis and enzyme release by cyclic nucleotides are somewhat conflicting. The process of macrophage proliferation appears to be stimulated by cyclic GMP and by agents which increase it, including acetylcholine and imidazole (62). A macrophage mitogenic factor (MMF), distinct from CSF and MIF, induces proliferation in association with discrete early changes in levels of cyclic GMP (see Ref. 53). Macrophage activation in terms of enhanced ability to kill intracellular bacterial pathogens is also induced by MMF but not by MIF, suggesting that both proliferation and activation of macrophages is mediated by cyclic GMP (53).

Cyclic Nucleotides in the Degranulation of Basophils, Mast Cells and Platelets

Basophils and mast cells bind IgE to their cell surface, rendering them susceptible to direct (antigen-induced) or indirect (anti-IgE antibody-mediated) immunologic activation which results in the generation and release of mediators such as histamine and SRS-A (slow-reacting substance of anaphylaxis) (see Refs. 45 and 46). The release of these inflammatory mediators involves a series of steps: (1) calcium-independent activation of serine esterase, involving metabolic energy, (2) synthesis of mediators, and (3) calcium-dependent release of both stored (histamine) and unstored mediators (SRS-A), which may involve cyclic GMP. A divalent cation ionophore can bypass the antigen requirement for activation of these cells. Agents elevating intracellular levels of cyclic AMP (e.g., β-adrenergic agents, histamine, and prostaglandin) inhibit the first phase of this process. Histamine, which regulates its own release from basophils and mast cells by an H-2 receptor-mediated stimulation of intracellular levels of cyclic AMP, may also have a role in modulating various lymphocyte responses. Cholinergic agents can reverse inhibition of SRS-A release by cyclic AMP, presumably by increasing intracellular levels of cyclic GMP, but cannot reverse the cyclic AMP-induced inhibition of SRS-A generation by immunologically activated mast cells.

Platelet degranulation and subsequent aggregation are modulated by cyclic nucleotides. Cyclic AMP and agents which elevate its intracellular levels inhibit, while cGMP and agents which increase its levels induce these platelet functions (see Ref. 72). The action of cyclic GMP has an absolute requirement for calcium. PGE_2, which increases intracellular levels of cyclic AMP, appears to be formed within the platelet during the aggregation process, and thus may modulate the event by exerting a negative feedback effect. Glucocorticoids inhibit the platelet aggregation which has been induced by cGMP-stimulating agents.

Cyclic Nucleotides and Immunopharmacology

The foregoing observations indicate that, in a spectrum of cell types involved in immune response, the cyclic nucleotide pathways represent important regulatory systems for mediating the expression of a variety of agents which influence cellular responses. The modulation of these pathways by a variety of hormonal and pharmacologic agents, which lead to a corresponding alteration in the cell function, suggests that cyclic GMP may play a positive role and cyclic AMP a negative role in the functions of lymphocytes, macrophages, granulocytes, and platelets. In undifferentiated lymphocytes, cyclic AMP appears to initiate the differentiation process. We envision a multitude of possibilities for the development of an immunopharmacology based upon manipulation of cyclic nucleotide levels in cells, using both pharmacologic and biologic agents.

The application of such an immunopharmacologic approach to the study of immunopotentiator action appears to be reasonable, since these pathways represent the most physiological mechanisms through which regulators and potentiators would be expected to act. The present chapter seeks to define the extent to which three prototypic immunopotentiators involve cyclic nucleotide mediation in effecting alterations of lymphocyte and macrophage function. The three agents selected (levamisole, poly A-poly U, endotoxin) have been demonstrated to modify T-cell-mediated immune response *in vivo* and *in vitro*, and have been linked to cyclic nucleotide mediation.

Levamisole

Levamisole, a phenylimidazothiazole, is an immunopotentiator which has been shown to be of benefit in the treatment of chronic or recurrent infections in immunodeficient patients and of patients with such diseases as rheumatoid arthritis, lupus erythematosus, and aphthous stomatitis (see Ref. 146).

In laboratory animals, levamisole given alone has been ineffective in the treatment of a variety of experimental tumors, whereas levamisole given after immunosuppressive chemotherapy or combined with active immunization (irradiated tumor cells) has increased immunological reactivity and survival of mice with spontaneous leukemia or transplanted solid tumors (25, 26, 87, 140, 146).

In cancer patients, levamisole has been observed to improve impaired immune functions (8, 18, 98, 128, 147, 149). Levamisole given after extirpation of all evident disease by surgery or radiation therapy, has been reported to increase survival and retard the onset of recurrence in patients with breast cancer (29, 128) or lung cancer (145). Another beneficial effect of levamisole is acceleration of regeneration of bone marrow following chemotherapy (102).

Levamisole treatment of mice augments the antibody response to bacterial infection (121, 126) and to T-cell-dependent antigens such as sheep erythrocytes (SRBC) (122), enhances the graft-versus-host reaction (GvH) (125), and increases nonspecific resistance to bacterial infections (126). A number of variables affect the response to levamisole. In mice that are immunodeficient because of genetic factors or old age, levamisole augments antibody production; in those with normal immunocompetence, it has little or no effect (123, 140). Higher doses of levamisole are required to enhance lymphocyte cytotoxicity to tumor cells than to potentiate humoral responses (106, 32).

Mouse spleen cells and thymocytes exposed to levamisole in vitro show increased DNA synthesis in the absence of antigenic stimuli and enhancement of mitogen- and alloantigen-induced DNA synthesis (109, 164). Human lymphocytes exposed to levamisole in vitro generally show only slight potentiation of blastogenic responses to mitogens (22, 49, 51, 100, 130) and to antigens or allogeneic cells (100, 114). Addition of levamisole to human lymphocytes in vitro has also been observed to potentiate mitogen-induced lymphokine production (157), to enhance E-rosette formation by T cells (148) and to increase T cell suppressor activity (130). In general, low doses are stimulatory; high doses, inhibitory. Lymphocyte responses in vitro to suboptimal stimuli are augmented more than those to optimal stimuli. Lymphocytes from immunosuppressed patients respond more markedly than those from normal individuals. The preponderance of evidence indicates that thymus-derived lymphocytes are preferentially responsive to levamisole.

Levamisole stimulates the murine reticuloendothelial system (RES), augmenting nonspecific resistance to infectious organisms, and enhancing the phagocytic and bactericidal capacity of peritoneal exudate macrophages exposed to the drug either in vivo or in vitro (38, 69, 112, 127, 150). In both normal and immunodeficient patients, levamisole increases the chemotactic responsiveness of neutrophils and monocytes (165).

Mechanisms of Action

Levamisole is an imidazole analog. The latter acts on cyclic nucleotide phosphodiesterases, inducing increased breakdown of cyclic AMP and decreased breakdown of cyclic GMP. Like levamisole, imidazole stimulates the proliferative responses of murine and human lymphocytes (51) and phagocytic activity of macrophages (112). Predictably, theophylline, which inhibits the breakdown of cyclic AMP, inhibits the enhancing effect of levamisole on anti-SRBC antibody production by murine spleen cells (124). Like levamisole, imidazole potentiates cytotoxicity of lymphocytes (143). Induction of increased intracellular levels of cyclic GMP by these agents has been found to parallel closely their effects on proliferation of lymphocytes (51) and on chemotactic responses of human monocytes (165).

It is of particular interest that levamisole overcomes the maturation-dependent functional deficiency of granulocytes and monocytes from newborn animals, as evidenced by the mobilization of polymorphonu-clear leukocytes to infectious sites in levamisole-treated suckling rats (39). This action of levamisole may be mediated by its stimulation of chemotactic responses of polymorphonuclear neutrophils and monocytes (165). In addition, levamisole may also augment the action of colony stimulating factor (CSF) which regulates proliferation and maturation of these two cell lines, since imidazole and other cyclic GMP-stimulating agents potentiate the action of CSF on granulocyte and macrophage colony formation in vitro (92).

Polynucleotides

The synthetic double-stranded complementary RNA homo-polymers (dsRNA) poly I:C and poly A:U stimulate specific and nonspecific immune responses in vivo and in vitro, augmenting antibody responses to SRBC (16) and stimulating the RES, as evidenced by increased phagocytic activity (16) and enhanced nonspecific resistance to viral and bacterial infections (37, 97). In rodents, dsRNA has been reported to delay the onset not only of spontaneous but also of transplanted tumors, and to reduce the rate of recurrence following surgical removal of such tumors (14, 33, 93, 94, 99, 103, 107, 131, 167).

Investigations into the therapeutic potential of dsRNA has shifted in recent years from poly I:C to poly A:U, because the latter is less toxic at doses required for immunopotentiating and antitumor activity.

In vivo treatment of mice with dsRNA modulates T cell-dependent antibody responses by several mechanisms. Administration of dsRNA simultaneously with antigen enhances antibody production and shortens the induction period to both immunogenic (13, 80) and subimmunogenic doses of antigens (13, 80, 91), enhances responses to weak immunogens (99), induces secondary antibody responses in the absence of antigen (13, 80), inhibits induction of tolerance to T-cell-dependent antigens (91), accelerates the development of immune competence in neonatal mice as effectively as adult peritoneal macrophages (5, 15, 162), and reverses the depression of humoral immune responses in aged mice and genetically low responder mice (11, 111).

In vitro addition of poly A:U modulates primary and secondary antibody production by lymphocytes in response to SRBC (28, 78). Poly A:U is thought to affect antibody production in vitro by potentiating T-cell-helper function, since it reduces the requirement for T helper cells to initiate a humoral response to SRBC (80).

Cell-mediated immune responses are also modulated by dsRNA. If given within 12 hours before antigen, dsRNA augments GvH and delayed skin hypersensitivity reactions (13, 20). In addition, dsRNA restores immune competence to T-cell-deficient mice by promoting the differentiation of residual T cells (80).

Addition of dsRNA to lymphocyte cultures modulates T cell responses in vitro by inducing splenic T cell precursors to express T cell-specific surface markers (132), augmenting secondary T cell responses to antigens and cytotoxic action on allogeneic cells (23, 50, 151), and inhibiting T cell responses to strong stimuli such as PHA (23). For both T and B cell responses, optimal concentrations of poly A:U are stimulatory; supraoptimal ones, inhibitory. Responses to suboptimal concentrations of antigen are potentiated whereas responses to optimal immunogenic concentrations of antigen are only slightly augmented. In general, lower concentrations of poly A:U are required for affecting T cell functions in vitro than for modulating humoral immune responses in vitro.

The stimulatory effects of dsRNA on the RES in vivo are reflected by increased nonspecific resistance to pathogenic microorganisms (23, 36, 37, 65), presumably due to enhanced phagocytosis and killing (16, 80). In vitro, dsRNA stimulates macrophages involved in primary antigen processing resulting in increased RNA synthesis by macrophages in vitro (84) and in increased antibody production when such stimulated macrophages are injected in vivo (80). Double-stranded RNA also activates macrophages directly as indicated by the development of selective cytotoxicity for tumor cells (2).

Mechanism of Action of dsRNA

Werner Braun and his associates postulated that the effects of poly A:U are mediated by cyclic AMP, based on their findings (12, 76, 77, 161) that cyclic AMP mimicks the actions of poly A:U on T cell-dependent antibody responses in vivo and in vitro, that the phosphodiesterase inhibitor theophylline potentiates the immunomodulatory effects of poly A:U, and that poly A:U increases adenylate cyclase activity in spleen cells. To date, the effect of in vivo administration of poly A:U or cyclic AMP itself on intracellular levels of cyclic AMP has not been investigated. However, it has been shown that injection of SRBC is associated with increased levels of cyclic AMP in spleen cells during the early stage of the immune response, probably reflecting initiation of T cell helper activity (166). Although poly A:U-induced changes in cyclic AMP levels have not been detected in vitro in unfractionated spleen cells (110), T cell differentiation can be demonstrated in mouse spleen cell fractions enriched in T cell precursors after treatment with poly A:U, cyclic AMP or agents that increase intracellular levels of cyclic AMP (132). In our experience, there is a direct correlation between elevation of intracellular levels of cyclic AMP and induction of T cell differentiation *in vitro* with poly A:U (Hadden, Scheid and Coffey, Unpublished). These findings suggest that poly A:U potentiates T cell-dependent antibody production by expanding the T helper cell compartment.

The mechanism of action of poly A:U on T and B cell proliferation and on macrophage functions have not been examined and can only be inferred on the basis of these observations. By analogy to LPS, it seems reasonable to suggest that the actions of poly A:U on these cellular functions may be linked to increased intracellular levels of cyclic GMP.

Lipopolysaccharides

Endotoxins of gram negative bacteria have markedly similar biological activities attributable to the common lipid A structure of their lipopolysaccharide component (LPS). The ability of LPS (itself a potent immunogen and tolerogen) to modulate nonspecific and specific immune responses to unrelated antigens and to induce necrosis and regression of established tumors in laboratory animals has long been documented. LPS may act as an immunostimulatory or as an immunodepressing agent *in vivo* (4, 34, 41, 64, 79, 135) and *in vitro* (19, 70, 113, 136, 152), depending on the experimental conditions. LPS modulates responses to both T cell-dependent and -independent antigens, enhances responses to weak antigens and to suboptimal doses of antigen (24), renders tolerogenic doses of antigen immunogenic (24), and restores impaired humoral immune competence in aged mice (141).

Cellular immune responses of mouse lymphocytes to SRBC are enhanced if LPS is injected after antigen (efferent arc) but inhibited if it is given before antigen (afferent arc) (95, 96). Under appropriate conditions, LPS augments GvH reactions, accelerates allograft rejection, and potentiates antibody-dependent cell-mediated cytotoxicity (1, 120, 139).

LPS is a polyclonal mitogen for B cells from some but not all tissue sources (44, 117, 154) and, although it is not mitogenic for T cells from murine thymus (44), it does modify T cell responses to mitogens by either direct or by macrophage-mediated actions (134). *In vitro*, LPS induces the expression of specific surface markers by B cell precursors from spleen and fetal liver (66, 89) and by T cell precursors from spleen (132). Addition of LPS to spleen cell cultures after antigen stimulates antibody production *in vitro*, but addition of LPS before or together with antigen is inhibitory (70, 113).

In vivo studies indicate that macrophages may mediate the adjuvant effect of LPS (123), and that LPS activates macrophages, as evidenced by increased proliferation (40) and acquisition of nonspecific tumoricidal capacity (2). LPS also activates macrophages *in vitro*, as manifested by increased lysosomal enzyme activity, augmented CSF production, enhanced glucosamine and cytophilic antibody uptake, secretion of a B cell-activating factor, and acquisition of selective tumoricidal activity (2, 129, 159, 160, 163).

Mechanism of Action of LPS on Cells of the Immune System

It is thought that, like hormones and lectin mitogens, LPS acts through cell surface receptors, although no specific receptors have yet been demonstrated. The possibility of a realtion of LPS to cell surface enzymes was first examined by Bitensky et *al.* (9) who demonstrated that lymphocytes and liver cells from mice given LPS *in vivo* showed increased membrane sensitivity to epinephrine, as measured by adenylate cyclase activity. This finding suggested that LPS activity could be mediated by increased intracellular levels of cyclic AMP in lymphocytes, liver cells, and possibly other cell types. While no LPS-induced increases in adenylate cyclase activity or cyclic AMP levels have been detected in unfractionated spleen cells (30), LPS has been demonstrated to induce T and B cell surface markers on precursor cells obtained by albumin gradient fractionation of spleen cells, a response comparable to that induced by cyclic AMP itself or cyclic AMP-elevating agents (66, 132). In our experience, concentrations of LPS required to induce T and B cell differentiation of gradient-fractionated splenic precursor cells also induce cyclic AMP accumulation in these cells (Hadden, Scheid, and Coffey, unpublished). This suggests that LPS-induced differentiation of T and B cell precursors is mediated by increased intracellular accumulation of cyclic AMP, presumably due to a LPS-initiated increase in membrane adenylate cyclase activity.

A number of activities induced by LPS are consonant with events generally associated with elevation of cyclic GMP. LPS-induced B cell proliferation is associated with increases in intracellular cyclic GMP in spleen lymphocytes (152; Hadden & Coffey, unpublished) and is mimicked by cyclic GMP (155). Other LPS-initiated phenomena, including activation and possibly also stimulation of proliferation of macrophages as well as aggregation of platelets, are mimicked by agents that increase levels of cyclic GMP in macrophages and platelets; the effects of LPS on cyclic GMP levels in these cases have not been examined. Cells which show increased levels of cyclic GMP in response to LPS invariably possess surface receptors for complement component C3, suggesting a relation of C3 to the cyclic GMP response to LPS.

Conclusion

In summary, in lymphocytes levamisole has been linked to cyclic GMP increases; poly A-poly U, to cyclic AMP increases, endotoxin, to both cyclic GMP and cyclic AMP increases. These agents offer a diversified spectrum of activities related to cyclic nucleotides. The correlation of the effects of these immunopotentiators on biological activities with changes in cellular levels of cyclic AMP and cyclic GMP indicates, but does not prove that the cyclic nucleotide is directly linked to the particular biological response. Further studies are needed to specifically address the question of whether the cyclic nucleotide actually mediates the action. The ability of these immunopotentiators to simulate the action of hormonal and hormone-like agents on cyclic nucleotide levels of the relevant cell population and also on the corresponding biological function, lends strong support to the concept that these three immunopotentiators may act principally through the cyclic nucleotides.

It seems reasonable to predict that, like the hormones endogenous to the immune system (e.g. thymopoietin), the molecular mediators involved in intercellular communication (e.g., lymphokines, transfer factor, interferon) will be found to act via the cyclic nucleotides.

We assume that like lectin mitogens and other cell surface ligands, antigens will be found to trigger lymphocyte proliferation and activation through cyclic nucleotide mechanisms. Within this theoretical framework, we can begin to predict by what mechanisms the more complex immunotherapeutic agents such as BCG, C. parvum, or mixed bacterial vaccines achieve their effects on cells of the immune system. While these mechanisms, of course, do not represent the only ones involved in immunopotentiator action, they do represent a good basis for designing new immunopotentiators which are less toxic, more potent and more specific, and for predicting and analyzing their effects.

REFERENCES

1. Al-Askari, W., Man, G., Lawrence, H. S., and Thomas, L. 1964. The effect of endotoxin on skin homografts in rabbits. J. Immunol. 93: 742–748.

2. Alexander, P., and Evans, R. 1971. Endotoxin and double-stranded RNA render macrophages cytotoxic. Nature New Biology 232: 76–78.

3. Allfrey, V. G., Inoue, A., Karn, J., Johnson, E. M., Good, R. A., and Hadden,

J. W. 1975. Sequence specific DNA binding by non histone proteins of the lymphocyte nucleus and evidence for their migration from cytoplasm to nucleus at times of gene activation. *Ciba Foundation Symposium* 28: 199–228.

4. Allison, A. C., and Davies, A. J. S. 1971. Requirement of thymus-dependent lymphocytes for potentiation by adjuvants and antibody formation. *Nature* 233: 330–332.

5. Argyris, B. F. 1968. Role of macrophages in immunological maturation. *J. Exp. Med.* 128: 459–467.

6. Bach, J. F., Dardenne, M., and Bach, M. 1973. Demonstration of a circulating thymic hormone in mouse and in man. *Transplant. Proc.* 5: 99–104.

7. Berridge, M. J. 1975. Control of cell division. *J. Cyclic Nuc. Res.* 1: 305–320.

8. Bimianov, M., and Ramot, B. 1975. In vitro restoration by levamisole of thymus-derived lymphocyte function in Hodgkin's disease. *Lancet* 1: 464.

9. Bitensky, M. W., Gorman, R. E., and Thomas, L. 1971. Selective stimulation of epinephrine-responsive adenyl cyclase in mice by endotoxin. *Proc. Soc. Exp. Biol. Med.* 138: 773–775.

10. Bourne, H. R., Lehrer, R. I., Cline, M. J., and Melmon, K. L. 1971. Cyclic 3'5' adenosine monophosphate in the human leukocyte: Synthesis degradation and effects on neutrophil candidacidal activity. *J. Clin. Invest.* 50: 920–927.

11. Braun, W. 1970. Some causes and repair of altered antibody formation in aged animals, in M. Sigel (ed.), *Tolerance, Autoimmunity and Aging*, pp. 166–180. C. C Thomas, Springfield, Ill.

12. Braun, W., and Ishizuka, M. 1971. Antibody formation: Reduced responses after administration of excessive amounts of non-specific stimulation. *Proc. Natl. Acad. Sci.* 68: 1114–1116.

13. Braun, W., Ishizuka, M., Yajima, Y., Webb, D., and Winchurch, R. 1971. Spectrum and mode of action of poly A:U in the stimulation of immune responses, in R. F. Beers, Jr., and W. Braun (eds.), *Biological Effects of Polynucleotides*, pp. 139–156. Springer-Verlag, New York.

14. Braun, W., Lampen, J. O., Plescia, O. J., and Pugh, L. 1963. Effects of nucleic acid digests on spontaneous and implanted tumors of C3H mice, in *Conceptual Advances in Immunology and Oncology*, pp. 450 456. Harper & Row, New York, New York.

15. Braun, W., and Lasky, L. J. 1967. Antibody formation in newborn mice initiated through adult macrophages. *Fed. Proc.* 26: 642.

16. Braun, W., and Nakano, M. 1967. Antibody formation: Stimulation by polyadenylic and polycytidylic acids. *Science* 157: 819–821.

17. Braun, W., Lichtenstein, L. N., and Parker, C. W. (eds.). 1974. *Cyclic AMP Cell Growth and the Immune Response*. Springer-Verlag, New York, New York.

18. Brugmans, J., Schuermans, V., de Cock, W., Thienpont, D., Janssen, P., Verhaegen, H., van Nimmen, L., Louwagie, A. C., and Stevens, E. 1973. Restoration of host defense mechanisms in man by levamisole. *Life Sci.* 13: 1499–1504.

19. Bullock, W. W., and Andersson, J. 1973. Mitogens as probes for immunocyte activation: Specific and nonspecific paralysis of B cell mitogens. *Ciba Foundation Symposium* 18: 173–188.

20. Casavant, C. H., and Youmans, C. P. 1975. The adjuvant activity of mycobacterial RNA preparations and synthetic polynucleotides for induction of delayed hypersensitivity to purified protein derivative in guinea pigs. *J. Immunol.* 114: 1014–1022.

21. Chambers, D. A., Martin, J. W., Jr., and Weinstein, Y. 1974. The effect of cyclic nucleotides on purine biosynthesis and induction of PRPP synthetase during lymphocyte activation. *Cell* 13: 375–380.

22. Chan, S. H., and Simons, M. J. 1975. Levamisole and lymphocyte responsiveness. *Lancet* 1: 1246–1247.

23. Cheers, C., and Cone, R. 1974. Effects of polyadenine:polyuridine on brucellosis in conventional and congenitally athymic mice. *J. Immunol.* 112: 1535–1539.

24. Chiller, J. M., Skidmore, B. J., Morrison, D. C. and Weigle, W. D. 1973. Relationship of the structure of bacterial lipopolysaccharides to its function in mitogenesis and adjuvanticity. *Proc. Nat. Acad. Sci.* 70: 2129–2133.

25. Chirigos, M. A., Fuhrman, F., and Pryor, J. 1975. Prolongation of chemotherapeutically induced remission of a syngeneic murine leukemia by L-2,3,5,6-tetrahydro 6-phenylimidazo (2,1-8) thiazole hydrochloride. *Cancer Res.* 35: 927–931.

26. Chirigos, M. A., Pearson, J. W., and Pryor, J. 1973. Augmentation of chemotherapeutically induced remission of a murine leukemia by a chemical immunoadjuvant. *Cancer Res.* 33: 2615–2618.

27. Coffey, R. G., Hadden, E. M., and Hadden, J. W. 1976. Norepinephrine stimulation of lymphocyte ATPase by an alpha adrenergic receptor mechanism. *Endocrine Res. Commun.* 2: 179–198.

28. Cone, R. E., and Marchalonis, J. J. 1972. Adjuvant action of poly A:U on T cells during the primary immune response *in vitro. Aust. J. Exp. Biol. Med. Sci.* 50: 69–77.

29. Debois, J. M. 1976. Preliminary experiences with levamisole in cancer patients, and particularly in breast cancer, in M. A. Chirigos (ed.), *Modulation of Host Resistance in the Prevention or Treatment of Induced Neoplasias,* Fogarty International Center Proceedings No. 28. U.S. Govt. Printing Office, Washington, D.C. (in press).

30. De Rubertis, F. R., Zenser, T. V., Adler, W. H., and Hudson, T. 1974. Role of cyclic adenosine 3′,5′-monophosphate in lymphocyte activity. *J. Immunol.* 113: 151–161.

31. Deviller, Y., Chille, Y., and Betuel, M. 1975. Guanyl cyclase activity of human blood lymphocytes. *Enzyme* 19: 300–319.

32. Dillon, P., Faanes, R. B., and Choi, Y. S. 1977. Levamisole augments the cytotoxic T cell response depending on the dose of drug and antigen administered. *Clin. Exp. Immunol.* 27: 502–506.

33. Drake, W. P., Cimino, E. F., Mardiney, M. R., Jr., and Sutherland, J. C. 1974. Prophylactic therapy of spontaneous leukemia in AKR mice by polyadenylic:polyuridylic acid. *J. Natl. Cancer. Inst.* 52: 941–944.

34. Dresser, D. W., and Phillips, J. M. 1973. The cellular targets for the action of adjuvants: T-adjuvants and B-adjuvants. *Ciba Foundation Symposium* 18: 3–28.

35. Estensen, R. D., Hill, H. R., Ovie, P. G., Hogan, N., and Goldberg, N. D. 1973. Cyclic GMP and Cell Movement. *Nature* 245: 458–460.

36. Fauve, R. M., and Hévin, M. B. Pouvoir bactéricide des macrophages spléniques et hépatiques de souris envers Listeria monocytogènes. *Ann. Inst. Pasteur* 120: 399–411.

37. Field, A. K., Tytell, A. A., Lampson, G. P., and Hilleman, M. R. 1967. Inducers of interferon and host resistance. II. Multistranded synthetic polynucleotide complexes. *Proc. Natl. Acad. Sci.* 58: 1004–1010.

38. Fischer, G. W., Podgore, J. K., and Bass, J. W. 1975. Immunopotentiation by levamisole. *Lancet* 1: 1137.

39. Fischer, G. W., Podgore, J. K., Bass, J. W., Kelley, J. L., and Kobayashi, G. Y. 1975. Enhanced host defense mechanism with levamisole in suckling rats. *J. Infect. Dis.* 132: 578–581.

40. Forbes, I. J. 1964. Induction of mitosis in macrophages by endotoxin. *J. Immunol.* 94: 37–39.

41. Franzl, R. W., and McMaster, P. O. 1968. The primary immune response in mice. I. Enhancement and suppression of hemolysin production by a bacterial endotoxin. *J. Exp. Med.* 127: 1087–1107.

42. Galant, S. P., and Remo, R. A. 1975. β-adrenergic inhibition of human T lymphocyte rosettes. *J. Immunol.* 114: 512–516.

43. Gale, R. P., and Zighelboin, J. 1974. Modulation of polymorphonuclear leukocyte med ated antibody dependent cellular cytotoxicity. *J. Immunol.* 113: 1793–1800.

44. Gery, J., Kruger, J., and Spiesel, S. Z. 1972. Stimulation of B-lymphocytes by endotoxin. Reactions of thymus-deprived mice and karyotypic analysis of dividing cells in mice bearing T6T6 thymus grafts. *J. Immunol.* 108: 1088–1091.

45. Gillespie, E. 1977. Pharmacologic control of mediator release from leukocytes, *in* J. W. Hadden, R. G. Coffey, and F. Spreafico (eds.), *Immunopharmacology*, pp. 101–112. Plenum Press, New York, New York.

46. Goetzl, E. J., and Austen, K. F. 1977. The generation, function and disposition of chemical mediators of the mast cell in immediate hypersensitivity, *in* J. W. Hadden, R. G. Coffey, and F. Spreafico (eds.), *Immunopharmacology*, pp. 113–124. Plenum Press, New York.

47. Goldberg, N. D., Haddox, M. K., Dunham, E., Lopez, C., and Hadden, J. W. 1974. Evidence for opposing influences in cyclic GMP and cyclic AMP regulation of cell proliferation and other biological processes, *in* B. Clarkson and R. Baserga (eds.), *Control of Proliferation in Animal Cells*, pp. 609–626. Cold Spring Harbor, New York.

48. Goldberg, N., Haddox, M., Hartle, D., and Hadden, J. 1973. The biological role of cyclic 3′,5′-guanosine monophosphate, *in Proceedings of the 5th International Congress of Pharmacology*, vol. 5, pp. 146–169. S. Karger, Basel, Switzerland.

49. Goyanes-Villaescusa, V. 1976. Mitogenic stimulation by levamisole on normal human lymphocytes and leukemic lymphoblasts. *Lancet* 1: 370.

50. Grazziano, K. D., Levy, C. C., Schmukler, M., and Mardiney, M. R., Jr. 1974. Additional characteristics of the amplification of immunologically induced lymphocyte tritiated thymidine incorporation by double-stranded synthetic

polynucleotides. *Cell. Immunol.* 11: 47–56.

51. Hadden, J. W., Coffey, R. G., Hadden, E. M., Lopez-Corrales, E., and Sunshine, G. H. 1975. Effects of levamisole and imidazole on lymphocyte proliferation and cyclic nucleotide levels. *Cell. Immunol.* 20: 98–103.

52. Hadden, J. W., Coffey, R. G., and Spreafico, F. 1977. *Immunopharmacology.* Plenum Press, New York.

53. Hadden, J. W., and England, A. 1977. Molecular aspects of macrophage activation and Proliferation, in J. W. Hadden, R. F. Coffey, and F. Spreafico (eds.), *Immunopharmacology,* pp. 87–100. Plenum Press, New York.

54. Hadden, J. W., Hadden, E. M., and Goldberg, N. D. 1974. Cyclic GMP and cyclic AMP in lymphocyte metabolism and proliferation, in W. Braun, L. M. Lichtenstein and C. W. Parker (eds.), *Cyclic AMP, Cell Growth and the Immune Response,* pp. 237–246. Springer-Verlag, New York.

55. Hadden, J. W., Hadden, E. M., and Good, R. A. 1971. Adrenergic mechanisms in human lymphocyte metabolism. *Biochim. Biophys. Acta* 237: 339–347.

56. Hadden, J. W., Hadden, E. M., and Good, R. A. 1971. Alpha adrenergic stimulation of glucose uptake in the human erythrocyte, lymphocyte, and lymphoblast. *Exp. Cell Res.* 68: 217–219.

57. Hadden, J. W., Hadden, E. M., Haddox, M. K., and Goldberg, N. D. 1972. Guanosine 3′,5′-monophosphate: A possible intracellular mediator of mitogenic influences in lymphocytes. *Proc. Natl. Acad. Sci.* 69: 3024–3027.

58. Hadden, J. W., Hadden, E. M., and Middleton, E. 1970. Lymphocyte blast transformation. I. Demonstration of adrenergic receptors in human peripheral blood lymphocytes. *J. Cell. Immunol.* 1: 583–595.

59. Hadden, J. W., Hadden, E. M., Sadlik, J. R., and Coffey, R. G. 1976. Effects of concanavalin A and a succinylated derivitive on lymphocyte proliferation and cyclic nucleotide levels. *Proc. Natl. Acad. Sci.* 73: 1717–1721.

60. Hadden, J. W., Hadden, E. M., Wilson, E. E., Good, R. A., and Coffey, R. G. 1972. Direct action of insulin on plasma membrane ATPase activity in human lymphocytes. *Nature New Biology* 235: 174–177.

61. Hadden, J. W., Johnson, E. M., Hadden, E. M., Coffey, R. G., and Johnson, L. D. 1975. Cyclic GMP and lymphocyte activation, in A. Rosenthal (ed.), *Immune Recognition,* pp. 359–389. Academic Press, New York.

62. Hadden, J. W., Leu, R., Goldberg, N. D., and Hadden, E. M. 1974. Possible mitogenic action of macrophage migration inhibitory factor. *Fed. Proc.* 33: 1677.

63. Haddox, M. K., Furcht, L. T., Gentry, S. R., Moser, M. E., Stephenson, J. H., and Goldberg, N. D. 1976. Periodate-induced increase in cyclic GMP in mouse and guinea pig splenic cells in association with mitogenesis. *Nature* 262: 146–148.

64. Hamaoka, T., and Katz, D. H. 1973. Cellular site of action of various adjuvants in antibody responses to hapten-carrier conjugates. *J. Immunol.* 111: 1554–1563.

65. Hamilton, L. D., Babcock, V. I., and Southam, C. M. 1969. Inhibition of herpes simplex virus by synthetic double-stranded RNA. *Proc. Natl. Acad. Sci.* 64: 878–883.

66. Hämmerling, U., Chin, A. F., Abbott, J., and Scheid, M. 1975. The on-

togeny of murine B lymphocytes. I. Induction of phenotypic conversation of Ia⁻ to Ia⁺ lymphocytes. *J. Immunol.* 115: 1425–1430.

67. Henney, C. S., and Lichtenstein, L. M. 1971. The role of cyclic AMP in the cytolytic activity of lymphocytes. *J. Immunol.* 107: 610–612.

68. Hirschhorn, R., Grossman, J., and Weissman, G. 1970. Effect of cyclic 3′,5′-adenosine monophosphate and theophylline on lymphocyte transformation. *Proc. Soc. Exp. Biol. Med.* 133: 1361–1363.

69. Hoebeke, J., and Franchi, G. 1973. Influence of tetramisole and its optical isomers on the mononuclear phagocytic system. Effect on carbon clearance in mice. *J. Reticuloendoth. Soc.* 14: 317–323.

70. Hoffman, M. K., Weiss, O., Koenig, S., Hirst, J. A., and Oettgen, H. F. 1975. Suppression and enhancement of the T cell-dependent production of antibody to SRBC in vitro by bacterial lipopolysaccharide. *J. Immunol.* 114: 738–741.

71. Hung-Sai, T., and Paetkau, V. 1976. Regulation of immune responses: The cellular basis of cyclic AMP effects on humoral immunity. *Cell. Immunol.* 24: 220–229.

72. Ignarro, L. J. 1977. Regulation of polymorphonuclear leukocyte, macrophage and platelet function, in J. W. Hadden, R. G. Coffey and F. Spreafico (eds.), *Immunopharmacology*, pp. 61–86. Plenum Press, New York.

73. Ignarro, I. J., and George, W. J. 1974. Mediation of immunologic discharge of lysosomal enzymes from human neutrophils by guanosine 3′,5′-monophosphage. Requirement of calcium and inhibition by adenosine 3′,5′-monophosphate. *J. Exp. Med.* 140: 225–238.

74. Illiano, G., Tell, G. P. E., Siegal, M. F., and Cuatrecasas, P. 1973. Guanosine 3′,5′-cyclic monophosphate and the action of insulin and acetylcholine. *Proc. Natl. Acad. Sci.* 70: 2443–2447.

75. *International Conference on Thymus Factors in Immunity.* 1975. *Ann. N.Y. Acad. Sci.* 249: 1–547.

76. Ishizuka, M., Braun, W., and Matsumoto, T. 1971. Cyclic AMP and immune responses. I. Influence of poly A:U and cyclic AMP on antibody formation in vitro. *J. Immunol.* 107: 1027–1035.

77. Ishizuka, M., Gafni, M., and Braun, W. 1970. Cyclic AMP effects on antibody formation and their similarities to hormone-mediated events. *Proc. Soc. Exp. Biol. Med.* 134: 963–967.

78. Jaroslow, B. N., and Ortiz-Ortiz, L. 1972. Influence of poly A:U on early events in the immune response in vitro. *Cell. Immunol.* 3: 123–132.

79. Jones, J. M., and Kind, P. D. 1972. Enhancing effect of bacterial endotoxins on bone marrow cells in the immune response to SRBC. *J. Immunol.* 108: 1453–1455.

80. Johnson, A. G., Cone, R. E., Friedman, H. M., Han, I. H., Johnson, H. G., Schmidtke, J. R., and Stout, R. D. 1971. Stimulation of the immune system by homopolyribonucleotides, in R. F. Beers, Jr., and W. Braun (eds.), *Biological Effects on Polynucleotides*, pp. 157–177. Springer-Verlag, New York.

81. Johnson, E. M., and Hadden, J. W. 1975. Phosphorylation of lymphocytic nuclear acidic proteins: Regulation by cyclic nucleotides. *Science* 65: 714–721.

82. Johnson, E. M., Hadden, J. W., Karn, J., and Allfrey, V. G. 1974. Effects of

acetylcholine and concanavalin A on phosphorylation of lymphocyte chromatin proteins. *Fed. Proc.* 33: 3030.

83. Johnson, E. M., Inoue, A., Crouse, L., Allfrey, V. G., and Hadden, J. W. 1975. Cyclic GMP modifies DNA binding by a calf thymus nuclear protein fraction. *Biochem. Biophys. Res. Comm.* 65: 614–621.

84. Johnson, H. G., and Johnson, A. G. 1971. Regulation of the immune system by synthetic polynucleotides. *J. Exp. Med.* 133: 649–664.

85. Johnson, L. D., and Hadden, J. W. 1975. Cyclic GMP and lymphocyte proliferation effects on DNA dependent RNA polymerase I and II activities. *Biochem. Biophys. Res. Comm.* 66: 1498–1505.

86. Johnson, L. D., and Hadden, J. W. 1977. Cyclic GMP-dependent regulation of isolated DNA-dependent RNA polymerases. *Nucleic Acids Res.* 4: 4007–4014.

87. Kassel, R. L. 1977. Levamisole plus antigen, and immunotherapy model, in M. A. Chirigos (ed.), *Modulation of Host Resistance in the Prevention or Treatment of induced Neoplasias,* Fogarty International Center Proceedings No. 28, pp. 347–348. U.S. Government Printing Office, Washington, D.C.

88. Katagiri, T., Terao, T., and Osawa, T. 1976. Activation of mouse spleenic lymphocyte guanylate cyclase by calcium ion. *J. Biochem.* 79: 849–852.

89. Kearney, J. F., and Lawton, A. R. 1975. B lymphocyte differentiation induced by lipopolysaccharide. I. Generation of cells synthesizing four major immunoglobulin classes. *J. Immunol.* 115: 671–681.

90. Komuro, K., and Boyse, E. A. 1973. *In vitro* demonstration of thymic hormone in the mouse by conversion of precursor cells into lymphocytes. *Lancet* 1: 740–743.

91. Kong, Y., and Capanna, S. L. 1974. Interference with tolerance induction in mice by poly A:U. *Cell. Immunol.* 11: 488–492.

92. Kurland, J. I., Hadden, J. W., and Moore, M. A. S. 1977. Cyclic nucleotides in the humoral regulation of haemopoietic progenitor cell proliferation. *Cancer Res.* 37: 4535–4538.

93. Lacour, F., Delage, G., and Chiniale, C. 1975. Reduced incidence of spontaneous mammary tumors in C3H/He mice following treatment with poly A • poly U. *Science* 187: 256–257.

94. Lacour, F., Spira, A., Lacour, J., and Prade, M. 1972. Polyadenylic-polyuridylic acid, an adjunct to surgery in the treatment of spontaneous mammary tumors in C3H/He mice and transplantable melanoma in the hamster. *Cancer Res.* 32: 648–649.

95. LaGrange, P. H., MacKaness, G. B., Miller, T. E., and Pardon, P. 1975. Effects of bacterial lipopolysaccharide on the induction and expression of cell-mediated immunity. I. Depression of the afferent arc. *J. Immunol.* 114: 442–446.

96. LaGrange, P. H., and Mackaness, G. B. 1975. Effects of bacterial lipopolysaccharide on the induction and expression of cell-mediated immunity. II. Stimulation of the efferent arc. *J. Immunol.* 114: 447–451.

97. Lampson, G. P., Tytell, A. A., Field, A. K., Nemes, M. M., and Hilleman, M. R. 1967. Inducers of interferon and host resistance. I. Double-stranded RNA from extracts of *Penicillium funiculosum. Proc. Natl. Acad. Sci.* 58: 782–789.

98. Levo, Y., Rotter, V., and Ramot, B. 1975. Restoration of cellular immune response by levamisole in patients with Hodgkin's disease. *Biomed.* 23: 198–200.

99. Levy, H. B., Law, L. W., and Rabson, A. S. 1969. Inhibition of tumor growth by polyinosinic-polycytidylic acid. *Proc. Natl. Acad. Sci.* 62: 357–361.

100. Lichtenfeld, J. L., Desner, M. R., Mardiney, M. R., Jr., and Wiernik, P. H. 1976. The modulating effects of levamisole on human lymphocyte response in vitro. *Cancer Chemother. Rep.* (in press).

101. Lies, R. B., and Peter, J. B. 1973. Cyclic AMP inhibition of cytotoxin ("lymphotoxin") elaboration by stimulated lymphocytes. *J. Cell. Immunol.* 8: 332–335.

102. Lods, J. C., Dujardin, P., and Halpern, G. M. 1976. Levamisole and bone marrow restoration after chemotherapy. *Lancet* 1: 548.

103. Lundy, J., Iritani, C. A., Wanebo, H. J., Wachtel, S. S., Tarnowski, G. S., and Old, L. J. 1973. Effect of poly A:U on transplanted mouse sarcoma. *Proc. Amer. Assoc. Cancer Res.* 14: 107.

104. MacManus, J. P., and Whitfield, J. F. 1969. Stimulation of DNA synthesis and mitotic activity of thymic lymphocytes by cyclic adenosine 3',5'-monophosphate. *Exp. Cell Res.* 58: 188–191.

105. MacManus, J. P., Whitfield, J. F., and Youdale, T. 1970. Stimulation by epinephrine of adenyl cyclase activity, cyclic AMP formation, DNA synthesis and cell proliferation in populations of rat thymic lymphocytes. *J. Cell Physiol.* 77: 103–116.

106. Mantovani, A., and Spreafico, F. 1975. Allogeneic tumor enhancement by levamisole, a new immunostimulatory compound: Studies on cell-mediated immunity and humoral antibody response. *Eur. J. Cancer* 11: 537–544.

107. Mathé, G., Hayat, M., Sakouhi, M., and Choay, J. 1971. L'action immunoadjuvante du poly I:C chez la souris et son application au traitement de la leucémie L1210. *C.R. Acad. Sci. (Paris)* 272 D: 170–173.

108. May, C. D. 1969. Inhibition of glycolysis in relation to chemical suppression of the proliferative response of lymphocytes stimulate *in vitro*. *J. Allergy* 43: 163.

109. Merluzzi, V. J., Badger, A. M., Kaiser, C. W., and Cooperband, S. R. 1975. Levamisole and murine lymphoid cell cultures: *In vitro* stimulation of murine lymphoid cell cultures by levamisole. *J. Clin. Exp. Immunol.* 22: 486.

110. Mozes, E., Shearer, G. M., Melmon, K. L., and Bourne, H. R. 1973. *In vitro* correction of antigen-induced immune suppression: Effects of poly (A) poly (U) and prostaglandin E. *Cell. Immunol.* 9: 226–233.

111. Mozes, E., Shearer, G. M., and Sela, M. 1970. Cellular basis of the genetic control of immune responses to synthetic polypeptides. I. Differences in frequence of splenic precursor cells specific for a synthetic polypeptide derived from multichain polyproline, (T,G)-Pro-L, in high and low responder inbred mouse strains. *J. Exp. Med.* 132: 613–622.

112. Oliveira Lima, A., Javierre, M. Q., Dias da Silva, W., and Sette Camara, D. 1974. Immunological phagocytosis: Effect of drugs on phosphodiesterase activity. *Experientia* 30: 945–946.

113. Ortiz-Ortiz, L., and Jaroslow, B. N. 1970. Enhancement by the adjuvant, endotoxin, of an immune response induced *in vitro*. *Immunology* 19: 387–399.

114. Pabst, N. F., and Crawford, J. 1975. L-tetramisole enhancement of human lymphocyte response to antigen. *Clin. Exp. Immunol.* 21: 468–473.

115. Pallavincini, M. G., and Nichols, W. K. 1975. Inhibition of lymphocyte blastogenesis by plasma from alloxan diabetic rats. *Fed. Proc.* 34: 760.

116. Parker, C. W., Sullivan, T. J., and Wedner, H. J. 1974. Cyclic AMP and the immune response, in P. Greengard and G. A. Robinson (eds.), *Advances in Cyclic Nucleotide Research*, pp. 1–80. Raven Press, New York.

117. Peavy, D. L., Adler, W. H., and Smith, R. T. 1970. The mitogenic effects of endotoxin and staphylococcal enterotoxin B on mouse spleen cells and human peripheral lymphocytes. *J. Immunol.* 105: 1453–1458.

118. Pick, E. 1977. Lymphokines: Physiological control and pharmacological modulation of their production and action, in J. W. Hadden, R. G. Coffey, and F. Spreafico (eds.), *Immunopharmacology*, pp. 163–202. Plenum Press, New York.

119. Prieur, A. M., and Grange, G. A. 1975. The effect of agents which modulate levels of the cyclic nucleotides on human lymphotoxin secretion and activity in vitro. *Transplantation* 20: 331–337.

120. Pudifin, D. J., Harding, B., and MacLennan, I. C. M. 1971. The differential effect of γ-irradiation on the sensitizing and effector stages of antibody-dependent lymphocyte-mediated cytotoxicity. *Immunology* 21: 853–860.

121. Renoux, G., and Renoux, M. 1971. Effet immunostimulant d'un imidothiazole dans l'immunisation des souris contre l'infection par *Brucella abortus*. *C.R. Acad. Sci. (Paris)* 272 D: 349–350.

122. Renoux, G., and Renoux, M. 1972. Action immunostimulante de derivés du phénylimidothiazole sur les cellules spléniques formatrices d'anticorps. *C.R. Acad. Sci. (Paris)* 274 D: 756–757.

123. Renoux, G., and Renoux, M. 1972. Restauration par le phénylimidothiazole de la response immunologique des souris agées. *C.R. Acad. Sci. (Paris)* 274 D: 3034–3035.

124. Renoux, G., and Renoux, M. 1972. Inhibition par la théophylline de la stimulation immunologique induite par le phénylimidothiazole. *C.R. Acad. Sci. (Paris)* 274 D: 3149–3151.

125. Renoux, G., and Renoux, M. 1972. Action du phénylimidothiazole (tétramisole) sur la réaction du greffon nontre l'hôte. Rôle des macrophages. *C.R. Acad. Sci. (Paris)* 274 D: 3320–3323.

126. Renoux, G., and Renoux, M. 1972. Antigenic competition and nonspecific immunity after a rickettsial infection in mice: Restoration of antibacterial immunity by phenylimidothiazole treatment. *J. Immunol.* 109: 761–765.

127. Renoux, G., Kassel, R. L., Fiore, N., Guillaumin, J.-M., and Palat, A. 1977. Immunomodulation by levamisole in normal and leukemic mice, in M. A. Chirigos (ed.), *Modulation of Host Immune Resistance in the Prevent on or Treatment of Induced Neoplasias*. Fogarty International Center Proceedings No. 28, pp. 45–52. U.S. Govt. Printing Office, Washington, D.C..

128. Rojas, A. F., Mickiewicz, E., Feierstein, J. N., Glait, H., and Olivari, A. J. 1976. Levamisole in advanced human breast cancer. *Lancet* 1: 211–215.

129. Ruscetti, R. W., and Chevernick, P. A. 1974. Release of colony-stimulating factor from monocytes by endotoxin and polyinosinic-polycytidylic

acid. *J. Lab. Clin. Med.* 83: 64–72.

130. Sampson, D., and Lui, A. 1976. The effect of levamisole on cell-mediated immunity and suppressor cell function. *Cancer Res.* 36: 952–955.

131. Sarma, P. S., Shui, G., Neubauer, R. H., Baron, S., and Heubner, R. Y. 1969. Virus-induced sarcoma of mice. Inhibition by a synthetic polyribonucleotide complex. *Proc. Natl. Acad. Sci.* 62: 1046–1057.

132. Scheid, M. P., Hoffmann, M. K., Komuro, K., Hämmerling, U., Abbott, J., Boyse, E. A., Cohen, G. H., Hooper, J. A., Schulof, R. S., and Goldstein, A. L. 1973. Differentiation of T cells induced by preparations from thymus and by nonthymic agents. *J. Exp. Med.* 138: 1027–1032.

133. Schmidtke, J. R., and Dixon, F. J. 1972. Immune response to a hapten coupled to a nonimmunogenic carrier. *J. Exp. Med.* 136: 392–397.

134. Schmidtke, J. R., and Najarian, J. S. 1975. Synergistic effects on DNA synthesis of phytohemagglutinin or concanavalin A and lipopolysaccharide in human peripheral blood lymphocytes. *J. Immunol.* 114: 742–746.

135. Schumm, D. E., Morris, H. P., and Webb, T. E. 1974. Early biochemical changes in phytohemagglutinin-stimulated peripheral blood lymphocytes from normal and tumor-bearing rats. *Eur. J. Cancer* 10: 107–113.

136. Sjöberg, O., Anderson, J., and Möller, G. 1972. Lipopolysaccharide can substitute for helper cells in the antibody response *in vitro*. *Eur. J. Immunol.* 2: 326–331.

137. Skopinska, E. 1972. Some effects of *Escherichia coli* endotoxin on the graft-versus-host reaction in mice. *Transplantation* 14: 432–437.

138. Smith, C. G. 1976. Approaches to drug discovery through the cyclic nucleotide regulatory system, *in Proceedings and Techniques of Human Research and Therapeutics* (in press).

139. Smith, J. W., Steiner, A. L., and Parker, C. W. 1971. Human lymphocyte metabolism: Effects of cyclic and noncyclic nucleotides on stimulation by phytohemagglutinin. *J. Clin. Invest.* 50: 442–449.

140. Spreafico, F., Vecchi, A., Mantovani, A., Poggi, A., Franchi, G., Anaclerio, A., and Garattini, S. 1975. Characterization of the immunostimulants levamisole and tetramisole. *Eur. J. Cancer* 11: 555–563.

141. Strausser, H. R., Bober, L. A., Bucsi, R. A., Shillock, J. A., and Goldstein, A. L. 1971. Stimulation of the hemagglutinin response of aged mice by cell-free lymphoid extracts and bacterial endotoxins. *Exp. Gerontol.* 6: 373–375.

142. Strom, T. B., Bear, R. A., and Carpenter, C. B. 1975. Insulin induced augmentation of lymphocyte mediated cytotoxicity. *Science* 187: 1206–1208.

143. Strom, T. B., Bear, R. A., Carpenter, C. B., and Merrill, J. P. 1974. Modulation of GVH proliferation by cyclic nucleotides. *J. Clin. Invest.* 53: 79.

144. Strom, T. B., Deisseroth, A., Morganroth, J., Carpenter, C. B., and Merrill, J. P. 1972. Alteration of the cytotoxic factor of sensitized lymphocytes by cholinergic agents and activators of adenylate cyclase. *Proc. Natl. Acad. Sci.* 69: 2995–2999.

145. Study Group for Bronchogenic Carcinoma. 1975. Immunopotentiation with levamisole in resectable bronchogenic carcinoma. A double-blind placebo-controlled trial. *Brit. Med. J.* 3: 461–464.

146. Symoens, J. 1977. Levamisole: An anti-anergic chemotherapeutic agent,

in M. A. Chirigos (ed.), *Modulation of Host Resistance in the Prevention or Treatment of Induced Neoplasias*, Fogarty International Center Proceedings No. 28, pp. 3–16. U.S. Government Printing Office, Washington, D.C..

147. Tripodi, D., Parks, L. C., and Brugmans, J. 1973. Drug-induced restoration of cutaneous delayed hypersensitivity in anergic patients with cancer. *New Engl. J. Med.* 289: 354–357.

148. Verhaegen, H., de Cree, J., Verbruggen, F., Hoebeke, J., de Brabander, M., and Brugmans, J. 1973. Immune responses in elderly cuti-negative subjects and the effect of levamisole. *Verhandl. Deutsch. Gesell. Inn. Med.* 79: 623–628.

149. Verhaegen, H., de Cock, W., de Cree, J., Verbruggen, F., Verhaegen-Declerq, M., and Brugmans, J. 1975. *In vitro* restoration by levamisole of thymus-derived lymphocyte function in Hodgkin's disease. *Lancet* 1: 978.

150. Versijp, G., van Zwet, T. L., and van Furth, R. 1975. Levamisole and functions of peritoneal macrophages. *Lancet* 1: 798.

151. Wagner, H., and Cone, R. 1974. Adjuvant effect of poly A:U upon T cell-mediated *in vitro* cytotoxic allograft responses. *Cell. Immunol.* 10: 394–403.

152. Watson, J. 1975. The influence of intracellular levels of cyclic nucleotides on cell proliferation and the induction of antibody synthesis. *J. Exp. Med.* 141: 97–111.

153. Watson, J., Epstein, R., and Cohn, M. 1973. bcyclic nucleotides as intracellular mediators of the expression of antigen-sensitive cells. *Nature* 246: 405–409.

154. Weber, W. T. 1973. The *in vitro* response of chicken B cell populations to lipopolysaccharide. *J. Immunol.* 111: 1277–1280.

155. Weinstein, Y., Chambers, D. A., Bourne, H. R., and Melmon, K. L. 1974. Cyclic GMP stimulates lymphocyte nucleic acid synthesis. *Nature* 251: 352–353.

156. Weissman, G., Zurier, R. B., and Hoffstein, S. 1974. Leucocytes as secretory organs of inflammation: Control by cyclic nucleotides and autonomic agonists, *in* W. Braun, L. M. Lichtenstein and C. W. Parker (eds.), *Cyclic AMP, Cell Growth, and the Immune Response*, pp. 176–188. Springer-Verlag. New York.

157. Whitcomb, M. E., Merluzzi, V. J., and Cooperband, S. R. 1976. The effect of levamisole on human lymphocyte mediator production *in vitro*. *Cell. Immunol.* 21: 272–277.

158. Whitfield, J. F., MacManus, J. P., Boynton, A. L., Gillan, D. J., and Isaacs, R. J. 1974. Concanavalin A and the initiation of thymic lymphoblast DNA synthesis and proliferation by a calcium dependent increase in cyclic GMP level. *J. Cell. Physiol.* 84: 445–458.

159. Wiener, E., and Levanon, D. 1968. The *in vitro* interaction between bacterial lipopolysaccharide and differentiating monocytes. *Lab. Invest.* 19: 584–590.

160. Wilton, J. M., Rosenstreich, D. L., and Oppenheim, J. J. 1975. Activation of guinea pig macrophages by bacterial lipopolysaccharide requires bone marrow-derived lymphocytes. *J. Immunol.* 114: 388–393.

161. Winchurch, R., Ishizuka, M., Webb, D., and Braun, W. 1971. Adenyl cyclase activity of spleen cells exposed to immunoenhancing synthetic oligo- and polynucleotides. *J. Immunol.* 106: 1399–1400.

162. Winchurch, R., and Braun, W. 1969. Antibody formation: Premature

initiation by endotoxin or synthetic polynucleotides in newborn mice. *Nature* 223: 843–844.

163. Wood, D. D., and Cameron, P. M. 1976. Stimulation of the release of B cell-activating factor from human monocytes. *Cell. Immunol.* 21: 133–145.

164. Woods, W. A., Siegal, M. J., and Chirigos, M. A. 1974. *In vitro* stimulation of spleen cell cultures by poly I: poly C and levamisole. *Cell. Immunol.* 14: 327–331.

165. Wright, D. G., Kirkpatrick, C. H., and Gallin, J. F. 1976. Effects of levamisole on normal and abnormal human leukocyte locomotion, in M. A. Chirigos (ed.), *Modulation of Host Immune Resistance in the Prevention or Treatment of Induced Neoplasias*, Fogarty International Center Proceedings No. 28. U.S. Government Printing Office, Washington, D.C. (in press).

166. Yamamoto, I., and Webb, D. R. 1975. Antigen stimulated changes in cyclic nucleotide levels in the mouse. *Proc. Natl. Acad. Sci.* 72: 2320–2324.

167. Youn, J. K., Barski, G., and Huppert, J. 1968. Inhibition de leucémigenèse virale chez la souris par traitement aux polynucléotides synthétiques. *C.R. Acad. Sci. (Paris)* 267: 816–819.

CHAPTER 6

IMMUNOADJUVANT, ANTIVIRAL, AND ANTITUMOR ACTIVITY OF SYNTHETIC POLYANIONS

A. M. Kaplan,
R. M. Ottenbrite,
W. Regelson,
R. Carchman,
P. Morahan,
A. Munson

Departments of Surgery,
Chemistry, Medicine,
Pharmacology, Microbiology,
and MCV/VCU Cancer Center
Medical College of Virginia
Virginia Commonwealth University
Richmond, Virginia 23298

Various synthetic polyanions have been shown to induce production of interferon and to have antiviral, antitumor, and reticuloendothelial stimulating activity. Both the biologic activity and toxicity of polyanions have been shown to be closely related to polymer molecular weight. Several lines of experimental evidence support the hypothesis that both the antitumor and antiviral activity of the polyanions are in part mediated by macrophage activation. The polyanions also represent a class of compounds with potent immunoadjuvant activity. These agents have potential as adjuvants with bacterial, viral, and tumor vaccines. The future of the polyanions in medicine rests in the synthesis of materials of defined molecular weight with reduced toxicity.

I. Introduction

Polymers are known to exhibit broad and varied activities with biological systems (23, 65, 70, 75, 77). Anionic and cationic polyelectrolytes of both natural and synthetic origin have been found to exhibit inhibitory effects on viruses, bacteria, tumors, and enzymes. Polyanions in particular have a wide range of biological activity and have received considerable attention in the areas of oncology and virology. The prolonged protective action of synthetic polyanions when given prior to virus inoculation also has significant clinical potential.

Most polyanions are water soluble which is significant not only for transport but also for systemic administration, since injection of suspensions into blood vessels can cause "colloido-clasmic shock" or "macromolecular syndrome" with major hypersensitive clinical toxicity (74). Water-soluble polyanionic polymers can distribute themselves in a living system by blood or lymphatic circulation, by cellular transport through the involvement of mobile phagocytic cells, or by absorption on cell surfaces. The role of polymers in the biology of organisms usually relates to their soluble or insoluble forms in tissue and tissue fluid (14). The compatibility of a polymer, or any substance for that matter, in blood, requires that it should not cause thrombosis or destroy cellular elements, alter plasma proteins, deplete electrolytes, nor cause acute or delayed toxic or immune allergic tissue damage.

Polyanions that enter into biological functions by distribution throughout the host behave similarly to certain proteins, glycoproteins, and polynucleotides which modulate a variety of biological responses related to bacteria and fungi, enhanced immune responsiveness, inhibition of adjuvant arthritis and, depending on polymer size, either depress or stimulate the functional phagocytic activity of the reticuloendothelial system. In relation to these immunologic and hormonal responses, inflammation, wound repair, blood clotting, and tissue damage are subject to the action of these macromolecules (72, 73). Perhaps the most significant role of polyanions is their mitotic inhibitory effects and their functional role in antineoplastic processes.

The toxicology of polyanions is of prime importance to their medical applicability. Initially polyanions were found to be too toxic and clinical testing of pyran copolymer as an antitumor agent was halted due to adverse side effects. Polyanions can cause anemias, leukocytosis, hepatosplenomegaly, and liver enzyme induction, and can sensitize biological systems to the lethal action of bacterial endotoxins (75). Further, they interfere with Type I and Type II drug metabolism mediated by liver microsomal systems by prolonging high levels of barbituates and aminopyrenes through blocking of detoxification (93). The biologic and clinical application of synthetic polyanions is again of major interest since recent evidence has shown that toxicity is in many instances related to higher molecular weight fractions (64).

II. Structures of Some Biologically Active Polyanions

Several synthetic anionic polymers have been tested for biological activity (38, 65, 73, 75). These studies indicate that the more important features of the carboxylic polymers for interferon induction, antiviral activity, and growth inhibition are a high density of carboxylate groups that are pendant to a longchain polymeric backbone. The molecular weight should be greater than 1000 and the carboxyl groups can be in alternate or adjacent positions. Polyanionic polymers, in general, have been found to be fairly stable and not readily biodegradable, which may account for their prolonged activity. Polymers with carboxylate functions bound by amidation or noncarboxylated polyethylenes of comparable dosages are inactive.

One of the most interesting and the most widely studied anionic polymers is pyran copolymer, which is prepared from 1:2 divinyl ether (DIVE) and maleic anhydride (MA) and often referred to in the literature as DIVEMA. This material was first prepared by Butler (16) using a radical catalyst. He proposed a cyclopolymerization mechanism to describe the formation of a six-membered pyran system. Since the tetrahydropyran ring is an integral part of the polymer chain, the polymer became widely known as "pyran copolymer" and is indexed in the medical literature as such.

Although this pyran structure has been widely accepted and analysis confirms the 1:2 copolymer ratio, no hard evidence for its existence has been produced. In fact, cyclopolymerizations reported to yield six-membered ring polymers have been under extensive studies recently and results indicate that primarily five-membered rings are formed. In many cases a mixture of five- and six-membered rings are obtained; the amounts of each appears to vary with experimental conditions. For example, polymerization of N-methyldimethylallylamine gave both types of ring systems and the proportions of six-membered polymer increased with increasing temperature (89). More recently, Samuels, by means of a quantitative evaluation, reported that divinyl ether-maleic anhydride copolymer was a five-membered ring structure (personal communication).

The complexity of the data appears to suggest the presence of both five- and six-membered rings. Other complications are also prevalent in the determination of this polymer's structures, for example, chain-branching in the polymer, since divinyl ethers can homopolymerize with radical catalysts (3). It is felt that simpler structures can be prepared, that are quantitatively and qualitatively more reproducible and as biologically active and possibly better therapeutically than pyran (DIVEMA).

Polyacrylic acid-maleic anhydride copolymer has similar biological activities to pyran but is not as biologically effective. It is prepared by 1:1 radical polymerization of acrylic acid and maleic anhydride. The resultant polymer on hydrolysis is a flexible straight-chain polymer with a ratio of 3 carboxyl groups for every 4 carbons in the polymer chain.

Maleic anhydride homopolymer is produced by high temperature and high concentrations of (2–4%) benzoyl peroxide to yield a molecular weight material (1000–100,000). This polymer was much less toxic than pyran but also much less effective against tumor growth and viruses (38).

Polyacrylic acid (64, 81), poly (methacrylic) acid (81), acrylic acid-maleic anhydride copolymer (64), and maleic anhydride-furan copolymer (64), are among the other purely synthetic polyanionic polymers which have been evaluated.

Several polysaccharide derivatives have been studied and the most active biologically was chlorite-oxidized amylose, known as COAM. This polymer is prepared by a two-step oxidation of the polysaccharide (21). The anhydropyranose units are first cleared with iodate and the resultant aldehyde groups are oxidized with sodium chlorite to the corresponding carboxylic acid functionality. These materials were developed to produce a polymer chain with a fairly high carboxylic group density polymer with an essentially biodegradable backbone. COAM has limited antiviral activity (8) and inhibits tumor growth (25). Although it appears to be relatively non-toxic, no clinical evaluation has been reported.

Another natural product-type polyanion is the double-stranded RNA polyinosinic-polycyticylic acid (poly I.C.). It possesses a broad spectrum of biologic activity and is a potent interferon inducer (58). Although laboratory tests were very encouraging, clinical anti-tumor activity has been disappointing (1). Aspartic acid–glutamic acid copolymer was also evaluated and found to be inactive (unpublished observations).

Several similarities in structure are apparent in the polymers just discussed. Among these are a fairly flexible polymer chain and a high density of carboxyl groups situated along the backbone of the polymer. It is conceivable that polyanions with better therapeutic indexes could be obtained from systematic studies involving alterations of these basic structures but incorporating the features that apparently evoke biological activity.

III. Effect of Molecular Weight of Polyanions on Pharmacological Activity

Most of the research with anionic polymers has been done without regard to either the average molecular weight or the molecular weight distribution of particular polymer samples. Polyanions have been tested and activity compared in many cases where the average molecular weight was as low as 1000 and as high as 500,000. Optimally the polymer should be of sufficient molecular weight so as to delay body clearance ($> 30,000$) but still be below the kidney threshold ($< 50,000$). Consequently, the molecular-weight distribution would be more critical than the average molecular weight since very large molecules can cause erythrocyte aggregation (74), and changes in platelet or leukocyte distribution or morphology. Another approach to this problem would be to fabricate biodegradable polymers that can retain their biologically active structure long enough to perform their task and then be converted to harmless metabolites which are readily eliminated. This latter concept has not been widely attempted, except in the development of degradable coatings for sustained drug release and prolonged drug activity.

A variety of fractionations, degradations, and synthetic techniques have been used to produce different molecular weight fractions of pyran with antitumor activity. Both degradation and large-scale fractionations of pyran on sand columns failed to give consistent and/or enough material for evaluation (13). Breslow (12) subsequently prepared pyran copolymer at low-temperature in acetone, using a free-radical initiator and tetrahydrofuran as a chain-transfer agent. This method appeared to provide controlled molecular weight polymers with narrow polydispersity. Regelson et al. (77, 79) evaluated these different molecular weight copolymers for biological activity. It was found that low molecular weight samples of pyran copolymer with narrow molecular weight distribution not only possessed lower toxicity but retained the antitumor activity exhibited by the higher molecular weight samples against both Ehrlich adrenocarcinoma and Lewis lung carcinoma in mice. Also, serum glutamic pyruvate transaminase levels and inhibition of drug metabolism increased with increasing polymer size, as did sensitization to endotoxin. Phagocytosis was stimulated by low molecular weight polymers and depressed by high molecular weight polymers.

In our laboratory we have isolated from the broad molecular weight range polymer, Hercules XA 124-177, pyran copolymer, two fractions with low molecular weight and narrow polydispersity. These fractions were obtained by membrane ultrafiltration techniques using PM-10 and PM-30 Amicon membrane filters. Table 1 compares the biological activities of the original XA 124-177 DIVEMA copolymer and the two lower molecular weight materials. It was observed that the parent pyran XA 124-177 caused hepatosplenomegaly, sensitization to endotoxin and inhibition of the microsomal enzymes as manifested by the increased hexobarbital sleeping time. However, the polymer fractions that were obtained by passing the polymer through the PM-10 and PM-30 filters showed much higher LD_{50}'s than the parent polymer, caused no hepatosplenomegaly, and did not sensitize to bacterial endotoxin. Both fractions contained antitumor activity but were devoid of antiviral activity. They did not inhibit the microsomal enzymes as measured by hexobarbital sleeping time. Both fractions were active against Lewis lung carcinoma but only the parent compound retained substantial activity against encephalomycarditis virus. In addition, similar to the parent pyran, both PM-10 and PM-30 fractions activated peritoneal macrophages to destroy tumor cells nonspecifically while not affecting normal cells. Both of these fractions increased the liver and spleen weight only slightly compared to the parent pyran compound and increased the LD_{50} (endotoxin) from 0.12 mg/kg for the parent polymer to > 15 mg/kg for each of these fractions. Consequently the use of discrete molecular weight fractions may have a decided effect on the toxicities of these polymers without loss of their antitumor activity.

Fractionation of polyacrylic acid-maleic anhydride copolymer (PAAMA) was carried out by the same technique. Table 2 compares the antitumor activity for the whole polymer PAAMA with the polymer which was passed through the PM-50 membrane filter. The antitumor activity of these two polymer preparations was similar as measured by primary tumor size and increased life span. Whole body weight loss caused by the lower molecular weight polymer was markedly less than that of the parent polymer. Further fractionation and biological studies of this polymer are in progress.

The significance of molecular-weight differences in polyanions could be important in relation to their ability to displace deoxyribonucleoprotein (DNP) from its binding position in the nucleus. DNA itself can be lethal to tumor cells (63) and apparently, irradiated tissue is more vulnerable to DNP displacement by polyanions. One area of projected clinical investigation for pyran is whether it can act as a synergist for radiation or radiomimetic induced tumor injury (51). Alternatively, the DNP displaced by polyanions (i.e., pyran) may be a critical factor that is responsible for some of pyran's adjuvant anti-tumor or antiviral action. This DNP

displacement induced by polyanions may also be crucial to cellular nuclear extrusion as a phenomenon.

The clinical future of polyanions lies with the separation of toxicity
from anti-tumor, anti-viral, RES, and immunologic effects. It is apparent
from data so far that in general the toxicity of polyanions increases with
molecular weight particularly over 50,000. Fortunately anti-tumor activity is retained in lower molecular weight fractions (< 10,000). These
fractions are relatively less toxic and are associated with macrophage
activation, however, they are devoid of anti-viral activity. It may be more
difficult to separate toxicity from anti-viral or immunologic stimulating
effects which apparently reside in molecular weights above 30,000.

IV. Antiviral Activity of Polyanions

Naturally occurring and synthetic polyanions have been investigated for antiviral activity in a number of systems. Regelson (72) has
reviewed the marked antiviral activity that many diverse polyanions exert
against virus replication in vitro. Polyanions also exert potent antiviral
effects against plant viruses (36), and polyanions are now being developed for purification of water from contaminating viruses. The
mechanism of antiviral activity in these systems has not been completely
defined, but may involve direct inactivation of viruses in some situations.

The one area of most interest has been in the protective effects observed against various animal virus infections in mammals. Pyran and
other polycarboxylate polyanions, ethylenemaleic anhydride copolymer,
acrylic   acid-maleic   anhydride   copolymer,   and   chlorite-oxidized
oxyamylose, exhibit a broad spectrum of antiviral activity (Table 3).
Polyanion treatment protects mice from mortality following lethal infection with both RNA or DNA cytopathic viruses. Treatment of mice with
polyanions also inhibits tumor formation and delays mortality after infection with DNA or RNA tumor viruses.

Our investigations have substantiated the importance of molecular
weight and specific polyanionic configuration. However, a complete
structure activity relationship in regard to antiviral activity still needs to
be performed. Greatest protection is observed with prophylactic treatment. Therapeutic treatment often does not alter the course of disease,
particularly with rapidly fatal infections. These results suggest that
polyanions may act very early during the viral infection, the drugs may
need to be activated by the animal, or the drugs may act through modulation of host responses. Greatest protection is observed when the drug is
administered at the same site where virus is subsequently injected. How-

Table 1. Pharmacologic studies of pyran fractions

	Control	Pyran XA 124-177 Whole Polymer	PM-10[a]	PM-30[b]
Intrinsic Viscosity	—	0.21	0.05	0.06
Toxicologic Properties				
LD_{50} (mg/kg)[c]		74(69–79)	120(105–135)	115(108–122)
Liver weight[d] % B.W.	5.4 ±0.4	7.8 ±0.2	5.1 ±0.2	5.9 ±0.8
Spleen weight[d] % B.W.	0.36 ±0.02	1.08 ±0.04	0.40 ±0.04	0.40 ±0.03
LD_{50}[e] (Endotoxin) mg/kg	25	0.12	>15	>15
Hexobarbital[f] sleeping time (min)	36.8 ±2.6	97.6 ±4.1	42.8 ±3.8	48.6 ±5.3

Antitumor and Antiviral Properties

Antitumor activity[g]				
Lewis lung % inhibition	0	76	69	64
Antiviral (EMC) % protection	0	89	0	30

a. PM-10 Filtrate of XA124-177 passed through Amicon PM-10 filter.

b. PM-30 Filtrate of XA124-177 passed through Amicon PM-30 filter.

c. LD_{50} (95%) confidence limits calculated by the method of Litchfield and Wilcoxon. Polymers administered intravenously. Mortality recorded after 24 hours.

d. Polymers administered in a dose of 25 mg/kg intravenously. Organ weights determined 7 days after drug injection and expressed as percent of total weight (Munson et al., J. Reticuloendothel. Soc. 7:375, 1970).

e. LD_{50} of S. typhosd 0904 lipopolysaccharide 24 hours after a single administration of 24 mg/kg of polymer. (Munson et a., Proc. Soc. Exp. Biol. Med. 137:553, 1971).

f. Group of NYLAR-A mice were inoculated with 25 mg/kg i.v. of the polymer (except ASP-Glun; 100 mg/kg). Twenty four hours later an anesthetic dose (80 mg/kg) of sodium hexobarbital was administered i.v. and duration of anesthesia recorded. (Munson et al., Proc. Soc. Exp. Biol. Med. 137:553, 1971).

g. BDF, mice were inoculated with 10^6 Lewis' lung cells into right-hind gluteus muscle. Polymers were administered daily by tne intraperitoneal route for 10 consecutive days following tumor implantation. Primary tumor size was determined on day 14 (% inhibition) and increased life span (% ILS) calculated from mean time to death.

Note: $P < 0.05$ mean ± S.E. derived from 8 mice per group. LD_{50} studies employed at least 100 animals.

Table 2. Comparison of antitumor activity for PAAMA-whole polymer with PAAMA-PM-50 polymer[a]

Treatment	Dose (mg/kg)	Body Weights Change[b]	Mean Survival Time (days)	Increase in Life Span (%)
Physiologic saline		+0.4	29.8 ± 1.4	
Whole polymer PAAMA	25	−0.4	40.7[c] ± 2.5	36.5
	50	−0.8	38.1[c] ± 2.4	27.9
	100	−1.2	43.9[c] ± 1.9	44
PM-50	25	+0.2	43.9[c] ±1.9	47
	25	+1.5	49.2[c] ± 2.1	65
	50	+1.3	44.1[c] ± 1.8	48

a. Groups of mice were inoculated im with 1×10^6 Lewis lung cells and treated ip for 10 days with polymer.

b. Whole body weight after 10 days of treatment (gms).

c. $P > 0.05$; mean ±S.E. derived from 8 mice per group.

ever, there often is significant protection when the virus is injected at other sites. For example, intravenous or intraperitoneal administration of pyran protects mice from lethal intravaginal infection with herpes simplex virus (57).

In contrast to standard antiviral chemotherapeutic agents, polyanions can provide prolonged protection. Mice treated with pyran were protected against subsequent picornavirus infection for two months (52), and were resistant to Friend leukemia virus infection for three weeks (85). This prolonged protection may be related to the slow degradation of most polyanions. Also in contrast to conventional chemotherapeutic drugs, polyanions provide a broad spectrum of antiviral resistance (Table 3).

Considerable emphasis has been directed toward defining the mechanism of antiviral action of polyanions, particularly for pyran and chlorite oxidized oxyamylose. The major modes of antiviral action that have been considered are listed in Table 4.

Polyanions can directly inactivate viruses (50, 52). However, the levels required are greater than those required for antiviral activity in vivo. Inhibition of virus replication by mechanisms similar to conventional antiviral chemotherapeutic drugs also does not appear to play an important part in polyanion resistance in vivo. Pyran does inhibit the RNA dependent DNA polymerase of avian myeloblastosis virus in vitro (66), but the enzyme is only present in oncornaviruses. Moreover, the

Table 3. Antiviral activity *in vivo* of pyran and similar polyanions

Virus	Virus Group	References
Cytopathic RNA viruses		
Encephalomyocarditis	Picornavirus	58
MM virus	Picornavirus	37, 69
Vesicular Stomatitis	Rhabdovirus	27
Foot and mouth disease	Picornavirus	49, 83, 87
Influenza	Orthomyxovirus	7, 17, 90
Mengo	Picornavirus	7, 9, 21, 52
Semliki forest	Togavirus	7
Hog cholera	Togavirus	49
Cytopathic DNA viruses		
Herpes simplex virus	Herpesvirus	7, 26, 50, 57
Vaccinia	Poxvirus	7, 10, 17, 21, 24, 26
RNA tumor viruses		
Friend leukemia	Oncornavirus	20, 60, 71, 85
Rauscher leukemia	Oncornavirus	20, 41
Gross leukemia	Oncornavirus	12
Moloney sarcoma	Oncornavirus	11, 35
Mammary tumor	Oncornavirus	25
DNA tumor viruses		
Polyoma	Papovirus	41
Adenovirus 12	Adenovirus	47

drug does not have a morphologically toxic effect on normal or transformed mammalian cells at doses far above the effective antiviral dose (61). Considerable effort has been directed toward determining whether induction of the antiviral protein, interferon, accounts for the antiviral action of polyanions (53). There is no clear evidence that systemic induction of interferon plays any role in the antiviral activity of pyran or chlorite oxidized oxyamylose (9, 26, 50, 58). Although pyran stimulates the

Table 4. Possible modes of antiviral action of polyanions

1. Direct inactivation of virus
2. Inhibition of virus replication
3. Interferon induction
4. Stimulation of phagocytosis and inflammation
5. Specific immunoenhancement of humoral or cell-mediated immune responses against the virus
6. Enhancement of macrophage antiviral functions

reticuloendothelial system, there is no correlation with antiviral activity. In fact, the lower MW compounds, which exert potent RES stimulating activity, do not exhibit antiviral activity (13, 77).

Because polyanions are immunomodulators for various humoral and cell mediated immunologic responses, attention has been directed toward specific immunoenhancement as the mode of antiviral action. Specific immunostimulation, however, at least in the case of pyran protection against herpes simplex virus, does not appear to play a prominent role in the antiviral activity. Pyran is an effective antiviral agent in animals depleted of thymus derived lymphocytes (26, 27, 40, 41), indicating that the drug probably acts independently of these immune cells. Moreover, animals protected by treatment with pyran possess none or low levels of protective antibody against the virus, and are not resistant to subsequent rechallenge with the same virus (unpublished observations). The polyanion appears to inhibit virus replication very early and efficiently (50), so that there is probably little virus antigen to stimulate an immune response.

Investigations that demonstrated no correlation between interferon induction and antiviral activity provided the first suggestions that activated macrophages might be involved in the antiviral action of polyanions (9, 58). Our recent data substantiate this hypothesis. Pyran activated peritoneal cells can transfer resistance to susceptible recipient mice to infection with herpes simplex virus or Friend leukemia virus (unpublished observations). Moreover, pyran activated peritoneal macrophages exhibit potent antiviral activity in vitro (59). Thus, we have demonstrated that activated macrophages have the capacity for antiviral activity; however, proof is still needed that these cells are the major mode of action in vivo in animals treated with polyanions.

Previous investigations have established that polyanions exert marked and broad spectrum antiviral activity. Some of the parameters of protection, and modes of action have been elucidated. However, prophylactic treatment with polyanions will not be clinically applicable on a large scale, except in special situations for immunosuppressed people at particular risk to various viral infections (e.g., cancer patients, renal transplant patients, other immunodeficient patients). In this regard, it is important to note that pyran treatment has proven effective in naturally immunodeficient neonatal animals (57, 84) in animals deficient in cell mediated immune responses (26, 27, 41), in animals suppressed by treatment with silica (11), and in animals treated with steroids (37).

Perhaps the greatest potential use for polyanions is in combination with virus vaccines. In this situation, the polyanion could act both in its antiviral capacity and as an immunoadjuvant. Campbell and Richmond, in a series of studies, have documented that polyanions increase the effectiveness of various foot and mouth disease virus vaccines (18). The new virus vaccines that are being currently advocated are those made of virus protein subunits, without the possibly cancer causing or otherwise deleterious virus nucleic acid. Unfortunately, these vaccines are not as effective as live attenuated virus or whole inactivated virus vaccines. However, in conjunction with polyanions, such vaccines might be prepared that possess adequate effectiveness.

Polyanions usually exert beneficial antiviral effects. Yet, treatment of animals with polyanions has also exacerbated tumor formation by Maloney sarcoma (35) and Friend leukemia viruses (85). We have demonstrated that protection of exacerbation of Friend leukemogenesis depends on the route of administration of pyran. In the protective regimen, the drug appears to activate the macrophage, while in the adverse regimen, the drug appears to stimulate the target cells in which the virus replicates (60). These investigations emphasize the "Yin-Yang" aspect of treatment with polyanions, and the absolute necessity to elucidate the parameters affecting metabolism and antiviral action of these compounds before a rationale for clinical treatment can be established.

V. Immunoadjuvant Activity of Polyanions

Synthetic polyanions, such as polacrylic acid, dextran sulfate and pyran copolymer, have been shown to have immunoadjuvant activity in several model systems. Polyacrylic acid, pyran copolymer and dextran sulfate have both been demonstrated to enhance the primary antibody response to sheep erythrocytes (sRBC) in vivo (4, 15, 31, 32, 58). Polyacrylic acid was found to increase background plaques in unimmunized animals (31), similar to what has been reported for lipopolysaccharide (LPS) (2, 42). In vivo administration of dextran sulfate or pyran on the other hand, did not stimulate the production of background plaques in unimmunized control mice (32, 58). If the adjuvant effect of pyran was a function of heightened antigen processing by macrophages or more effective presentation of antigen to B cells, administration of pyran after antigen should have produced less enhancement than if it was given at earlier times. This interpretation was consistent with the observation of Pierce and Benacerraf (68) that the primary antibody response to sRBC in vitro was independent of macrophages after 24 hours. However, varying the time of pyran administration with respect to that of antigen (from 1 day prior to 2 days after) made no difference in the potentiation of the antibody response to sRBC by pyran.

The adjuvanticity of dextran sulfate was felt to be a function of the polyanionic nature of the agent, as neutral dextran had no effect on the

antibody response while a positively charged derivative, diethyl-
aminoethyl (DEAE)-dextran, had an inhibitory effect (32). Inoculation of
polyacrylic acid or dextran sulfate with sRBC into thymectomized, irradiated, bone marrow reconstituted (TxBM) mice resulted in an enhanced antibody response as measured by plaque-forming cells and
hemolysin titers, compared to TxBM mice which had received sRBC alone
(34). However, the antibody response in immunomodulator treated TxBM
mice never reached that seen in normal immune mice. These results
suggested that these polyanionic immunomodulators were able to partially replace thymus cell function in T-depleted mice (34). However,
definitive experiments which would differentiate between replacement of
thymic function and enhancement of residual T cell function have not
been performed. In contrast, pyran was unable to enhance the specific
activity (plaques/10^6) spleen cells in TxBM mice (4). Moreover, the inability of pyran to enhance the antibody response to a thymic independent antigen, E. coli lipopolysaccharide (LPS) suggested that pyran did
not act directly on B lymphocytes (4).

Dextran sulfate has also been shown to enhance both the primary and
secondary antibody responses in mice which were primed and challenged
with suboptimal doses of sRBC (33). Enhancement of the primary antibody response by dextran sulfate did not result in a decreased secondary
response after challenge with a suboptimal dose of sRBC. These results
suggested that in addition to increasing the number of plaque-forming
cells, dextran sulfate was also able to increase the number of B-memory
cells (33). In addition, splenic uptake of ^{51}Cr-labeled sRBC was found to be
enhanced after treatment with dextran sulfate, and increased antigen uptake correlated with adjuvant activity (29).

Pyran was capable of enhancing the secondary response to sRBC
suggesting that this immunoadjuvant acted to expand the number of antibody producing B cells or memory T cells in this T-dependent response.
However, the inability of pyran to enhance the antibody response to the
T-independent antigen, LPS, suggested that pyran did not act directly on
B lymphocytes. Neither the antibody response to sRBC in TxBM mice nor
the antibody response to LPS in normal mice was increased in specific
activity after treatment of mice with pyran although both responses
showed an increase in total plaques/spleen. These results were consistent
with nonspecific blastogenesis of the entire spleen cell population; this
concept was supported by the blastogenesis data obtained in TxBM mice
in which pyran was shown to be mitogenic in vivo for both T and B
lymphocytes (5). If pyran induced blastogenesis of only specific antigen
stimulated cells, an increase in both specific activity as well as plaques/
spleen should have been seen. All of these experiments were consistent

with the hypothesis that the cellular site of action of pyran in the antibody response was the T lymphocyte.

Dextran sulfate has also been shown to be mitogenic for mouse lymphoid cells in vitro (30). Lymphocyte activation was immunologically nonspecific and caused induction of polyclonal antibody synthesis (22). DNA synthesis was stimulated in spleen cells obtained from normal, TxBM and athymic mice, which suggested that dextran sulfate was mitogenic for B lymphocytes (30). Normal thymus cells failed to respond to dextran sulfate although cortisone resistant thymus cells gave a small but significant response. Therefore, it could not be excluded that dextran sulfate might also have some effect on T lymphocytes (30). Furthermore, investigation of the mitogenic activity of other polyanions revealed that although adjuvanticity and mitogenicity were not strictly correlated, they were related (28, 91).

In general, compounds which stimulated DNA synthesis of B cells in vitro were also able to enhance the antibody response to suboptimal doses of sRBC (28, 91). Although Diamantstein et al. reported that unsubstituted dextrans lacked mitogenic (91) and adjuvant activity (32), Coutinho et al. (22) found that unsubstituted dextrans did have mitogenic activity, although the molecular weight had to be greater than 7×10^4 daltons. Above this molecular weight threshold, mitogenicity was found to correlate with the log of the molecular weight (22). Sulfate substitution of dextrans was found to enhance greatly mitogenicity, and to a lesser extent, adjuvanticity. Mitogenicity of the sulfonated dextrans was independent of molecular weight (22). Although the polymeric structure of the active compounds was not a requirement for mitogenicity, it seemed to enhance mitogenicity by providing multipoint binding to low-affinity receptors (22).

With regard to T cell reactivity as measured by cell mediated cytotoxicity, pyran treatment prior to allogeneic tumor cells caused a decrease in spleen cell cytolytic activity in addition to delaying the time of the peak response (4). Since the induction of cell mediatec cytotoxicity is macrophage dependent (92), this inhibition in cytotoxicity might have been due to macrophage inhibition during the inductive process.

A single intravenous injection of pyran was shown to depress significantly the in vitro blastogenic response of spleen cells to PHA as measured by counts per minute at various times 2–14 days after in vivo administration (4). This was similar to data that Scott (86) has presented for the biological immunopotentiator, Corynebacterium parvum. However, 5 days after pyran administration, thymidine incorporation in mitogen treated cultures of pyran treated cells were significantly higher than that of normal cells with mitogen. As this corresponded to the time of the peak increase in mitogen independent incorporation of ^{3}H-thymidine, it was possible that pyran primed spleen cells were more susceptible to the action of phytohemagglutinin or LPS and more resistant to the inhibitory effect of activated macrophages.

Similar to experiments reported by Scott (86), in which he found that the inhibition of the response to PHA was dependent on macrophages, we have found that pyran-induced inhibition of blastogenesis was also macrophage dependent (6). Peritoneal exudate cells from pyran treated animals were more effective than were normal macrophages in abrogating the PHA or LPS response of normal spleen cells (5, 6). Removal of glass adherent cells from the spleens of pyran-treated mice restored the response to PHA and LPS (5).

These results were consistent with a dual action of pyran on T lymphocytes and macrophages in the modulation of the immune response. The enhancement of the antibody response to sRBC and the inability to obtain comparable enhancement of the antibody response to a T-independent antigen (LPS) or a T-dependent antigen (sRBC) in TxBM mice was compatible with a direct action on thymus-derived lymphocytes. The inhibitory effect of pyran on cell mediated cytotoxicity could be due to a direct action on T cells, or an indirect effect mediated by macrophages. Further experiments are needed to clarify these results. The inhibitory effects of pyran on PHA and LPS blastogenesis were macrophage mediated (5, 6).

In summary, polyanions are capable of eliciting numerous effects on various parameters of immune reactivity. Polyanions have been described which mediated their effects by direct action on thymus-derived lymphocytes, bone marrow-derived lymphocytes or macrophages. Moreover, it is likely that some of the immunomodulators discussed, act on more than one cell type. The target cell for a specific polyanion is probably to a certain extent dependent on the model system used to determine immune reactivity. The effects of other immunomodulators on certain target cell populations have been determined to be mediated indirectly by an effect on a different cell type or by the production of soluble mediators. For example, administration of pyran has been shown to depress T lymphocyte functions in vitro and in vivo, and this effect has been demonstrated to be mediated by macrophages which have been activated by pyran treatment (5, 6).

Many of the studies designed to determine the cellular site or mechanism of action of a given immunomodulator were performed by different investigators using various strains of mice and a variety of antigens to assess immune reactivity. It is probable that a number of the apparent inconsistencies in the data presented by various investigators resulted from the use of different test systems. However, as the present review indicates, polyanions are capable of producing a wide spectrum of effects on immune reactivity, and the effect of a given immunomodulator on the response to a given antigen may be even more complex than anticipated. The data indicate that polyanions represent a class of compounds with potent immunoadjuvant activity. These agents have potential as adjuvants with bacterial, viral, and tumor vaccines and as general stimulators of the immune response in clinical situations where immunologic inhibition is present.

VI. Antitumor Activity of Polyanions

The action of polyanions as mitotic inhibitors and their functional role in neoplastic processes have been reviewed recently by Ottenbrite and Regelson (65). A possible mechanism for the activity of polyanions on tumor growth may be related to coupling of the polyanion to tumor antigen. However, the action of polyanions on a wide range of enzymes, alteration of the isoelectric point of proteins, displacement of nucleohistone, macrophage activation, and antiviral action all indicate possible alternative concepts of antitumor action.

Synthetic polyanions such as pyran, ethylene maleic anhydride (E/MA) and polyacrylic acid have been tested for antitumor activity (81). Polymers with MW of 1,000–100,000 or higher were tested against a variety of subcutaneous rodent tumors (71, 73). In each case, systemic drug administration was associated with significant tumor regression without excessive weight loss. The higher the molecular weight of the polymer, the more toxic the E/MA copolymer was in both the mouse and dog: Optimum activity was obtained in the series where carboxamide and ionizable carboxyl groups were interdispersed along the polymer backbone. Monomers were inactive and when all carboxyl groups were converted to carboxamides, significant tumor-inhibitory activity was lost. This was similar to observations on the antiviral action of these compounds (62). The most effective regimen with E/MA polymers was prophylactic treatment. Adequate treatment of mice with E/MA polymers prior to tumor inoculation resulted in inhibition of tumor growth, even when tumor was inoculated as long as 1 week following drug injection (71, 73).

In an effort to evaluate the antitumor activity of other polyanions we conducted a comparative study of maleic anhydride homopolymer and acrylic acid-maleic anhydride copolymer with pyran copolymer. The results are listed in Table 5. Acrylic acid-maleic anyhdride copolymer was as effective as pyran in both suppressing tumor growth (50–77%) as compared to pyran (59–77%) as well as causing an increase in mean survival

Table 5.   Comparison of antitumor activity of polyanionic polymers

	Dose (mg/kg)	Days After Tumor Implant[a]		MST
		15	24	
Control		1304 ± 104	4627 ± 317	29.4 ± 1.0
Maleic anhydride homopolymer	25	1074 ± 184 (18%)	2078 ± 724	
	50	774 ± 200 (41%)	2387 ± 492 (49%)	30.2 ± 1.5
	75	390 ± 99 (70%)	1505 ± 234 (78%)	33.8 ± 2.6
Acrylic acid-maleic anhydride copolymer	25	856 ± 130 (34%)	2309 ± 446 (50%)	39.4 ± 1.3
	50	322 ± 60 (75%)	1576 ± 271 (66%)	37.0 ± 2.5
	75	337 ± 141 (74%)	1053 ± 359 (77%)	39.1 ± 2.8
Pyran copolymer	25	546 ± 130 (58%)	1889 ± 353 (59%)	36.4 ± 3.5
	50	473 ± 106 (76%)	2125 ± 468 (54%)	37.2 ± 1.1
	75	319 ± 109 (76%)	1542 ± 284 (77%)	41.0 ± 2.3

a. Tumor weight derived from tumor measurements, mean ± S.E. derived from 15 control mice and 8 treated mice per group, polymers administered i.p. on days 1–10 after tumor transplantations.
  b. (% inhibition).

time by 33%. Although maleic anhydride homopolymer was effective in suppressing tumor size 49–78% it did not change the mean survival time to any significant extent.

Of all the polyanions pyran has received the greatest attention with respect to its antitumor activity. Pyran has minimal *in vitro* toxicity to tumor cells in contrast to alkylating or other chemotherapeutic agents (61). Treatment given prior to inoculation with Friend leukemia virus, the allogeneic sarcoma 180 or Ehrlich ascites tumor inhibits subsequent tumor growth (71). Pyran also inhibits tumors induced by Rasucher leukemia virus, polyoma virus, and Gross leukemia virus in normal or thymectomized, immunosuppressed mice (19, 41). Pyran treatment of mice bearing the LSTRA lymphoma produces apparent cures if the tumor burden is reduced by prior treatment with an alkylating agent (67).

The route of pyran administration is important. Intravenous pyran can stimulate Friend leukemia virus activity in contrast to intraperitoneal pyran, which is inhibiting (60, 85). Paradoxically, certain murine sarcoma virus induced tumors are stimulated by pyran as well as other interferon inducers (35). This stimulation may be related to the ability of pyran, in a manner similar to other maleic anhydride copolymers, to induce hepatosplenomegaly or splenomegaly in normal mice. Pyran also causes accelerated development of benzo(a)pyrene-induced skin tumors in mice (46) and this raises the important point that immunopotentiators as a class of compounds can often inhibit or enhance tumor growth, depending on a variety of factors (35, 60, 85).

Pyran also inhibited the growth of the first generation transplant of the mammary carcinoma, the Lewis lung carcinoma and B16 melanoma syngeneic tumors (41, 81). This antitumor action of pyran was not correlated with phagocytic stimulation or interferon-inducing capacity (78, 80) and recent work indicated that the antitumor action correlated with an increased macrophage-killing capacity (39, 44, 56).

Pyran was effective even when its administration was delayed until 8 days after tumor implantation, a time when the tumors have already metastasized (61). Moreover, systemic treatment with pyran after surgical removal of the Lewis lung carcinoma, resulted in a 50% reduction in the mice dying of metastatic tumor (45). The antitumor activity of pyran is apparently not due to direct cytotoxicity. Studies of in vitro cytotoxicity have shown that above 1 mg/ml of drug is required to destroy 50% of either tumor cells or normal cells, in contrast to nitrogen mustard which at concentrations of 9.5 μg/ml destroyed 50% of the cells (61).

Our observations that pyran was not cytotoxic for tumor cells (61) coupled with its known reticuloendothelial stimulating activity suggested that pyran's antitumor activity might be mediated by macrophages. Moreover, when several preparations of pyran and polyacrylic acid were tested for antitumor activity against the Lewis lung carcinoma only those preparations which activated macrophages had antitumor activity (56). Several direct lines of experimental evidence have supported the hypothesis that pyran's antitumor activity was mediated by macrophages: (1) peritoneal macrophages taken from mice treated with pyran intraperitoneally were cytotoxic to tumor cells in vitro; normal macrophages had no effect (44, 79); (2) systemic treatment of tumor bearing mice with pyran caused an increased infiltration of tumors with histiocytes (88); and (3) pyran activated peritoneal macrophages mixed with tumor cells in vitro and transplanted into syngeneic recipients inhibited tumor growth (43, 56).

Previous investigations have established that polyanions exert marked and broad-spectrum antitumor activity. Part or all of the antitumor effect of pyran appears to be related to macrophage activation, however, additional experiments will be necessary to define pyran's role in potentiating tumor specific immunity (55). The effectiveness of pyran in inhibiting tumor metastasis in animals treated with surgery and in combination with drug therapy is exciting and needs to be better understood mechanistically before clinical application is appropriate. A systemic evaluation of polyanions with potential antitumor activity and the isolation of polyanions with defined molecular weight already demonstrated to have antitumor activity should be pursued.

VII. Clinical Effects of Polyanions

The initial clinical and animal toxicity studies were done with the lyophilized hydrolysate of pyran (76, 82). The initial animal toxicity studies were performed with material of average 30,000 molecular weight (MW) while the clinical studies (NSC 46015) were done with pyran of average MW of 18,000 or 23,000. In the initial study, pyran copolymer was given to advanced cancer patients who were no longer responsive to other treatment modalities (76, 82). Survival had to be estimated at one month and patients had to be off other forms of chemotherapy or radiotherapy at least 2 weeks without signs of marrow depression or active sepsis and liver disease. Pyran copolymer was then given to 62 patients and the consistent limiting toxicity of pyran was transient thrombocytopenia. Cytoplasmic inclusions were seen in circulating leukocytes, nucleated marrow cells and phagocytic cells of liver and spleen after administration. Although not dose limiting, fever was seen in 50% of patients (76, 82).

Apart from thrombocytopenia and fever, the major limiting toxicity for pyran has been vascular in nature, associated with the unpredictable development of hypotension in six cases, seizure in two patients, and impairment of vision in three, with complete loss of vision in one case who expired in shock. Vision fully returned within 2 to 48 hours in the other two patients. Other significantly toxic side effects have included facial edema, onset of angina with myocardial infarction in another and confusion and somnolence in three patients.

Significant antitumor activity of NSC 46015 pyran with objective and subjective improvement was seen in one patient with myxomatous ovarian cancer (76, 82). However, a sufficient number of patients were not treated in any tumor category and almost all patients in the study were in the preterminal phases of their disease with treatment limited to a median of 9–14 days.

At this time, however, clinical formuation (the lyophilized hydrolyzed salt and the acid hydrolysate of pyran copolymer (m.w. average 18–23,000) (NSC 46015) is too toxic for continued intravenous trial. This is based on observation of hypotension, blindness and sclerosis of blood vessels. In contrast to vascular effects, pyrexia, thrombocytopenia, leukopenia and anti-coagulant effects are not seriously limiting toxicities. These effects are readily reversible and/or symptomatically controlled. Pyran had dose related in vitro and in vivo anticoagulant effects, however, prolonged anticoagulant activity (block to fibrin formation) was not associated with clinical hemorrhage as no clinical bleeding was encountered with pyran administration despite a mild increase in bleeding time. In adults, intravenous NSC 46015 at 12 mg/kg/day or a single dose up to 18 mg/kg did not produce evident hemolysis. Schizontocyte ("helmet") cells and renal toxicity have not been seen at this dosage in contrast to reported pediatric experience (48).

Pyran should be looked at as an adjuvant to the development of effective antitumor and antiviral vaccines in view of the experience of Campbell and Richmond in the foot and mouth disease model (18, 83) and in view of the experience of the Chirigos group (54, 55) with pyran's effect on prolonging remission following chemotherapeutic response to BCNU with and without the simultaneous administration of irradiated tumor cells. It should be emphasized that while toxicity of the current clinical formulation precludes further broad based intravenous clinical testing, it should stimulate renewed interest in the formulation of less toxic fractions, and their use in adjuvant antitumor and antiviral programs. Consequently, future clinical studies should involve: development of low molecular weight clinical material of improved therapeutic index; adjuvant use at lower dosage of NSC 46015 on a weekly or biweekly schedule; and regional or intratumoral use in subcutaneous, intrapleural, or intraperitoneal recurrences.

ACKNOWLEDGMENTS

Supported in part by U.S.P.H. Grants CA 1537, AI 11561, and AI 16193, and contract CB-43877. We thank Betty West for excellent secretarial assistance.

REFERENCES

1. Adamson, R. H., Levy, H. B., and Baron, S. 1972. Search for new drugs, in A. Rubin (ed.), *Medicinal Research,* pp. 292–311. Marcel Dekker, New York.

2. Anderson, J., Sjöberg, O., and Möller, G. 1972. Induction of immunoglobulin and antibody synthesis in vitro by lipopolysaccharide. *Eur. J. Immunol.* 2: 349–353.

3. Aso, C., Ushio, S., and Sogabe, M. 1967. Studies on the polymerization of bifunctional monomers. XI. The cyclic polymerization of divinyl ether and the structure of the polymer. *Makromol. Chem.* 100: 100–116.

4. Baird, L. G., and Kaplan, A. M. 1975. Immunoadjuvant activity of pyran copolymer. I. Evidence for direct stimulation of T-lymphocytes and macrophages. *Cell. Immunol.* 20: 167–176.

5. Baird, L. G., and Kaplan, A. M. 1977. Macrophage regulation of mitogen

induced blastogenesis. I. Demonstration of inhibitory cells in the spleens and peritoneal exudates of mice. *Cell. Immunol.* 28: 22–35.

6. Baird, L. G., and Kaplan, A. M. 1977. Macrophage regulation of mitogen induced blastogenesis. II. Mechanism of inhibition. *Cell. Immunol.* 28: 36–50.

7. Billiau, A., Desmyter, J., and DeSomer, P. 1970. Antiviral activity of chlorite oxidized oxyamylose, a polyacetal carboxylic acid. *J. Virol.* 5: 321–328.

8. Billiau, A., Muyembe, J., and DeSomer, P. 1971. Effect of chlorite-oxidized oxymylose on influenza virus infection in mice. *Appl. Microbiol.* 21: 580–584.

9. Billiau, A., Muyembe, J. J., and DeSomer, P. 1971. Mechanism of antiviral activity in vivo of polycarboxylates which induce interferon production. *Nature New Biol.* 232: 183–186.

10. Billiau, A., Muyembe, J. J., and DeSomer, P. 1972. Interferon inducing polycarboxylates mechanism of protection against vaccinia virus infection in mice. *Infec. Immun.* 5: 854–857.

11. Billiau, A., Leyten, R., Vandeputte, M., and DeSomer, P. 1971. Inhibition of development of mammary tumors in C3H mice. *Life Sci.* 10: 643–647.

12. Breslow, D. S. 1976. Biologically active synthetic polymers. *Pure Appl. Chem.* 46: 103–113.

13. Breslow, S., Edwards, E., and Newburg, N. 1973. Divinyl ether-maleic anhydride (pyran) copolymer used to demonstrate the effect of molecular weight on biological activity. *Nature* 246: 160–162.

14. Brown, J. W., and Firshein, W. 1967. Biodynamic effects of oligonucleotides. *Bacteriol. Rev.* 31: 83–94.

15. Brown, W., Regelson, W., Yajima, Y., and Ishizuko, M. 1970. Stimulation of antibody formation by pyran copolymer. *Proc. Soc. Exp. Biol. Med.* 131: 171–175.

16. Butler, G. B. 1960. Recent developments in polymerization by an alternating intra-intermolecular mechanism. *J. Polym. Sci.* 48: 279–289.

17. Came, P. E., Lieberman, M., Pascale, A., and Shimonaski, G. 1969. Antiviral activity of an interferon inducing synthetic polymer. *Proc. Soc. Exp. Biol. Med.* 131: 443–446.

18. Campbell, C. H., and Richmond, J. Y. 1973. Enhancement of primary antigen-specific resistance in infant mice with divinyl ether-maleic anhydride. *Infec. Immun.* 7: 199–204.

19. Chirigos, M. A. 1970. Current studies on the therapy of experimental leukemia, in R. M. Dutcher (ed.), *Comparative Leukemia Research. Bibl. Haemat.*, Vol. 36, pp. 278–292. Karger, Basel.

21. Claes, P., Billiau, A., DeClerq, E., Desmyter, J., Schonne, E., Vanderhaeghe, H., and DeSomer, P. 1970. Polyacetal carboxylic acids: a new group of antiviral polyanions. *J. Virol.* 5: 313.

22. Claes, P., Billiau, A., DeClerq, E., Desmyter, J., Schonne, E., Vanderhaeghe, H., and DeSomer, P. 1970. Polyacetal carboxylic acids; a new group of antiviral polyanions. *J. Virol.* 5: 313–320.

23. Coutinho, A., Moller, G., and Richter, W. 1974. Molecular basis of B-cell activation. I. Mitogenicity of native and substituted dextrans. *Scand. J. Immunol.* 3: 321–328.

24. DeClerq, E. 1972. Future possibilities of interferon inducers in human medicine. *Tijdschp. Gennesk,* 28: 307–318.

25. DeClerq, E., and DeSomer, P. 1969. Prolonged antiviral protection by interferon inducers. *Proc. Soc. Exp. Biol. Med.* 132: 699–703.

26. DeClerq, E., and DeSomer, P. 1972. Effect of chlorite-oxidized oxyamylose on Moloney sarcoma virus-induced tumor formation in mice. *Eur. J. Cancer* 8: 535–540.

27. DeClerq, E., and DeSomer, P. 1973. Protection of rabbits against local vaccinia virus infection by *Brucella abortus* and polyacrylic acid in the absence of systemic interferon production. *Infec. Immun.* 8: 669–673.

28. DeClerq, E., and Merigan, T. C. 1969. Local and systemic protection by synthetic polyanionic interferon inducers in mice against intranasal vesicular stomatitis virus. *J. Gen. Virol.* 5: 359–368.

29. Diamantstein, T., and Blitztein-Willinger, E. 1975. Relationship between biological activities of polymers. I. Immunogenicity, C3 activation, mitogenicity for B cells and adjuvant properties. *Immunology* 29: 1087–1092.

30. Diamantstein, T., Meinhold, H., and Wagner, B. 1971. Stimulation of humoral antibody formation by polyanions. V. Relationship between enhancement of sheep red blood cell uptake by the spleen and adjuvant action of dextran sulfate. *Eur. J. Immunol.* I: 429–432.

31. Diamantstein, T., Vogt, W., Ruhl, H., and Bochert, G. 1973. Stimulation of DNA synthesis in mouse lymphoid cells by polyanions *in vitro*. I. Target cells and possible mode of action. *Eur. J. Immunol.* 3: 488–493.

32. Diamantstein, T., Wagner, B., Beyse, I., Odenwald, M. V., and Schultz, G. 1971. Stimulation of humoral antibody formation by polyanions. I. The effect of polyacrylic acid on the primary immune response in mice immunized with sheep red blood cells. *Eur. J. Immunol.* 1: 335–340.

33. Diamantstein, T., Wagner, B., Beyse, I., Odenwald, M. V., and Schultz, G. 1971. Stimulation of humoral antibody formation by polyanions. II. The influence of sulfate esters of polymers on the immune response in mice. *Eur. J. Immunol.* 1: 340–343.

34. Diamantstein, T., Wagner, B., Odenwald, M. V., and Schultz, G. 1971. Stimulation of humoral antibody formation by polyanions. IV. The effects of dextran sulfate on the kinetics of secondary immune response in mice. *Eur. J. Immunol.* I: 426–429.

35. Diamantstein, T., Wagner, B., L'Age-Stehr, J., Beyse, I. Odenwald, M. V., and Schultz, G. 1971. Stimulation of humoral antibody formation by polyanions. III. Restoration of the immune response to sheep red blood cells by polyanions in thymectomized the lethally irradiated mice protected with bone marrow. *Eur. J. Immunol.* 1: 302–304.

36. Diamantstein, T., Wagner, B., Odenwald, M. V., and Schultz, G. 1971. Stimulation of humoral antibody formation by polyanions. IV. The effects of dextran sulfate on the kinetics of secondary immune response in mice. *Eur. J. Immunol.* 1: 426–429.

37. Gazdar, A. F., Steinberg, A. D., Spahan, G. F., and Baron, S. 1972. Interferon inducers: Enhancement of viral oncogenesis in mice and rats. *Proc. Soc. Exp.*

Biol. Med. 139: 1132–1137.

38. Gianinazzi, S., and Kassanis, B. 1974. Virus resistance induced in plants by polyacrylic acid. J. Gen. Virol. 23: 1–9.

39. Giron, D. J., Allen, P. T., Pindak, F. F., and Schmidt, J. P. 1971. Inhibition by estrone of the antiviral protection and interferon elicited by interferon inducers in mice. Inf. Immun. 3: 318–322.

40. Goodell, E. M., Ottenbrite, R. M., and Munson, A. E. Polymaleic anhydride: Effect on the immune system and Friend leukemia disease. J. Reticuloendothel. Soc., (in press).

41. Harmel, R. P., and Zbar, B. 1975. Tumor suppression by pyran copolymer: Correlation with production of cytotoxic macrophages. J. Natl. Cancer Inst. 54: 989–992.

42. Hirsch, M. S., Black, P. H., Wood, M. L., and Monaco, A. P. 1970. Immunosuppression, interferon inducers, and leukemia in mice. Proc. Soc. Exp. Biol. Med. 134: 309–313.

43. Hirsch, M. S., Black, P. H., Wood, M. L., and Monaco, A. P. 1973. Effects of pyran copolymer on leukemogenesis in immunosuppressed AKR mice. J. Immunol. 111: 91–95.

44. Hoffman, M. K., Weiss, O., Koenig, S., Hirst, J. A., and Oettgen, H. F. 1975. Suppression and enhancement of the T-cell dependent production of antibody to sRBC in vitro by bacterial lipopolysaccharide. J. Immunol. 114: 738–741.

45. Kaplan, A. M., and Morahan, P. S. 1976. Macrophage mediated tumor cell cytotoxicity. Ann. N.Y. Acad. Sci. 276: 134–145.

46. Kaplan, A. M., Morahan, P. S., and Regelson, W. 1974. Induction of macrophage mediated tumor-cell cytotoxicity by pyran copolymer. J. Natl. Cancer Inst. 52: 1919–1923.

47. Kaplan, A. M., Oyler, S. D., Regelson, W., and Morahan, P. S. 1975. Effect of immunopotentiator treatment pre- and post-tumor excision on the occurrence of metastasis in Lewis lung carcinoma. J. Reticuloendothel. Soc. 18: 1a.

48. Kripke, M. L., and Borsos, T. 1974. Accelerated development of benzo (a) pyrene-induced skin tumors in mice treated with pyran copolymer. J. Natl. Cancer Inst. 53: 1409–1410.

49. Larson, V. M., Clark, W. R., and Hilleman, M. R. 1969. Influence of synthetic (poly I:C) and viral double-stranded ribonucleic acids on adenovirus 12 oncogenesis in hamsters. Proc. Soc. Exp. Biol. Med. 131: 1002–1011.

50. Leavitt, T. J., Merigan, T. C., and Freeman, J. M. 1971. Hemolytic-uremic-like syndrome following polycarboxylate interferon induction. Amer. J. Dis. Child. 121: 43–47.

51. Leunen, J., Desmyter, J., and DeSomer, P. 1971. Effects of oxyamylose and polyacrylic acid on foot and mouth disease and hog cholera virus infections. Appl. Microbiol. 21: 203–208.

52. McCord, R. S., Breinig, M. K., and Morahan, P. S. 1976. Antiviral effect of pyran against systemic infection of mice with herpes simplex virus type 2. Antimicrob. Ag. Chemoth. 10: 28–33.

53. Matyasoua, J., Skalka, M., and Cejkova, M. 1974. The importance of molecular weight of inorganic polyphosphates for their interaction with deoxyribonucleoprotein of animal tissues. Folia. Biologica (Praha) 20: 193–204.

54. Merigan, T. C., and Finkelstein, M. S. 1968. Interferon stimulating and in vivo antiviral effects of various synthetic anionic polymers. Virology 35: 363–374.

55. Merigan, T. C., and Regelson, W. 1967. Interferon induction in man by a synthetic polyanion of defined composition. New Engl. J. Med. 277: 1283–1287.

56. Mohr, J., Chirigos, M. A., and Fuhrman, F. S. 1975. Pyran copolymer as an effective adjuvant to chemotherapy against a murine leukemia and solid tumor. Cancer Res. 35: 3750–3754.

57. Mohr, S. J., Chirigos, M. A., Smith, G. T., and Fuhrman, F. S. 1976. Specific potentiation of L1210 vaccine by pyran copolymer. Cancer Res. 36: 2035–2039.

58. Morahan, P. S., and Kaplan, A. M. 1976. Macrophage activation and antitumor activity of biologic and synthetic agents. Int. J. Cancer 17: 82–89.

59. Morahan, P. S., Kern, E. R., and Glasgow, L. A. 1977. Immunomodulator induced resistance against herpes simplex virus. Proc. Soc. Exp. Biol. Med. 154: 615–620.

60. Morahan, P. S., Regelson, W., and Munson, A. E. 1972. Pyran and polyribonucleotides: Differences in biological activities. Antimicrob. Ag. Chem. 2: 16–22.

61. Morahan, P. S., Glasgow, A., Crane, J. L., and Kern, E. R. 1977. Comparison of antiviral and antitumor activity of activated macrophages. Cell. Immunol. 28: 404–415.

62. Morahan, P. S., Schuller, G. B., Snodgrass, M. J., and Kaplan, A. M. 1976. Paradoxical effects of immunopotentiators on tumors and tumor viruses. J. Inf. Dis. Suppl. 133: A249–A255.

63. Morahan, P. S., Munson, J. A., Baird, L. G., Kaplan, A. M., and Regelson, W. 1974. Antitumor action of pyran copolymer and tilorone against Lewis lung carcinoma and B-16 melanoma. Cancer Res. 34: 506–511.

64. Niblick, J. R., and McCreary, M. B. 1971. The relationship of biological activities of poly I:C to homopolymer molecular weights. Nature New Biol. 233: 52–53.

65. Olick, J. L. 1967. The specificity of inhibition of tumor cell viability by DNA. Cancer Res. 27: 2338–2341.

66. Ottenbrite, R. M., Goodel, E. M., and Munson, A. E. A comparative study of anti-toxicologic properties of related polyanions. Polymer (in press).

67. Ottenbrite, R. M., and Regelson, W. 1977. Biological activity of water-soluble polymers, in N. M. Bakales (ed.), Encyclopedia of Polymer Science & Technology, Supplement, Vol. 2 (in press).

68. Papas, T. S., Pry, T. W., and Chirigos, M. A. 1974. Inhibition of RNA-dependent DNA polymerase of avian myeloblastosis virus by pyran copolymer. Proc. Natl. Acad. Sci. 71: 367–370.

69. Pearson, J. W., Chirigos, M. A., Chaparas, S. D., and Sher, N. A. 1974. Combined drug and immunostimulation therapy against a syngeneic murine leukemia. J. Natl. Cancer Inst. 52: 463–468.

70. Pierce, C. W., and Benacerraf, B. 1969. Immune Response in vitro: Independence of "activated" lymphoid cells. Science 166: 1002–1003.

71. Pindak, F. F., Schmidt, J. P., Giron, D. J., and Allen, P. T. 1971. Interferon levels and resistance to viral infection associated with selected interferon induc-

ers. *Proc. Soc. Exp. Biol. Med.* 138: 317–321.

72. Razvodovskii, E. F. 1972. Synthetic polymers in pharmacology. *Uspekhi Khimii i Fiziki Polimerov* 302–328.

73. Regelson, W. 1967. Prevention and treatment of Friend leukemia virus infection by interferon inducing synthetic polyanions. The Reticuloendothelial System and Atheroslcerosis. *Adv. Exp. Med. Biol.* 1: 315–332.

74. Regelson, W. 1968. Anionic polyelectrolytes as antimitotic agents. *Adv. Chemotherap.* 3: 303–371.

75. Regelson, W. 1968. The growth regulating activity of polyanions. *Adv. Cancer Res.* 11: 223–303.

76. Regelson, W. 1968. Thrombocytopenic and related physiologic effect of heparin and heparinoids: A macromolecular induced syndrome? *Hematologic Rev.* 1: 193–227.

77. Regelson, W. 1973. The biologic activity of water soluble polymers, in N. M. Bikales (ed.), *Water Soluble Polymers,* pp. 161–177. Plenum, New York.

78. Regelson, W. 1977. The biological activity for the synthetic polyanion, pyran copolymer and the heterocyclic bis deae fluorenone derivative, tilorone and congeners: Clinical and laboratory effects of these agents as modulators of host resistance, in A. C. Sartorelli (ed.), *International Encyclopedia of Pharmacology and Therapeutics.* Pergamon Press (in press).

79. Regelson, W., Morahan, P., and Kaplan, A. 1975. The role of molecular weight in pharmacologic and biologic activity of synthetic polyanions, in A. Rembaum and E. Selegny (eds.), *Polyelectrolytes and Their Applications* Vol. II, Reidel Publishing, Holland.

80. Regelson, W., Munson, A., and Wooles, W. 1970. Biologic activity of synthetic polymers: Interferon inducers and reticuloendothelial response; polyanion prophylaxis against microorganisms and alterations of drug metabolism. Int. Symp. Stand. Interferon & Interferon Inducers, London, 1969. *Symp. Series Immunobiol. Stand.* Vol. 14, pp. 227–236. Karger, Basel/New York.

81. Regelson, W., Morahan, P. S., Kaplan, A. M., Baird, L. G., and Munson, J. A. 1974. Synthetic polyanaions. Molecular weight, macrophage activation, and immunologic response, in W. H. Wagner and H. Hahn (eds.), *Activation of Macrophages,* pp. 97–110. Excerpta Medica, Amsterdam.

82. Regelson, W., Munson, A. E., Wooles, W. R., Lawrence, W., and Levy, H. 1970. Reticuloendothelial action of interferon inducers. The biphasic action of pyran copolymer and polynucleotides on phagocytic and immunologic response. *Interferon* 6: 381–385.

83. Richmond, J. Y. 1971. Mouse resistance against foot and mouth disease virus induced by injections of pyran. *Infec. Immun.* 3: 249–253.

84. Richmond, J. Y., and Campbell, C. H. 1974. Enhancement of primary antigen-specific resistance in infant mice, with divinyl ether-maleic anhydride. *Infec. Immun.* 10: 1029–1033.

85. Schuller, G. B., Morahan, P. S., and Snodgrass, M. 1975. Inhibition and enhancement of Friend leukemia virus by pyran copolymer. *Cancer Res.* 35: 1915–1920.

86. Scott, M. T. 1972. Biological effects of the adjuvant *Corynebacterium*

parvum. II. Evidence for macrophage T-cell interaction. *Cell. Immunol.* 5: 469–479.

87. Sellers, R. F., Herniman, K. A. J., and Hawkins, C. W. 1972. The effect of pyran on development of foot and mouth disease in guinea pigs, cattle, and pigs. *Res. Vet. Sci.* 13: 339–341.

88. Snodgrass, M. J., Morahan, P. S., and Kaplan, A. M. 1975. Histopathology of the host response to Lewis Lung Carcinoma: Modulation by pyran. *J. Natl. Cancer Inst.* 55: 455–462.

89. Solomon, D. H. 1975. Cylopolymerization. *J. Polym. Sci. Symp.* 49: 175–190.

90. Ter-Pogosyan, R. A., Vartevanyan, Z. T., Kamalyan, L. A., Dubovik, B. V., Kartasheva, A. L., and Etlis, V. S. 1976. Antiviral effect of pyran copolymers. *Chem. Abst.* 85: 40739.

91. Vogt, W., Ruhl, H., Wagner, B., and Diamantstein, T. 1973. Stimulation of DNA synthesis in mouse lymphoid cells by polyanions *in vitro*. II. Relationship between adjuvant activity and stimulation of DNA synthesis by polyanions. *Eur. J. Immunol.* 3: 493–496.

92. Wagner, H., Feldman, M., Boyle, W., and Schrader, J. W. 1972. Cell mediated immune response *in vitro*. III. The requirement of macrophages in cytotoxic reactions against cell-bound and subcellular alloantigens. *J. Exp. Med.* 136: 331–343.

93. Wooles, W., and Munson, A. E. 1971. The effect of stimulants and repressants of reticuloendothelial activity on drug metabolism. *J. Reticuloendothel. Soc.* 9: 108–119.

CHAPTER 7

IMMUNO-STIMULATORY EFFECTS OF LEVAMISOLE IN HUMANS WITH CANCER

William L. Donegan
Lyle R. Heim
George C. Owen
Derek Sampson

Department of Surgery
The Medical College of Wisconsin,
and the American Cancer Society
Department of Microbiology,
The Medical College of Wisconsin,
and Department of Laboratory Medicine,
Columbia Hospital,
Department of Medicine,
The Medical College of Wisconsin,
and Columbia Hospital,
Department of Surgery,
The Medical College of Wisconsin,
Milwaukee, Wisconsin 53233

Levamisole, a synthetic derivative of thiazole originally used as an antihelminthic but with immunologic effects, may prove useful for the treatment of cancer. The property of primary interest is its ability to stimulate cell-mediated immunity without appreciably affecting humoral immunity. Attractive features of the drug are its ability to be administered orally and its mild side effects. Rather than producing true potentiation, the drug's action is to restore depressed cell-mediated immunity to normal. Levamisole's most promising application in cancer therapy, therefore, is in clinical situations characterized by depressed cellular immunity or when depression can be anticipated as during systemic chemotherapy or irradiation.

Introduction

Levamisole is the levo-rotary form of tetramisole, a synthetic antihelminthic first described by Thienpont *et al.* in 1966 (138). In 1971
Renoux and Renoux reported that mice given tetramisole were afforded
greater protection by Brucella vaccine than animals that did not receive
the drug (106). This report provided an impetus for an intense effort to
evaluate tetramisole and levamisole as stimulants of host defense
mechanisms. Levamisole and tetramisole are nearly identical chemically
and pharmacologically and both have the same antihelminthic spectra,
except that levamisole is effective at a lower dose level (39). Although
levamisole has been most studied, the two imidazol compounds similarly
affect host defense mechanisms and this report will not distinguish between them (15, 21, 110).

Since Drs. Gerard and Micheline Renoux serendipitously discovered
that levamisole stimulated the immunologic systems of laboratory animals, a vast literature has accrued and its immunostimulatory effects have
been the subject of major conferences. Levamisole is primarily effective in
restoring deficient host defense mechanisms (25, 81, 112). Unlike many
nonspecific immunostimulants, it does not stimulate immunologic responses to excessive levels or affect the responses of immunologically
normal individuals. Consequently, levamisole is not an immunostimulant, or an immunomodulator in conventional terms; rather it is best described as an antianergic.

In an effort to augment flagging immunologic surveillance, various
substances have been employed as nonspecific immunostimulants in
animals and in man (11, 17, 89). Among those most extensively investigated, *Mycobacterium bovis*, Bacillus Calmette-Guérin (BCG), *Corynebacterium parvum*, Glucan, and levamisole have had the most favorable
therapeutic trials in man (10, 65, 86, 95, 112, 153). Although immunostimulants such as BCG have been promising in treatment of neoplasias,
they have a number of disadvantages not shared by levamisole (10, 65, 89,
90, 95, 129, 153). Among these are difficulty of standardization,
generalized infection by the antigenic agent, and lack of specificity for
cell mediated immunologic stimulation (8, 90).

The precise mechanism of levamisole's action on the immunologic
response is not known, but much evidence points to influences on T
lymphocytes and T-B lymphocyte interactions (2, 15, 19, 21, 54, 75, 78,

87, 102, 104, 107, 110, 140, 143, 155). Generally, levamisole stimulates depressed cell mediated immunity without significantly influencing humoral immunity. An impressive body of evidence implicates influences exerted upon the macrophage monocyte population, with macrophages in turn exerting a regulatory influence on lymphocytes (1, 2, 16, 25, 36, 37, 56, 82, 98, 100, 120, 121, 126, 131, 139, 142, 144, 155). In phagocytes and lymphocytes alterations of cyclic-nucleotide metabolism have been implicated. Several intracellular processes modulate the levels of cyclic 3′,5′-guanosine monophosphate (cGMP) and cyclic 3′,5′-adenosine monophosphate (cAMP). Specific cGMP or cAMP phosphodiesterases catalyze hydrolysis, respectively, converting cGMP or cAMP to non-cyclic nucleotide. Various substances influence intracellular cAMP and cGMP levels through inhibition or stimulation of specific anabolic or catabolic enzymes. Agents with the ability to inhibit cAMP phosphodiesterase activity inhibit antigen-induced release of histamine and slow reacting substances from leukocytes (72, 79). Isoproterenol and epinephrine interact with specific beta receptors to activate membrane-bound adenyl cyclase and to increase the cAMP level (135). Methylxanthine derivatives such as aminophylin inhibit cAMP phosphodiesterase to increase the cAMP level (69, 136). By contrast, alpha-adrenergic agents such as phenylephrine, decrease levels of cAMP and enhance immunologic responses (69). A second group of "messengers" composed of cholinergic stimulators that increase cGMP levels also enhance immunologic responses (68).

Levamisole increases the cGMP level of T lymphocytes and decreases the cAMP level with a dose response of cAMP and cGMP levels that correlates with lymphocyte responses to mitogen (54). This relationship, similar to that of cholinergic agents that increase cGMP levels, is associated with proliferation, lymphokine production and lymphocytotoxicity (53, 55, 134).

Agents that increase cGMP levels in macrophages also enhance macrophage proliferation and immunologic phagocytosis (98). Immunologic phagocytosis involves attachment of macrophages to and engulfment of antigenic material that has been coated with specific antibody. Macrophage membranes have receptors specific for the Fc-portion of antibody that has combined with antigen. Macrophages activated by receptor-Fc union undergo intracellular alterations that include reduction of cAMP and increase of cGMP.

In summary, metabolic events in macrophages and lymphocytes suggest that cellular functions mediated by cGMP and cAMP account for the antianergic activity of levamisole and that its activation of lymphocytes is regulated by macrophages (38).

Chemistry, Pharmacology, and Metabolism

Levamisole (R12,564) is ordinarily used as the hydrochloride salt of (S)-(-)-2,3,5,6-tetrahydro-6-phenylimidazo (2,1-b)-thiazole (Fig. 1). This white crystalline powder (molecular weight of 240.75) is stable. The hydrochloride salt of levamisole is soluble in methanol, water, and most organic solvents. In water it is freely soluble and can hydrolize, the rate of hydrolysis being increased with increased pH or temperature. At a pH of 4 or less, 3-18% aqueous solutions of levamisole have remained stable for more than 40 months. At 37C and increased pH, solutions decompose approximately 5 times as rapidly as at 23C. Levamisole promptly precipitates from solution at pH 7.5. Upon hydrolysis 1-(2-Mercaptoethyl)-5-phenyl-2-imidazolidinone is formed, which in oxidizing conditions can be converted to a double structure with a disulfide bridge, 1,1'-(dithiodi-2,1-ethanediyl) bis(4-phenyl-2-imidazolidinone). Neither is very water soluble.

Levamisole has a mild stimulatory effect on autonomic ganglia, the basis for its antihelminthic property. It also increases heart rate and strength of contraction. Levamisole has no direct effect upon bacteria, viruses or fungi, and in vitro it is not cytotoxic to normal or neoplastic cells (78, 101). Levamisole's effects on cell function are produced both in vitro and in vivo (25, 35, 43, 51, 54, 56, 78, 98, 101, 111, 116, 119, 130, 154, 155, 158). The drug can be administered orally or parenterally, but only oral administration is used in man. It is rapidly absorbed from the alimentary tract and peak plasma levels are attained 2–4 hours after administration. The plasma half-life is 4 hours. Within three days of oral administration approximately 70% of levamisole is excreted in the urine unchanged or as metabolites; about 4% of the total is excreted in the feces (50). The primary site of levamisole metabolism is the liver where 24 hours after drug administration the highest residual level is found (48, 49,

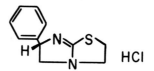

Fig. 1.   Levamisole.

59). Wynates *et al.* developed a gas chromatographic assay for quantitation of levamisole in body fluids and tissue (156).

In Vitro Effects of Levamisole upon Immune Responses

There is now general agreement that the immunopotentiating properties of levamisole can be demonstrated in several *in vitro* immunological models. Most studies have been concerned with the effect of the drug on lymphocyte function and, clearly, it is with this population of cells that the most important clinical application of the drug might be derived.

Lichtenfeld has shown that the drug is able to amplify the response of lymphocytes to mitogens such as phytohamagglutinin (PHA) or to allo antigen in mixed lymphocyte culture (77). The effect was dose dependent, but at the optimum drug dose level of approximately 1.0 μg/ml, thymidine uptake was increased three to four times. In controls the drug was without effect on unstimulated lymphocyte cultures. Al-Ibrahim determined that the proliferative response of sensitized lymphocytes to specific antigen *in vitro* is influenced by the concentration of specific antigen and of levamisole (2). At optimal antigen concentration, levamisole did not significantly alter radiothymidine incorporation. Lymphocytes incubated with sub-optimal antigen concentration, however, significantly increased thymidine uptake in the presence of levamisole. Similar observations were observed when PHA was used to stimulate lymphocytes.

These observations were confirmed by Kimura and his colleagues using PHA and pokeweed (PWM) mitogen as stimulators (58). A similar amplification of the response to antigens derived from candida, measles virus, or PPD was demonstrated by Pabst and co-workers (101). However, a study by Copeland failed to demonstrate immunopotentiation of responses to PHA, PWM, streptokinase-streptodornase, streptolysin-0 or in MLC (24). The most likely explanation for the discrepancy of these observations is that in the latter study the dose response was performed using concentrations of the drug increased by logarithmic increments, hence the optimum dose may have been missed. As will be discussed later, the dose of levamisole employed in both *in vitro* and *in vivo* studies is critically important.

Chan and Simons have shown that the immunopotentiation of the lymphocyte response to PHA is most marked when the cells are hyporesponsive to this mitogen (18). This observation is of considerable importance when one considers the impaired responses of some patients with cancer. In a study involving patients with either acute lymphoblastic leukemia or chronic lymphocytic leukemia, Goyanes-Villaescusa demonstrated that levamisole could, even in these patients, potentiate the responses of peripheral blood leucocytes to PHA (45).

Sampson and Lui confirmed that levamisole can indeed amplify the response of peripheral blood lymphocytes to PHA, PWM, and Concanavalin A (Fig. 2), and observed similar effects on mixed lymphocyte cultures (Fig. 3) (119). However, the effects were clearly dose dependent and, in fact, at high doses; that is, in excess of 2.0 μg/ml, the drug was immunosuppressive rather than a potentiator. The optimum dose level was similar to that reported by Lichtenfeld (77).

This phenomenon of suppression at higher dose levels must be taken into account in the design of clinical trials with levamisole, since there is a very real risk of increasing the spread of cancer rather than inhibiting growth if high doses are given.

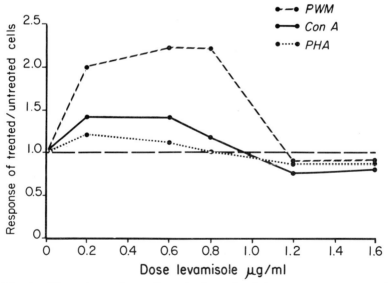

Fig. 2. The ratio on the ordinate is the ratio of the counts per minute for the cell cultures with levamisole compared with the counts per minute without the drug. Augmentation of the responses to all three mitogens is seen, but at higher dose the drug tends to be immunosuppressive. The points are the means of six experiments. (Reproduced with kind permission of editors of *Cancer Research*, Williams and Wilkins, Baltimore, Maryland.)

EFFECT of LEVAMISOLE on MLC

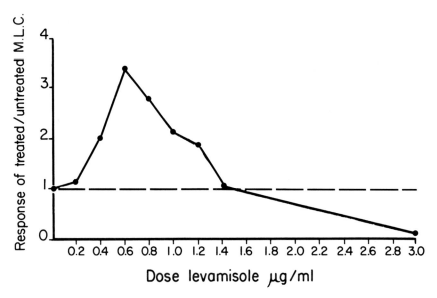

Fig. 3. Augmentation of the mixed lymphocyte culture is seen, similar to that for the mitogen responses shown in Figure 1. Again, immunosuppression is seen at the higher doses of levamisole. Each point is the mean of between 3 and 18 observations. (Reproduced with kind permission of editors of *Cancer Research,* Williams and Wilkins, Baltimore, Maryland.)

The functions of lymphocytes alluded to so far have been those of the thymus derived or T cell population, and it is apparent that levamisole restores or increases impaired function of the T lymphocyte rather than the bone marrow derived or B lymphocyte. Thus, in a group of patients with Hodgkins disease, in whom there was a defect of peripheral blood T cell function as shown by a low level of E-rosette formation with sheep red blood cells, the addition of levamisole to peripheral blood lymphocytes markedly increased the number of E-rosettes formed to normal levels. In this study by Biniaminov and Ramot, there was no effect on the level of E-rosette formation when the blood of normal volunteers was used (13). However, in a later series of experiments by Verhaegen and co-workers, not only was levamisole shown to be capable of increasing the proportion of E-rosette formation in the peripheral blood of cancer patients, but this effect could also be observed in normal controls (143). Further, these workers were able to show that levamisole could restore the impaired function of the T cell population which was brought about by the incubation of lymphocytes with the immunosuppressive drug, azathioprine. Cells incubated with this drug had impaired T cell function as evidenced by the low level of E-rosette formation when they were incubated with sheep red blood cells, but this was returned to normal levels when levamisole was added. This phenomenon has also been employed clinically in order to modify the toxicity of drugs given to cancer patients.

The effects of levamisole on monocyte and polymorphonuclear chemotactic responses have been described by Pike and Snyderman (103). They found that the drug could increase chemotactic migration of monocytes in response to endotoxin activated human serum, to lymphocyte derived chemotactic factor, and to an active polypeptide. They elegantly showed that this augmentation of chemotaxis required binding of levamisole to the cell membrane. Snyderman, Daniels and Pike also showed that in vitro levamisole treatment of monocytes reversed the depressed chemotactic responsiveness produced by influenza virus infection (126). However, levamisole was unable to potentiate the chemotactic response of polymorphonuclear cells, and again its activity seemed to be lymphocyte specific.

Levamisole is able to increase phagocytic activity in both man and animals and this can be demonstrated in an in vitro system. DeCree and his colleagues have shown that incubation of whole blood with levamisole significantly stimulated the phagocytosis of yeasts (25). The levamisole dose for enhancement of phagocytosis in vitro is 2.5-10μg/ml with maximum enhancement at 5 micrograms/ml (126). Phagocytic enhancement was not related to presence of Levamisole during phagocytosis. Although enhancement of phagocytosis was observed after 48 hours of incubation with levamisole, maximum enhancement was obtained after 72 hours and prolonged incubation did not further increase phagocytosis. The degree of enhancement was generally in the range of 130–150% that of unincubated cells.

Another cell type which has been shown to be susceptible to the potentiating effects of levamisole is the suppressor T cell. This cell, which is thought to be a regulator of immune responses, is normally found in the spleen and thymus. In an attempt to explain the potentiation of immune responses by levamisole, Sampson and Lui hypothesized that the drug worked by selective impairment of suppressor cell function, thus removing inhibition of immune responses. In a series of experiments splenic suppressor cells were incubated with levamisole (119). Contrary to expectation, suppressor function was not impaired by the drug but was, in fact, potentiated (Fig. 4). Thus, it seems that levamisole is a non-specific potentiator of T lymphocytes irrespective of their function. This observation,

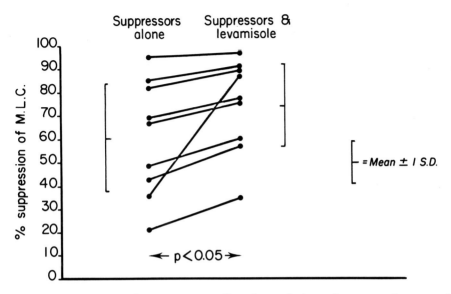

Fig. 4. Treatment of suppressor cells obtained from human spleens with levamisole consistently augmented the ability of the cells to inhibit a mixed lymphocyte reaction. p was derived from a paired t test. (Reproduced with kind permission of editors of *Cancer Research*, Williams and Wilkins, Baltimore, Maryland.)

too, has clinical implications in that the satisfactory response of systemic lupus erythematosus to levamisole reported by Gordon and Keenan has, in part, been ascribed to the restoration of deficient T cell suppressor function by this drug (44).

Effects of Levamisole on the Immune Response In Vivo

a. ANIMALS. The *in vitro* immunopotentiating capacity of levamisole has naturally led to investigation of its ability to increase immune responses *in vivo*. Thus, Renoux and Renoux (1973) have shown that subcutaneous injection of levamisole could potentiate the immunity given by vaccination with *Brucella melitensis* (109). In this study clear protection against subsequent infection with *Brucella abortus* was demonstrated, but interestingly, no increase in production of antibody to this organism could be demonstrated. This observation is consistent with the hypothesis that levamisole is primarily a potentiator of cell mediated immunity rather than humoral immunity. In a later study (1974), the same investigators showed that levamisole could increase the immune reactivity of mice to sheep red blood cells, and again demonstrated that there was no increase in antibody production to this antigenic stimulus, but rather the effect was mediated via an increase in T cell responsiveness (110).

Further confirmation of the ability of levamisole to increase cell mediated immunity *in vivo* was provided in a study by Woods and coworkers in which the drug was shown to increase DNA synthesis in spleen cells obtained from mice (154). They also demonstrated that the drug could reverse the depression of DNA synthesis induced by the antitumor drug BCNU. However, stimulation of reactivity to allo-antigen in mixed lymphocyte culture was very inconsistent in these experiments.

In a study using mice Irwin and Knight showed that not only was cell mediated immunity to *Corynebacterium pseudotuberculosis* increased by levamisole administration but, in addition, humoral immunity, as judged by levels of the immunoglobulins G_2 and A, was decreased (64a). They concluded from the study that resistance to *C. pseudotuberculosis* was basically cell mediated. Similar results were obtained in a different model by Fischer and his colleagues (38a). In this system rats were subjected to the induction of encephalitis by the intraperitoneal injection of herpes type 2 virus. They found that subcutaneous injections of levamisole gave considerable protection against development of the disease, but they could not detect antibody to HSV2 virus.

In contrast to these studies, Potter has demonstrated that levamisole administration can result in increased antibody production to influenza virus in the hamster, and Kulkarni has shown that the drug was able to increase antibody production to Newcastle disease virus vaccine in chickens (72a, 103a).

Reference has already been made to the fact that levamisole is able to increase phagocytic activity *in vitro*, and this phenomenon has also been observed *in vivo*. Hoebeke and Franchi have shown that levamisole given to mice increases the rate at which carbon is cleared from the circulation, especially when this function is impaired by age or prior steroid therapy (56).

b. HUMANS.   Both the immunopotentiation by levamisole which has been observed *in vitro*, and that seen in animals *in vivo*, has been demonstrated in man in clinical studies. Tripodi and his collaborators have shown that oral administration of levamisole to cancer patients can result in stimulation of cell mediated responses as judged by the fact that patients who did not respond to DNCB or PPD were able to do so after treatment with the drug (140). These patients had a variety of advanced cancers, but it was not possible to demonstrate any effect of the drug on the tumors.

These results were essentially confirmed by Verhaegen in patients with and without cancer, but in addition Verhaegen showed that macrophage function was also stimulated in the patients given levamisole as demonstrated by an increased rate of clearance of intravenously injected lipid emulsions (142). He also noted that an increased serum hemolytic complement was associated with the immunostimulatory effects of levamisole.

In another clinical study, levamisole was used by Schuermans to treat rheumatoid arthritis (122). In addition to marked clinical improvement, he noted a marked fall in the erythrocyte sedimentation rate and in some patients a conversion from positive to negative for rheumatoid factor. These results could not be confirmed by Dinai and Pras; however, they did observe restoration of cutaneous delayed hypersensitivity (27a). Webster and Hughes in treating carcinoma of the gastrointestinal tract found a similar increase in cell mediated immunity as judged by skin testing (149).

The increase in serum hemolytic complement induced by levamisole which was reported by Verhaegen was not confirmed in a study of a small number of patients with rheumatoid arthritis described by Engels and his co-workers (33). They observed decreased total hemolytic complement and clinical improvement in their patients. They showed a clear increase in the number of E-rosette forming cells in the peripheral blood of their patients following therapy with the immunostimulant, again providing evidence that levamisole acts primarily on the T cell population.

Some encouraging results from the treatment of breast cancer with levamisole have been reported by Rojas and his colleagues who showed decreased recurrence and increased survival for the treated group of patients (114). As have others, they noticed an increase in the number of positive reactions to skin testing with DNCB, Candida, and PPD and, in addition, they reported an increase of the absolute lymphocyte count in the treated patients. It seems that some protection against radiation induced leukopenia was afforded by treatment with levamisole. However, Rosenthal and collaborators have shown that levamisole can result in a sporadic leucopenia, and this was associated with development of leucocyte-agglutinating antibodies (115). This effect was seen in two patients out of a series of 48 patients with various rheumatic diseases.

The conflicting reports on the value of levamisole in rheumatic disease states can, in part, be explained by the observations of Yaron and his group (157). They showed that one of the most important effects of the drug was a decrease in hyaluronic acid production by synovial fibroblasts exposed to levamisole. They propose that the beneficial effects might not be immunologically mediated at all, but may be due to this biochemical property. They also suggest that a good clinical response might depend on accumulation of the drug within the synovium and that consequently long term treatment is required before the effect of the drug can be truly assessed.

It is likely, however, that the protection afforded by levamisole against radiation leucopenia will be an important effect. A similar protection against drug induced leucopenia has been observed in a series of cancer patients reported by Lods and his group (83). They noted that they were able to give courses of chemotherapy much more frequently in a group of patients receiving levamisole compared with a control group in whom bone marrow depression prevented the frequent administration of the chemotherapeutic agents.

It might be expected that levamisole would be of most value in the treatment of immune deficiency diseases. Evidence that this is so has been provided by Lieberman and Hsu who have shown in six patients that administration of the drug resulted in both clinical improvement and an improvement in cell mediated immunity as judged by increase in the leukocyte migration inhibition test (80). These workers stress that for maximal effect, the drug must be given simultaneously with suboptimal doses of recall antigens. This condition may well have implications for the use of the drug in the treatment of cancer patients.

The Effects of Levamisole on Experimental Tumors

There can be little doubt that levamisole must be regarded as an effective potentiator of cell mediated immunity whether in vitro or in vivo, and in both animals and in man. In view of its low toxicity and the above considerations, it would seem an ideal agent for the treatment of malignancy, assuming that host immune defenses play an important part in controlling the growth and spread of tumors. It is somewhat surprising then, that there is little information on the value of levamisole in experimental tumor systems, and that the information available is highly contradictory.

Renoux reported in 1972 that subcutaneously administered levamisole could inhibit the growth of Lewis lung (3LL) tumor transplanted to C57B1 mice (108). He showed that not only were some mice cured of their disease but even if the drug was given after the tumors were established, regression could still be induced by levamisole. The effects were exerted both on primary tumors and on pulmonary metastases. In a different system, Chirigos and his group were able to show that levamisole was of value in the treatment of mice with a transplanted Moloney lymphoid leukemia cell line LSTRA (21). They noted that survival could be improved when the levamisole was given during remissions induced by BCNU, however, levamisole alone was without effect. They incidentally confirmed the T cell immunopotentiating effect of levamisole by demonstrating that mice given this drug were able to reject allografts of skin more rapidly than untreated animals. Sadowski and Rapp have demonstrated that levamisole is of value in the inhibition of the growth of metastases from tumors resulting from the transformation of hamster cells by HSV2 virus and ultraviolet irradiation (118). Such cells produce tumors at the inoculation site and these tumors metastasize. These workers found that in levamisole treated animals, higher doses of inoculated cells were required to produce tumors, and the frequency of metastasis was reduced in the treated animals.

In contrast to the encouraging results reported above, Johnson and his group found that levamisole was without effect on several transplantable syngeneic murine tumors (67). There was no effect against L1210 leukemia, P388 leukemia, B16 melanoma, Madison 109 lung tumor and Lewis lung carcinoma. There was variable protective effect on rhabdomyosarcomas following injection of Moloney sarcoma virus. Similarly, Fidler and Spitler showed that levamisole did not protect mice against B16 melanoma and adenocarcinoma 15091 (35). While inconsistent results from the use of levamisole in experimental tumors seem confusing, it is almost certainly due to variations in the antigenicity of the tumors employed, in the timing and dosage regimes of the levamisole, and in host immunocompetence.

The critical nature of this dose of levamisole has already been referred to in in vitro studies, and experiments using the in vivo tumor model in our laboratory (Sampson, Peters, and Lewis, unpublished data) have confirmed that dose is of overriding importance. In this study, breast cancer was induced in rats by the injection of dimethyl benzanthrine (DMBA). Beginning at the time of DMBA injection, the animals were treated orally with levamisole in doses of 2, 4, and 8 mg/kg body weight/day. A control group did not receive levamisole. Table 1 indicates the survival of the animals, the number that developed tumors, the rate of tumor regression and the average tumor size after six months of treatment. It will be seen that the optimum dose of levamisole was 4 mg/kg/day. Concern, based on in vitro studies, that higher doses might be detrimental appear to be confirmed in the group of animals that received 8 mg/kg/day (119). Firstly,

Table 1. The effect of levamisole on rats with DMBA-induced breast cancer after treatment for six months

Treatment	Number in Group	Alive at 6 Months	Alive with Tumor	Number with Tumor	Number with Regression	Dead with Tumor	Average Size Tumor (cm)
None	30	10	9	1	0	11	8.5
Levamisole 2 mg/kg	30	21	10	9	12	6	1.6
Levamisole 4 mg/kg	30	23	10	9	9	2	1.2
Levamisole 8 mg/kg	30	23	23	0	0	2	6.9

The growth retarding effects of levamisole upon DMBA-induced tumors are highly dose dependent, with optimum effects at 2–4 mg/Kg.

Source: Sampson, Peters, and Lewis, previously unpublished data.

a much higher percentage of animals developed tumors after DMBA injection, and although the animals appeared to survive reasonably well, the average size of their tumors was almost that of untreated controls. In addition, there was no tumor regression.

To summarize, levamisole does appear to have antitumor activity in experimental systems but its effects are variable. Caution is required in extrapolating the results of these animal studies to man, and when levamisole is used clinically, it is important that patients are monitored by immunological assay systems to be sure that the dosage regimes employed do, in fact, produce the full immunopotentiation of which levamisole is capable.

Experience with Levamisole in Clinical Cancer

a. CANCER OF THE BREAST.   Because of its frequency among women and its importance as a cause of death, the immunologic aspects of cancer of the breast have received detailed attention clinically and in the laboratory. Much evidence exists for a host immune response against breast cancer in humans. Sparks and associates found antibody against antigen prepared from allogeneic breast cancer cells substantially more often among women with breast cancer than among healthy controls, i.e., 39% versus 13% (129). Cellular immunity against allogeneic breast cancer antigen is also evident in migration inhibition assays using leucocytes of patients with the disease, the reaction being more marked in lymphocytes from regional lymph nodes than in circulating lymphocytes (31). Host immunologic competence measured by a variety of parameters is generally related inversely to the stage of the disease. In early operable stages little or no impairment is detected in comparison with healthy controls (96, 132, 146). Immune competence is not reduced by metastasis to axillary nodes in clinically early stages, nor by dissemination that is clinically inapparent, but patients with clinically evident dissemination, recurrence after mastectomy, and with terminal disease regularly have depressed cellular immunity (96). Using crossed-serum experiments Whittaker and Clark were able to attribute the defect, at least in part, to an abnormality in the patient's serum (151). These investigators as well as Stein and associates pointed out that maintenance of immunity in the presence of early dissemination and its deterioration later suggests that tumor spread is the cause rather than the result of changing immunologic status (132). In operable cases Wanebo, et al. found only mitogenic response to PHA reflective of risk for recurrence (146). It was not correlated with delayed cutaneous sensitivity to antigens, absolute lymphocyte levels, T lymphocyte proportions, or to other mitogens.

The lasting reduction of leukocyte count, particularly the disproportionate depletion of T lymphocytes, produced by postoperative irradiation, has evoked concern insofar as it might promote dissemination and postsurgical recurrence. Stjernswärd found T lymphocytes reduced to 45% in irradiated patients compared with a normal of 60% (133). However, concern appears to be unfounded since lymphocyte counts and T cell fractions have little correlation with risk of recurrence; patients irradiated are so treated because they are already at high risk, and immunologic status after treatment is not a reliable predictor of long term cure or lack of it (132).

Clinical trials presently in progress employing various immunostimulants as adjuvants in the treatment of operable breast cancer have yet to substantiate the value of immunotherapy alone or in combination with chemotherapy for breast cancer. In view of the fact that patients with early operable stages of breast cancer, including those with clinically occult axillary metastases manifest little evidence of impaired immunity, it might be expected that levamisole would be of little benefit as a single agent. Its most appropriate use for early disease would be as a concomitant of adjuvant chemotherapy or irradiation to prevent the anticipated immunodepression associated with treatment, or in advanced stages of breast cancer when immunologic restitution is needed.

The reports of therapeutic experience with levamisole are limited. Apropos of advanced disease, occasional regressions of cancer are observed. Ward reported that one of five patients with postoperative chest wall recurrence had temporary disappearance of tumor nodules on therapy with levamisole (147). Also observed in 5/9 cases was temporary, generally partial regression of enlarged axillary nodes that appeared after mastectomy.

The most encouraging study to date is a randomized prospective trial reported by Rojas et al. in which levamisole was used as an adjuvant to irradiation for locally advanced breast cancer (114). Patients with inoperable State III (UICC) cancers were rendered disease free by cobalt irradiation to the breast, supraclavicular, and axillary regions and then alternatively treated with levamisole (150 mg orally/day for 3 consecutive days every other week) until evidence of progression. Controls received no levamisole or other adjuvant. Five of 48 patients were lost to follow-up, but all patients were observed for at least 21 months. Compared to 23 controls, 20 patients treated with levamisole in this fashion between 1972 and 1976 had significant prolongation of median disease free interval (25 vs 9 months) and survival (90% vs 35% alive at 30 months). Twenty-one controls developed metastases in contrast with only eleven treated patients. Among those who developed metastases, the median interval was three months longer for treated patients than controls, i.e., 12 months versus 3 months. Curiously, despite the overall reduction in dissemination associated with levamisole, pulmonary metastases tended to predominate, possibly suggesting that irradiated lung did not share the resistance of other tissues. According to the investigators the improved results were accompanied by increased frequency and intensity of skin response to recall antigens and DNCB and with increased absolute lymphocyte counts. The dramatic improvement in results attributed to levamisole in this small study warrants confirmation.

Hortobagyi *et al.* studied 110 patients with metastatic breast cancer who were treated with 5-fluorouricil,adriamycin, cyclophosphamide and levamisole (62). They reported that patients treated with combination chemotherapy (FAC) plus levamisole had remission rates identical to those obtained with FAC alone or with BCG. The duration of remission and survival were identical to those obtained with FAC plus BCG, but significantly prolonged as compared to FAC alone. The results while suggestive and encouraging are too preliminary to be conclusive.

b. LUNG CANCER. In contrast to other patients with solid tumors, patients with lung cancer appear to be especially prone to immunodepression, and it develops early in the disease (60). The degree of immunodepression associated with lung cancer bears a relation to the stage of neoplasia, its resectability and the potential for survival (26, 60, 150).

Little information is available relative to the immunogenicity of carcinoma of the lung (9, 148, 150). Several reports, however, suggest benefit from immunotherapy (46, 92, 113, 123). A beneficial effect has been ascribed to postoperative bacterial infection which might be the consequence of immunologic reactions enhanced by the infecting bacteria (92, 113). Ruckdeschel *et al.* postulated that the host's specific immunologic reaction to bacteria promotes non-specific destruction of tumor cells (113). Numerous lymphokines may be operative. Macrophage activating factor (MAF), a product of lymphocyte antigen interaction, is capable of creating "angry" macrophages with elevated levels of lysosomal enzymes, increased intracellular bacteriocidal capacity, increased mitoses and increased endocytosis (85). Activated macrophages could conceivably cause tumor cell death as an incidental event. Alternatively, macrophages could act at the tumor cell surface via lysosomal enzyme release, exposing tumor-specific antigens that have been hidden by other surface materials, this exposure permitting tumor specific immunologic responses to destroy tumor cells.

Several investigations are in progress to determine the efficacy of levamisole in lung cancer. The most complete reports are of a long term multi-center study headed by Amery (3–6). The initial report concerned 111 patients with primary bronchial carcinoma who were subjected to surgery (3). Seventy-one had squamous cell carcinoma, 21 adenocarcinoma, 17 had other types and for two patients histologic diagnoses were not available. Tumors were equally distributed in right and left lungs and slightly more than 50% were peripheral. Lobectomy was performed in 68 cases, pneumonectomy in 33 cases and a more limited operation in one patient; in 9 cases the type of surgery was not specified. In double-blind fashion levamisole or placebo was randomly administered orally as 50 mg 3 times a day for three days before surgery with repeat 3 day courses at two week intervals thereafter for at least two years. The follow-up at the time of the report was continuing. Similar side effects were noted in the two treatment groups, but with slightly greater occurrence of gastric disturbance, nervousness and fever in the recipients of levamisole. In the group that received levamisole ten of 51 were suspected or proved to have tumor recurrence, and 7 (13.7%) had died at time of the report. The group of 60 placebo recipients had 23 suspected recurrences of which 20 were proved; 12 (20%) were dead. Twelve patients that received levamisole and 14 placebo recipients died from causes other than cancer. The differences in recurrence and mortality from cancer were not statistically significant, but appeared to indicate a trend.

It was of interest that tumors recurred in 21.2% of the levamisole patients who smoked more than 10 cigarettes per day and in 47.5% of similarly categorized placebo receeipients (p = 0.027). The respective disease mortalities of levamisole and placebo recipients were 18.2% and 27.5% (p > 0.05) among the smokers of more than ten cigarettes per day (3).

More than any other factor, characteristics of the tumor appeared to influence the effectiveness of levamisole. Suspected recurrence of squamous cell carcinoma was more common in placebo recipients than in levamisole recipients (p = 0.035), but the differences between proved recurrence and death from metastases were not significant.

Regardless of histologic type levamisole was most effective when tumors were large (Table 2). Distant metastases (bone, brain, and liver) were fewer in the levamisole group (4 or 7.8% versus 13 or 21.7% p = 0.06). The interval between surgery and recurrence was not altered by levamisole. Reporting on 82 levamisole recipients and 96 placebo treated patients, the same group reported continuation of the earlier trends (5). An important aspect of the updated study was identification of a relationship between levamisole effect and body weight. No significant difference was seen in patients with initial body weights greater than 70 kg, but those weighing 70 kg or less appeared to derive benefit from levamisole.

Table 2. Primary tumor size related to recurrence and death from cancer of the lung[a]

	Levamisole			Placebo		
Tumor Size	Suspected Recurrence	Proved Recurrence	Death	Suspected Recurrence	Proved Recurrence	Death
< 3 cm	16.7	16.7	11.1	18.2	13.6	4.6 (p>0.5)
4–6 cm	21.1	21.1	15.8	55.6 (p<0.045)	50.0	27.8
>7 cm	14.3	14.3	0.0	81.8	72.7	54.5 (p>0.005)

Therapy with levamisole was associated with reduced recurrence and death after pulmonary resection for carcinoma of the lung. The most notable changes accompanied treatment of large tumors.

a. Amery (3–6).

Nine months after surgery, a significant difference was observed between recurrence in the levamisole group (10%) and the placebo group (28%) $p < 0.05$. This difference progressively increased and peaked at 18 months (levamisole 18%, placebo 49%) ($p < 0.001$). Survival became significantly different at 15 months (levamisole 92%, placebo 70%) ($p < 0.05$), the greatest difference appearing at 21 months.

On the basis of these results, it was concluded that the appropriate dose of levamisole was 2.1 to 2.8 mg per kg (median 2.4 mg per kg). Amery strongly recommends use of 2.5 mg per kg daily divided into 2–3 doses (7). In patients with extended resectable tumors, levamisole appeared to be especially effective in decreasing bloodborne metastases, but changes in intrathoracic relapse was only marginal.

Among lung cancer patients treated with levamisole, Holmes & Golub observed augmentation of lymphocyte responses to mitogen in vitro (61). Those with unresectable disease who received levamisole demonstrated an increase in skin reactivity to dinitrochlorobenzine (DNCB), but the difference did not reach significant proportions.

Thus, while levamisole appears to hold promise for increasing disease free interval after pulmonary resections for lung cancer and survival of lung cancer patients, additional clinical trials are clearly necessary for confirmation of these trends.

c. MALIGNANT MELANOMA. Malignant melanoma constitutes a small fraction of all malignant neoplasia but is of considerable interest because of the evidence that host immunologic resistance has a significant influence upon its clinical course. Melanoma along with neuroblastoma and hypernephroma is among the more frequent of tumors to undergo spontaneous regression, possibly as a result of immunologic rejection (34). The blood of patients who have had a spontaneous remission is also sometimes capable of producing regression in other patients with melanoma (134a). Melanoma cells are now known to have identifiable tumor associated antigens and to elicit delayed cutaneous hypersensitivity reactions characteristic of cellular type immunity. Shibata and co-workers reported that individually specific antitumor membrane antibody present in early stages of the disease correlated with the prognosis of patients with melanoma and disappeared when the tumor disseminated (124).

There is much, therefore, to recommend melanoma as a logical tumor system with which to conduct trials of immunotherapy. Much work has involved nonspecific immunostimulation with Bacillus Calmette-Guerin (BCG) with or without concomitant chemotherapy (28, 47). Intralesional injection of BCG has been effective in producing regression of cutaneous nodules and occasionally of uninjected nodules, but rarely is an effect upon visceral metastases observed; any alteration of clinical course is questionable (71, 89). Nadler and Moore as well as Jewell and associates reported clinical remissions following cross transfusion of sensitized leukocytes between paired melanoma tumor implant recipients (66, 94a). Objective tumor regressions have followed specific immunotherapy with homogenates of allogeneic melanoma cells and irradiated tumor cell vaccines (66, 91).

Levamisole has had limited use against melanoma to date. Of interest are its capacities to sustain spontaneous tumor specific antibodies and to potentiate the stimulatory effects of BCG. Shibata et al. used levamisole in doses of 150 mg/day for 3 days weekly in 8 week courses to treat patients with malignant melanoma and used antitumor antibody and lymphocyte cytotoxicity to monitor effects (124). The results with levamisole were generally similar to those observed with oral BCG. Levamisole increased antitumor antibody in 3/15 patients and produced small increases in lymphocyte cytotoxicity in 5/12. After immunization with autochthonous or allogeneic tumor cells, levamisole prolonged the specific antitumor antibody response in 3/6 patients and increased cytotoxicity in 2/5. In contrast with BCG, levamisole had a marked adjuvant effect if given immediately prior to immunization with tumor cells. Furthermore, of six patients who received no tumor cells and who failed to be stimulated by oral BCG, four showed significant antibody responses when given levamisole. Three had increased lymphocyte cytotoxicity.

Thus levamisole may be an effective adjuvant to specific immunologic stimulation of melanoma patients and a synergist with other nonspecific immunostimulants. In one of the few therapeutic trials to date, Ward reported a temporary (2 months) partial regression of a 4 cm subcutaneous mass of tumor in one of four patients with disseminated melanoma during treatment with levamisole (50 mg daily continuously) (147).

d. LYMPHOMAS. Deficiency of cell-mediated immunologic responsiveness in patients with Hodgkin's disease is variable, and its nature is not understood (23, 32, 41, 76, 159). Whether the depression is caused by the disease or therapeutic agents, it is an important aspect of patient welfare and perhaps of disease control (20, 27, 32, 52, 76, 93, 94, 127). Although studies concerning the ability of levamisole to restore flagging cellular immunologic responsiveness in patients with Hodgkin's disease are limited, the results are encouraging (13, 70, 75, 104, 143). Biniaminov and Ramot reported that levamisole in vitro significantly increased the proportion of E-rosette forming cells of peripheral blood (13). Lymphocytes from control subjects formed 50.8% and 44.4% E-rosettes, respectively, before and after levamisole treatment ($p < 0.01$). By contrast, 37.7% of lymphocytes from Hodgkin's disease patients formed E-rosettes before levamisole, and after treatment 62.9% formed rosettes ($p < 0.0005$). These results are in accord with other studies which show that the absolute number of T-lymphocytes is normal in Hodgkin's disease, but that a qualitative defect is present (70).

Verhaegen et al. confirmed that levamisole increased the E-rosette forming cells in Hodgkin's disease. They also showed that levamisole reversed or inhibited azathioprine induced reduction of E-rosette forming cells, in vitro, by incubating cells with levamisole after or before azathioprine exposure (143).

Administering levamisole to a heterogeneous group of patients with Hodgkin's disease, Levo et al. found that dermal reactivity to a battery of antigens (PPD, mumps, Candida and SK-SD) was significantly increased. 52% of patients with negative skin tests converted to positive reactions after levamisole treament (75). In addition, patients with positive reactions before treatment had greater areas of skin reaction after levamisole treatment. A few reports indicate that responses of cancer patients to PPD and DNCB increase after levamisole treatment, but the possibility exists that the increase is the result of stimulation by repeated applications of the antigens (140, 142). In the study of Levo et al., levamisole treament was followed by a significant increase in the total peripheral blood leukocyte count, a major contributor being an increase in E-rosette or T-lymphocytes (75). The lymphocyte count before levamisole (1373/mm^3) increased to 1965/mm^3 after levamisole, representing a 43% increase. The proportion of E-rosette forming cells increased from 19% before treatment to 41% after treatment; T-lymphocyte counts of 214/mm³ increased to 664/mm³, a 210% rise. T-lymphocyte counts decreased within 6 months of treatment. Administration of another 3 day course of levamisole (150 mg/day) promptly increased the number of E-rosette forming cells; this increase persisted for at least 2 months. Using in vitro treatment, Ramot et al. showed that while the in vivo response to levamisole was in effect, in vitro treatment with levamisole did not further augment lymphocyte responses (104).

The mechanism by which cell-mediated immunologic functions are depressed in Hodgkin's disease patients is not understood, nor is it known how levamisole overcomes the immunologic depression. In a recent report, Ramot et al. presented data that provides some insight (105). A radiolabeling technique showed that lymphocytes from patients with Hodgkin's disease have surface associated proteins not present on lymphocytes from normal individuals. In vitro treatment of lymphocytes with levamisole removed 85% of the protein; lymphocytes from patients that had received levamisole or from untreated normal individuals did not have appreciable surface associated protein. Immunoprecipitation of the lymphocyte surface associated protein identified it as mainly ferritin. Further identification of the protein as the factor responsible for blocking lymphocyte responsiveness was provided in the study of Ramot et al.

Lymphocytes from normal individuals do not ordinarily adhere to a nylon column, but some lymphocytes from Hodgkin's disease patients do adhere. When the latter were mechanically dislodged for comparison with nonadherent cells and with non-filtered lymphocytes, the adherent cells were identified as those that become E-rosette forming cells after levamisole exposure. Furthermore, the nylon adherent cells could be eluted from the nylon by exposure to levamisole. Additional information relating ferritin to lymphocytes was provided by "reconstitution" experiments (105). Lymphocytes from patients were successively incubated with levamisole (which increased the E-rosetteing capacity), incubated with ferritin (which reduced the rosette-forming capacity to levels seen before the levamisole treatment), and incubated a second time with levamisole to restore the E-rosette forming capacity to that seen after the initial levamisole treatment. Similar treatment of lymphocytes from normal subjects did not alter these activities.

In summary, these investigations identified a subpopulation of lymphocytes in Hodgkin's disease patients that had a surface associated protein that consisted mainly of ferritin (105). This protein was not present on lymphocytes with a levamisole-induced increase of E-rosette forming capacity. Re-incubation of treated cells with ferritin reduced the E-rosette forming capacity, but with a second levamisole treatment it was restored.

Lymphocytes from normal individuals did not display these characteristics, thus a qualitatively unique sub-population of lymphocytes appears to be present in patients with Hodgkin's disease. Preliminary studies suggest that the lymphocyte abnormalities persist after radiotherapy but are reduced by chemotherapy.

Mediation of the effects on lymphocytes via cAMP and cGMP is a reasonable explanation for the prompt effect of levamisole on mononuclear cells *in vitro*. Ramot *et al.* detected an elevated level of cAMP in lymphocytes from Hodgkin's disease patients as compared to normal subjects (104).

Lymphomas in general have been the subject of few immunotherapeutic trials. Patients with Stage Ia or IIa disease treated for cure with radiotherapy have received treatment with BCG (128). Randomly assigned controls had a mean remission duration of 10.6 months whereas BCG therapy was associated with a 25.9 month remission (P < 0.01). In a study of Burkitt's lymphoma relapse after complete remission on cyclophosphamide occurred in 46% of BCG treated patients and 64% of controls with remission durations of 30 and 36 weeks, differences not statistically significant (160). Hoerni *et al.* reported disease free intervals of one year for 79% of 15 patients with advanced Hodgkin's disease treated with BCG and 53% of 12 control patients, again not a statistically significant difference (57).

With respect to the use of levamisole in Hodgkin's disease one may state that its effects on immunologic responses have been measured, but there are no indications that it has clinically beneficial effects.

e. LEUKEMIA. Only one report has been made on a trial of levamisole for treatment of acute myeloid leukemia, an interim report not readily available (14). Levamisole (2.5 mg/kg/day given 3 days alternate weeks) or placebo was given in a double-blind manner together with intermittent cytostatic chemotherapy. The median durations of remission were 16 months and 10 months, respectively, for levamisole and placebo recipients. As the groups were composed of 12 patients each, the difference was not significant.

f. IMMUNOBLASTIC LYMPHADENOPATHY. Immunoblastic lymphadenopathy is a recently described, poorly understood morphological entity frequently identified erroneously as Hodgkin's disease (40, 84). It is thought to be a disorder of the B-cell system, but their immunologic characteristics are not clearly delineated. Two patients with this disorder have been treated with levamisole (12, 30). Both were anergic to recall antigens SK/SD and DNCB until treated with levamisole. Moreover, in both patients, the pre-treatment level of T-cells was decreased and the number of B-cells was increased. Normal levels returned after treatment with levamisole.

g. CANCER OF THE HEAD AND NECK.

Cancers of the head and neck are predominantly epithelial in origin and squamous in type. They are also closely associated with tobacco use and excessive consumption of alcohol. Patients with squamous cancers of the head and neck regularly have impaired cellular immunity. Olkowski and associates found both the mean percentages and the absolute levels of circulating lymphocytes in 46 patients with squamous cancer of the head and neck significantly lower than those of 51 healthy controls (99). Others have reported skin reactivity to recall antigens and lymphocyte response to PHA stimulation deficient as well (99). Wanebo and co-workers found 30% of patients with early resectable lesions unresponsive to DNCB skin challenge and 40% with impaired response to lymphocyte mitogens (Concanavallin A and PHA) (146).

As tobacco and alcohol are implicated in the etiology of these cancers, it is of interest that no difference was found by Silverman and associates in lymphocyte blastogenesis between smokers and nonsmokers, nor was any acute effect of smoking on in vitro lymphocyte reactivity evident (125).

In alcoholics Wanebo et al. did observe decreased reactivity of lymphocytes to Con A and PHA as well as reduced T cell levels, but skin reactivity to DNCB was normal as was lymphocyte response to pokeweed mitogen and skin reactivity to recall antigens (146). Thus, the evidence that impaired immunity preceeds the disease in high risk individuals is not impressive. A considerable body of evidence relates the immunologic status of patients with squamous cancer of the head and neck to their prognosis; T cell levels and mitogen responses of lymphocytes correlate inversely with the stage of the disease prior to treament (146). After apparently successful conventional treatment DNCB skin reactivity improves and T cell levels rise, but the immunologic deficits of cured and uncured patients with squamous cancer tend to continue and to remain correlated with the extent of disease prior to treatment (99, 125, 141). Continued immunologic depression after successful treatment is a characteristic peculiar to patients with head and neck cancers of the squamous type and is not shared by patients with sarcomas, adenocarcinomas, and melanomas in this region (141). Twomey and associates attributed this continuing impairment to a serum factor which depressed lymphocyte reactivity (141).

As might be expected from their association with advanced clinical stage, depressed pre-operative lymphocyte blastogenesis and DNCB anergy tend to be predictive of early recurrence after treatment. In a series observed for three years after definitive operations, Chretien and associates reported recurrences in six of ten patients with low reactivity to DNCB and one of two with high reactivity (22). Wanebo *et al.* correlated DNCB reactivity with recurrence and survival; if cancers were small and clinically localized (T 1–2 NO MO), 44% of anergic patients had early recurrence and 36% survived for two years. Analogous figures for reactors were 22% and 86% (146).

The influence of levamisole upon the clinical course of patients with head and neck cancer is as yet uncertain, but its ability to restore immunologic competence is evident. Tripodi *et al.* demonstrated that levamisole is capable of restoring cutaneous cell mediated immunity in anergic patients with a variety of head and neck cancers (140). Six of nine patients with advanced cancers given levamisole in the dose of 150 mg per day for 3 days reacted with increased responses to DNCB skin tests, and six manifested heightened responses to tuberculin challenge (PPD). Among four controls with comparable cancers who received no levamisole, only one reacted weakly to DNCB challenge, and none showed increased sensitivity to PPD.

Cancers of the head and neck are heterogeneous and prognostically diverse; for this reason they pose a poor therapeutic proving ground for levamisole. Nevertheless, insofar as immunologic competence may determine the course of the disease rather than reflect it, the capacity of levamisole to restore the cellular immunity of patients with cancers of the head and neck is of considerable import.

Toxicity and Side Effects

In animal trials levamisole in high doses rapidly produces convulsions and death (52). Levamisole has an LD_{50} dose level in mice of 28.2 mg/kg I.V., 121 mg/kg subcutaneously, and 285 mg/kg orally. Except for a higher LD_{50} oral dose, i.e., 545 mg/kg, rats react practically the same. Daily doses of 10–40 mg/kg for 13 weeks produces decreased weight gain and decreased food consumption in female rats but no change in behavior and no fetal loss. At 160 mg/kg these effects as well as decreased organ weight are observed in both sexes. When given during early pregnancy (6–15 day) levamisole results in decreased litter size and a reduction in the number of live fetuses. No such alterations occur if it is administered late in pregnancy.

In humans levamisole is given only by the oral route. A daily standard dose of 150 mg has been used in most studies, but great variation is encountered in the number of days per week this dose is repeated and the overall duration of therapy. A single dose of 1–5 mg/kg (avg 2.5) is effective as an antihelminthic.

Generally levamisole is well tolerated; side effects are mild and tran-

Table 3.   Side effects observed in 146 patients
treated with levamisole

Side Effect	Percent of Patients
Bitter taste	40
Queasiness	37
Nausea	37
Abdominal cramps	17
Diarrhea	17
Tiredness	17
Vomiting	23
Insomnia	17
Light-headedness	13
Headache	10
Eructation	10
Dizziness	3
Pruritis	3

Dose and schedule of levamisole: 150 mg p.o. daily
for 3 days every 2 weeks.

The side effects of levamisole are varied but are usually
mild. In addition to those listed in this table, a flu-like syndrome and leucopenia have been observed. The latter are discussed in the text.

Source: Oettgen et al., 1976.

sient. A single oral dose of 2.5–3.5 mg/kg produces symptoms in only
3.3% of patients (73, 74). The most frequent symptoms are nausea, vomiting, and abdominal pain. Vertigo, fever, and headache also occur. At
recommended antihelminthic doses no hepatic or renal toxicity has been
observed (64). Side effects in childran and adults are similar. In some
comparative trials in children placebo treatment has produced more side
effects than levamisole (42). At Memorial Sloan-Kettering Cancer Center
in New York 146 adult cancer patients treated with daily doses of 150–750
mg by mouth three times a week had mild and infrequent side effects (97).
No change in hematological or biochemical parameters were noted. The
symptoms and signs associated with 150 mg daily for 3 days every two
weeks are shown in Table 3. The frequency of undesirable drug effects
increases with the dose (52); dizziness, lethargy and gastrointestinal
symptoms are the most bothersome.

In summarizing experience with various treatment schedules involving 1,439 patients, and including intermittent treatment for up to three
years, the Janssen Company found reports of nausea, gastric intolerance,

and anorexia as well as nervousness, irritability, insomnia, and alterations of taste and smell (137). Encountered was a flu-like syndrome with fatigue, muscle and joint pains, fever, chills, shivering, and malaise (124). Skin rashes characterized as papulovesicular and sometimes urticarial occurred in 26 patients variably after a few days to a few months of therapy, and transient granulocytopenia occurred in 7.

Leukopenia is an unusual but potentially serious complication of levamisole therapy. It has most often accompanied treatment of rheumatic diseases and prolonged therapy. According to Rosenthal et al. two of 48 such patients treated with 150 mg daily × 4 weeks and 150 mg 3 × weekly thereafter developed leukopenia after 3–6 weeks of treatment (115). Recovery was complete 10–20 days after discontinuing the drug and no effect upon red blood cells or platelets was observed. Leukocyte agglutinating antibodies could be demonstrated in the patient's serum in the presence of levamisole.

Ruuskanen et al. reported two cases of lethal agranulocytosis in children with rheumatoid arthritis while on treatment with levamisole (117). The adverse reaction was noted after 5 and 10 doses of the drug at daily doses of 2.5 mg/kg and 3.5 mg/kg. These 3- and 5-year-old females were on intermittent schedules. Both had previously had leukopenic reactions to anti-inflammatory drugs and were taking corticosteroids concurrently. It is possible that these circumstances warrant caution.

Preliminary results reveal no adverse effects of levamisole upon human pregnancies (73, 74).

Summary

Levamisole is a synthetic low molecular weight derivative of thiazole originally used as an antihelminthic but with recently discovered immunologic effects that may prove useful for the treatment of cancer. The property of primary interest is its ability to stimulate cell mediated immunity without appreciably affecting humoral immunity. This is an important differential since the former is presently considered the chief mechanism of host resistance to neoplasia, while humoral immunity may enhance tumor growth.

Attractive features of the drug are its ability to be administered orally, the fact that it is not a biological preparation with attendant problems of standardization and infectivity, and its mild side effects compared to other non-specific immunostimulants. Disagreeable reactions are generally limited to anorexia, nausea, irritability, nervousness, skin rashes and fatigue, although agranulocytosis is occasionally noted.

The mechanism by which levamisole activates thymus dependent lymphocytes and macrophages is uncertain, but is probably by increasing intracellular levels of cyclic GMP. Rather than producing true potentiation, the drug's action is to restore depressed cell mediated immunity to normal.

Evidence from *in vitro* work and from animal tumor models indicate that dose level is critical for optimal effects; too little or too much of the drug can be ineffective. It is also evident that levamisole's most appropriate application in cancer therapy is in clinical situations characterized by depressed cellular immunity or in which depression can be anticipated such as during systemic chemotherapy or during therapeutic irradiation. A promising application is in conjunction with specific antigens. Levamisole's ability to restore cellular immunity to normal in cancer patients is becoming increasingly well established; the numerous clinical trials in progress designed to determine its therapeutic value are as yet largely inconclusive and its use at the present time must be considered investigational.

ACKNOWLEDGMENTS

This work was supported in part by the Stanley and Polly Stone Fund, the Cudahy Foundation, and the Gladys Stone Wirth Fund of Immunology Research Foundation, Inc.

Levamisole for the author's (D. S.) *in vitro* and animal studies referred to in this work was supplied through the courtesy of Janssen R & D, Inc.

REFERENCES

1. Al-Ibrahim, M. S. *In vitro* effects of levamisole on human mononuclear phagocytes, in Proceedings of the Third Conference on Modulation of Host Immune Resistance in the Prevention or Treatment of Induced Neoplasias, 1976 (in press).

2. Al-Ibrahim, M. S., Holzman, R. S., and Lawrence, H. S. 1977. Levamisole concentrations required for enhanced proliferation of human lymphocytes and phagocytosis by macrophage. *J. Infectious Dis.* (in press).

3. Amery, W., *et al.* 1975. Immunopotentiation with levamisole in resectable bronchogenic carcinoma: A double-blind controlled trial. *Brit. Med. J.* 3: 461–464.

4. Amery, W. 1976. Double-blind levamisole trial in resectable lung cancer. *Ann. N.Y. Acad. Sci.* 277: 260–268.

5. Amery, W. K. 1976. A placebo-controlled levamisole study in resectable lung cancer. Presented at International Conference on Immunotherapy of Cancer: Present Status of Trials in Man. Raven Press, New York.

6. Amery, W. Double-blind trial with levamisole in resectable lung cancer, in Proceedings of the 9th International Congress of Chemotherapy, 1976. Plenum Publishing, New York (in press).

7. Amery, W. K. 1976. Levamisole as an immunotherapeutic agent. *World J. Surg.* (in press).

8. Aungst, C. W., Sokal, J. E., and Jager, B. V. 1973. Complications of BCG vaccination. *Proc. Amer. Assoc. Cancer Res.* 14: 108.

9. Baldwin, R. W., Embleton, M. J., Jones, J. S., *et al.* 1973. Cell-mediated and humoral immune reactions to human tumors. *Int. J. Cancer* 12: 73–83.

10. Bast, R. C., Jr., Zhor, B., Borsos, T., and Rapp, H. J. 1974. BCG and Cancer. *N. Engl. J. Med.* 290: 1413–1420 and 1458–1469.

11. Bast, R. C., Jr., Bast, B. S., and Rapp, H. J. 1976. Critical review of previously reported animal studies of tumor immunotherapy with nonspecific immunostimulants. *Ann. N.Y. Acad. Sci.* 277: 60–93.

12. Bensa, J. C., Faure, J., Martin, H., Sotto, J. J., and Schaerer, R. 1976. Levamisole in angio-immunoblastic lymphadenopathy. *Lancet* 1: 1081.

13. Biniaminov, M., and Ramot, B. 1975. *In vitro* restoration by levamisole of thymus-derived lymphocyte function in Hodgkin's disease. *Lancet* 1: 464.

14. Brincker, H. Prolongation of the duration of remission in acute myeloid leukemia (AML) with levamisole. Presented at Spring meeting of Scandinavian Hoematologists, Aarhus, Denmark, 1976.

15. Brugmas, J., Schuermans, V., DeCock, W., Thienport, D., Janssen, P., Verhaegen, H., van Nimmen, L., Louwagine, A. C., Stevens, E. 1973. Restoration of host defense mechanisms in man by levamisole. *Life Sciences* 13: 1499–1504.

16. Bruley-Rosset, M., Florentin, I., and Mathe, G. 1976. *In vivo* and *in vitro* macrophage activation by systemic adjuvants. *Agents and Actions* 6: 251–255.

17. Burnet, F. M. 1970. The concept of immunological surveillance. *Prog. Exp. Tumor Res.* 13: 1–27.

18. Chan, S. A., Lee, S. K., and Simons, M. J. 1976. Levamisole augmentation of lymphocyte hyporesponsiveness to phytohemagglutinin in patients with pulmonary tuberculosis. *Proc. Soc. Exp. Biol. Med.* 151: 716–719.

19. Chan, S. H., and Simons, M. J. 1975. Levamisole and lymphocyte responsiveness. *Lancet* 1: 1246–1247.

20. Cheever, A. W., Valsamis, M. P., and Rabson, A. S. 1965. Necrotizing toxoplasmic encephalitis and herpetic pneumonia complicating treated Hodgkin's disease. *N. Engl. J. Med.* 272: 26–29.

21. Chirigos, M. A., Pearson, J. W., and Pryor, J. 1973. Augmentation of chemotherapeutically induced remission of a murine leukemia by a chemical immuno-adjuvant. *Cancer Res.* 33: 2615–2618.

22. Chretieu, P. B., Crowder, W. C., Gartner, H. R., Sample, W. F., and Catalona, W. J. 1973. Correlation of preoperative lymphocyte reactivity with the clinical course of cancer patients. *Surgery Gynecol. Obstet.* 136: 380–384.

23. Churchill, W. H., Rocklin, R. R., Moloney, W. C., and David, J. R. 1973. *In vitro* evidence of normal lymphocyte function in some patients with Hodgkin's disease and negative delayed cutaneous hypersensitivity. *Natl. Cancer. Inst. Monogr.* 36: 99–106.

24. Copeland, D., Stewart, T., and Harris, J. 1974. Effect of Levamisole (NSC-177023) on *in vitro* human lymphocyte transformation. *Cancer Chemotherapy Rep.* 58: 167–170.

25. DeCree, J., Verhaegen, H., DeCock, W., *et al.* 1974. Impaired neutrophil phagocytosis. *Lancet* 2: 294.

26. Dellon, A. L., Potoin, C., and Chretien, P. B. 1975. Thymus-dependent lymphocyte levels in bronchogenic carcinoma: Correlations with histology, clinical stage, and clinical course after surgical treatment. *Cancer* 35: 687.

27. Denton, P. M. 1973. Immune responsiveness in Hodgkin's disease. *Brit. J. Cancer* 28: Suppl. I, 119.

27a. Dinai, Y., and Pras, M. 1975. Levamisole in rheumatoid arthritis. *Lancet* 2: 556.

28. Eilber, F. R., and Morton, D. L. 1970. Impaired immunologic reactivity and recurrence following cancer surgery. *Cancer* 25: 362–367.

29. Eilber, F. R., Morton, D. L., Holmes, E. C., Sparks, F. C., and Ramming, K. P. 1976. Adjuvant immunotherapy with BCG in treatment of regional lymph node metastases from malignant melanoma. *N. Engl. J. Med.* 294: 237–240.

30. Ellegaard, J., Boesen, A. M. 1976. Restoration of defective cellular immunity by levamisole in a patient with immunoblastic lymphadenopathy. *Scand. J. Haematol* 17: 36–43.

31. Ellis, R. J., Wernick, G., Zabriskie, J. B., and Goldman, L. I. 1975. Immunologic competence of regional lymph nodes in patients with breast cancer. *Cancer* 35: 655–659.

32. Eltringham, J. P., and Kaplan, H. S. 1973. Impaired delayed-hypersensitivity responses in 154 patients with untreated Hodgkin's disease. *Natl. Cancer Inst. Monogr.* 36: 107–115.

33. Engels, H., Sonck, W. 1975. The effect of levamisole in 5 patients suffering from rheumatoid arthritis. Interim report. Clinical Res. Report. Serial No. R12564/29—Janssen Research Products Information Service.

34. Everson, T. C. 1964. Spontaneous regression of cancer. *Ann. N.Y. Acad. Sci.* 114: 721–735.

35. Fidler, I. J., and Spitler, L. E. 1975. Effects of levamisole on *in vivo* and *in vitro* murine host response to syngeneic transplantable tumor. *J. Natl. Canc. Inst.* 55: 1107–1112.

36. Fischer, G. W., Oi, V. T., Kelley, J. L., Podgore, J. K., Bass, J. W., Wagner, F. S., and Gordon, B. L., II. 1974. Enhancement of host defense mechanisms against gram-positive pyogenic coceal infections with Levo-telrom isole (levamisole) in neonatal rats. *Ann. Allergy* 33: 193–198.

37. Fischer, G. W., Podgore, J. K., Bass, J. W., Kelley, J. W., and Kobayashin, G. Y. 1975. Enhanced host defense mechanisms with levamisole in suckling rats. *J. Inf. Dis.* 132: 578–581.

38. Fischer, G. W., Cromrine, M. H., Balk, M. W., Chang, S. P., Hokana, Y., Heu, P., and Chou, S. C. 1976. The effect of levamisole on suckling rat spleen cells: Evidence for macrophage regulation, *in* Proceedings of the Third Conference on Modulation of Host Immune Resistance in the Prevention or Treatment of Induced Neoplasias, 1976 (in press).

38a. Fischer, G. W., Balk, M. W., Cromrine, M. H., and Bass, J. W. 1976. Immunopotentiation and antiviral chemotherapy in a suckling rat model of herpesvirus encephalitis. *J. Infec. Dis.* 133: A217–A220.

39. Forsyth, B. A. 1968. The antihelminthic activity of the optical isomers of tetramisole in sheep and cattle. *Aust. Vet. J.* 44: 395–400.

40. Frizzera, G., Moran, E. M., Rappaport, H. 1974. Angioimmunoblastic lymphadenopathy with dysproteinemia. *Lancet* 1: 1070–1073.

41. Gaines, J. D., Gilmer, M. A., and Remington, J. S. 1973. Deficiency of lymphocyte antigen recognition in Hodgkin's disease. *Natl. Cancer Inst. Monogr.* 36: 117–121.

42. Gatti, F., Krubwa, F., Vandepitte, J., and Thinepont, D. 1972. Control of intestinal nematodes in African school children by the trimestrial administration of levamisole. *Ann. Soc. Belg. Med. Trop.* 52: 19–32.

43. Ginckel, van, R. F., and Hoebeke, J. 1976. Effects of levamisole on spontaneous rosette-forming cells in murine spleen. *Eur. J. Immunol.* 6: 305–307.

44. Gordon, B. L., and Keenan, J. P. 1975. The treatment of systemic lupus erythematosus (SLE) with the T-cell immunostimulant drug levamisole: A case report. *Ann. Allergy* 35: 343–355.

45. Goyanes-Villaescusa, V. 1976. Mitogenic stimulation by levamisole on normal human lymphocytes and leukemic lymphoblasts. *Lancet* 1: 370.

46. Graham, E. A., and Singer, J. J. 1933. Successful removal of an entire lung for carcinoma of the bronchus. *JAMA* 101: 1371–1374.

47. Gutterman, J. U., Mavligit, G., Bottlieb, J. A., Burgess, M. A., McBride, C. E., Einhorn, L., Freireich, E. J., and Hersh, E. M. 1974. Chemoimmunotherapy of disseminated malignant melanoma with dimethyl triazeno inidaxole carboxamide and Bacillus Calmette-Guerin. *N. Engl. J. Med.* 291: 592–597.

48. Heykants, J., Dominicus, J., Marsboom, R. 1974. Plasma and tissue levels of levamisole in cattle after intramuscular administration. Unpublished Biological Report, Janssen Research Products Information Service, October.

49. Heykants, J., Dominicus, J., and Marsboom, R. 1974. Plasma and tissue levels of levamisole (R12564) in the pig after a single intramuscular dose of 10 mg/kg. Unpublished Biological Report, Janssen Research Products Information Service, December.

50. Heykants, J., Wynants, J., and Scheijgrond, H. 1975. The absorption, excretion, and metabolism of levamisole in man. Janssen Clinical Research Report, November (unpublished).

51. Hill, H. R., and Quie, P. G. 1975, in J. A. Bellanti and D. H. Dayton (eds.), *The Phagocytic Cell in Host Resistance*, p. 262. Raven Press, New York.

52. Hirshaut, Y., Pinsky, C. M., Wanebo, H. J., and Oettgen, H. F. 1976. Design of Phase-I trials of immunopotentiators for cancer therapy: Levamisole and *Corynebacterium parvum*. *Ann. N.Y. Acad. Sci.*, pp. 252–259.

53. Hodden, J. W., Hodden, E. M., and Goldberg, W. D. 1974. *In* Braun, Whichtenstein, L. M., and Dorker, C. W. (eds.), *Cyclic AMP, Cell Growth, and the Immune Response*, p. 237. Springer-Verlag, New York.

54. Hodden, J. W., Coffey, R. G., Hodden, E. M., Lopes-Corrales, E., and Sunshine, G. H. 1975. Effects of levamisole and imidozole on lymphocytoproliferation and cyclic nucleotide levels. *Cell. Immunol.* 20: 98–103.

55. Hodden, J. W., Hodden, E. M., Coffey, R. G., Johnson, E. M., and Johnson, L. D. 1975. in A. S. Rosenthal (ed.), *Immune Recognition*, p. 359. Academic Press, New York.

56. Hoebeke, J., and Franchi, G. 1973. Influence of tetramisole and its optical

isomers on the mononuclear phagocytic system: Effect on carbon clearance in mice. *J. Reticuloendothial Soc.* 14: 317–323.

57. Hoerni, B., Chauvergne, J., Hoerni-Simon, G., Durand, M., and LaGarde, C. 1974. Immunotherapic non specifique de la maladie de Hodgkin por BCG. *Acta Haematol.* 52: 214–219.

58. Hokama, Y., Kimura, L., Perreira, S., and Palumbo, N. 1974. Effects of levamisole and C-reactive protein on mitogen stimulated lymphocytes *in vitro* and on the C-reactive protein response *in vivo*. *Fed. Proc.* 33: 650.

59. Holbrook, A., and Scales, B. 1967. Polarographic determinants of tetramisole hydrochloride in extracts of animal tissue. *Analyt. Biochem.* 18: 46–53.

60. Holmes, E. C., and Golub, S. H. 1976. Immunologic defects in lung cancer patients. *J. Thorac. Cardiovasc. Surgery* 71: 161–167.

61. Holmes, E. C., and Golub, S. H. The effect of levamisole on cell mediated immunity in patients with lung cancer, in Proceedings of the Third Conference on Modulation of Host Immune Resistance in the Prevention or Treatment of Induced Neoplasias, 1976 (in press).

62. Hortobagyi, D. N., Gutterman, J. U., Blumenschein, G. R., Tashima, C. K., Buzdar, A. U., and Hersh, E. M. Levamisole in the treatment of breast cancer, in Proceedings of the Third Conference on Modulation of Host Immune Resistance in the Prevention or Treatment of Induced Neoplasias, 1976 (in press).

63. Humphrey, L. J., Lincoln, P. M., Griffen, W. O., Jr. 1968. Immunologic response in patients with disseminated cancer. *Ann. Surg.* 168: 374–381.

64. Huys, J., Kayihigi, J., Freyers, P., and Vandenberghe, G. Treatment of infection with levamisole, in *Basic Medical Information*, Levamisole (R 12,564) Janssen R & D, Inc., New Brunswick, New Jersey.

64a. Irwin, M. R., and Knight, H. D. 1975. Enhanced resistance to corynebacterium pseudotuberculosis infections associated with reduced serum immunoglobulin levels in levamisole-treated mice. *Infect. Immun.* 12: 1098–1103.

65. Israel, L., Edelstein, R., Depierre, A., and Dimitrov, N. 1975. Daily intravenous infusions of *Corynebacterium power* in twenty patients with disseminated cancer: A preliminary report of clinical and biological findings. *J. Natl. Cancer Inst.* 55: 29–33.

66. Jewell, W. R., Thomas, J. H., Sterchi, J. M., Morse, P. A., and Humphrey, L. J. 1976. Critical analysis of treatment of stage II and stage III melanoma patients with immunotherapy. *Ann. Surgery* 183: 543–549.

67. Johnson, R. K., Houchens, D. P., Gaston, M. R., and Goldin, A. 1975. Effects of levamisole (NSC-177023) and tetramisole (NSC-102063) in experimental tumor systems. *Cancer Chemotberapy Rep.* 59: 697–705.

68. Kaliner, M. A., Orange, R. P., Laraia, P. J., and Austen, K. F. 1972. Cholinergic enhancement of the immunologic release of histamine and slow reacting substance of anophylaxis (SRS-A) from human lung. *Fed. Proc.* 31: 748.

69. Kaliner, M. A., Orange, R. P., and Austen, K. F. 1972. Immunological release of histamine and slow reacting substance of anophylaxis from human lung. IV. Enhancement by cholinergic stimulation. *J. Exp. Med.* 136: 556–567.

70. Kaplan, H. S., Babrove, A. M., Fuks, Z., and Strober, S. 1974. Letter to the editor. *N. Engl. J. Med.* 290: 971.

71. Karakousis, C. P., Douglass, H. O., Jr., Yeracaris, P. M., and Holyoke, E. D.

1976. BCG immunotherapy in patients with malignant melanoma. *Arch. Surg.* 111: 716–718.

72. Koopman, W. J., Orange, R. P., and Austen, K. F. 1970. Immunochemical and biologic properties of rat IgE.III. Modulation of the IgE mediated release of slow reacting substance of anophylaxis by agents influencing the level of cyclic 3',5'-adenosine monophosphate. *J. Immunol.* 105: 1096–1102.

72a. Kulkarni, V., Mulbagal, B., and Paranjape, V. L. 1973. Immunostimulating effect of tetramisole on antibody formation against Newcastle disease virus in chicks. *Indian Vet. J.* 50: 225.

73. Levamisole (R12564) Basic Medical Information. 1970. Janssen Pharmaceutica, Research Laboratoria. Beerse Belgium, January.

74. Levamisole (R12564) II. 1970. Janssen R & D, New Brunswick, New Jersey.

75. Levo, Y., Ratler, V., and Ramot, B. 1975. Restoration of cellular immune response by levamisole in patients with Hodgkin's disease. *Biomedicine* 23: 198–200.

76. Levy, R., and Kaplan, H. S. 1974. Impaired lymphocyte function in untreated Hodgkin's disease. *N. Engl. J. Med.* 290: 181–186.

77. Lichtenfeld, J. L., Desner, M., Mardiney, M. R., Jr., Wiernik, P. H. 1974. Amplification of immunologically induced lymphocyte ^{3}H thymidine incorporation by levamisole. *Fed. Proc.* 33: 790.

78. Lichtenfeld, J. L., Desner, M. R., Wiernik, P. H., and Mardiney, M. R., *et al.* 1976. Modulating effects of levamisole (NSC-177023) on human lymphocyte response *in vitro. Cancer Treatment Rep.* 60: 571–574.

79. Lichtenstein, L. M., and Margolis, S. 1968. Histamine release *in vitro.* Inhibition by catecholamines and methylxanthines. *Science* 161: 902–903.

80. Lieberman, R., and Hsu, M. 1976. Levamisole-mediated restoration of cellular immunity in peripheral blood lymphocytes of patients with immunodeficiency disease. *Clin. Immun. Immunopath.* 5: 142–146.

81. Lima, A. O., Javierre, M. Q., da Silva, W. D., *et al.* 1974. Immunological phagocytosis: Effects of drugs on phosphodiesterose activity. *Experientia* 30: 945–946.

82. Lods, J. C., Dujardin, P., and Halpern, G. 1975. Action of levamisole on antibody protection after vaccination with antityphoid and para-typhoid A and B. *Ann. Allergy* 34: 210–212.

83. Lods, J. C., Dujardin, P., and Halpern, G. M. 1976. Levamisole and bone-marrow restoration after chemotherapy. *Lancet* 1: 548.

84. Lukes, R. J., and Tindle, B. H. 1975. Immunoblastic lymphadenopathy. *N. Engl. J. Med.* 292: 1–8.

85. Mackoness, G. B. 1969. The influence of immunologically comitted lymphoid cells on macrophage activity *in vivo. J. Exp. Med.* 129: 973–992.

86. Mansell, P. W. A., DiLuzio, N. R., McNamee, R., Rowden, G., and Proctor, J. W. 1976. Recognition factors and nonspecific macrophage activation in the treatment of neoplastic disease. *Ann. N.Y. Acad. Sci.* 277: 20–44.

87. Mantovani, A., and Spreafico, F. 1975. Allogeneic tumor enhancement by levamisole, a new immunostimulatory compound: Studies on cell-mediated immunity and humoral antibody response. *Eur. J. Cancer* 11: 537–544.

88. Mastrangelo, M. J., Bellet, R. E., Berkelhammer, J., and Clark, W. H., Jr.

1975. Regression of pulmonary metastatic disease associated with intralesional BCG therapy of intracutaneous melanoma metastases. *Cancer* 36: 1305–1308.

89. Mastrangelo, M. J., Berd, D., and Bellet, R. E. 1976. Critical review of previously reported clinical trials of cancer immunotherapy with nonspecific immunostimulants. *Ann. N.Y. Acad. Sci.* 277: 94–123.

90. Mathe, G. 1971. Experimental basis and first clinical controlled trials of leukemia active immunotherapy, in B. Amos (ed.), *Progress in Immunology,* p. 959. Academic Press, New York.

91. McCarthy, W. H., Cotton, G., Carlon, A., Milton, G. W., and Kossard, S. 1973. Immunotherapy of malignant melanoma, a clinical trial. *Cancer* 32: 97–103.

92. McKneally, M. F., Mauer, C., Kansel, H. W., and Alley, R. 1976. Regional immunotherapy with intrapleural BCG for lung cancer. *J. Thorac. Cardiovasc. Surg.* 72: 333–338.

93. Mikus, J. P., Carrington, C. B., and Gaensler, E. A. 1974. Rapidly fatal cytomegalovirus pneumonia in Hodgkin's disease. *Respiration* 31: 439–448.

94. Muller, S. A. 1967. Association of Zoster and malignant disorders in children. *Arch. Dermatol.* 96: 657–664.

94a. Nadler, S. H., and Moore, G. E. 1969. Immunotherapy of malignant disease. *Arch. Surg.* 99: 376.

95. Nathanson, L. 1974. Use of BCG in the treatment of human neoplasia, a review. *Sem. Oncol.* 1: 337 350.

96. Nemoto, T., Han, T., Minowada, J., Angkur, V., Chamberlain, A., and Dao, T. L. 1974. Cell-mediated immune status of breast cancer patients: Evaluation by skin tests, lymphocyte stimulation, and counts of Rosette-forming cells. *J. Natl. Cancer Inst.* 53: 641–645.

97. Oettgen, H. F., Pinsky, C. M., and Delmonte, L. 1976. Treatment of cancer with immunomodulators. *Med. Clin. N. A.* 60(3): 511–537.

98. Oliveira Lima, A., Javierre, M. Q., Dias da Silva, W., and Camara, S. D. 1974. Immunological phagocytosis: Effect of drugs on phosphodiesterose activity. *Experientia* 30: 945.

99. Olkowski, Z. L., and Williams, S. A. 1975. T-lymphocyte levels in the peripheral blood of patients with cancer of the head and neck. *Ann. J. Surg.* 130: 440–444.

100. Oss, van, C. J., and Gillman, C. F. 1972. Phagocytosis as a surface phenomenon. I. Contact angles and phagocytosis of nonopsomized bacteria. *J. Reticulo Soc.* 12: 283–292.

101. Pabst, H. F., and Crawford, J. A. 1974. Enhancement of *in vitro* cellular immune response by L-tetramisole. *Pediat. Res.* 8: 416.

102. Pabst, H. F., and Crawford, J. 1975. L-tetramisole, enhancement of human lymphocyte response to antigen. *Clin. Exp. Immunol.* 21: 468–473.

103. Pike, M. C., and Snyderman, R. 1976. Augmentation of human monocyte chemotactic response by levamisole. *Nature* 261: 136–137.

103a. Potter, C. W., Carr, I., and Jennings, R. 1974. Levamisole inactive in treatment of four animal tumours. *Nature* 249: 567.

104. Ramot, B., Biniaminov, M., Shoham, C., and Rosenthal, E. 1976. Effect of levamisole on E-rosette-forming cells *in vivo* and *in vitro* in Hodgkin's disease. *N. Engl. J. Med.* 294: 809–811.

105. Ramot, B., Biniaminov, M., and Rosenthal, E. The unblocking effect of levamisole on a subpopulation of T-lymphocytes in Hodgkin's disease, in Proceedings of the Third Conference on Modulation of Host Immune Reactions in the Prevention or Treatment of Induced Neoplasias, 1976 (in press).

106. Renoux, G., and Renoux, M. 1971. Effet immunostimulant d'un imidothiazole dans l'immunization des souris contre l'infection por Brucella abortos. C. R. Hebdomad. Séances l'Acad. Sci. (Paris) 272: 349–350.

107. Renoux, G., and Renoux, M. 1972. Antigenic competition and non-specific immunity after a Rickettsial infection in mice: Restoration of antibacterial immunity by phenyl-imidothiazole treatment. J. Immunol. 109: 761.

108. Renoux, G., and Renoux, M. 1972. Levamisole inhibits and cures a solid malignant tumour and its pulmonary metastases in mice. Nature New Biol. 240: 217–218.

109. Renoux, G., and Renoux, M. 1973. Stimulation of antibrucella vaccination in mice by tetramisole, a phenyl-imidothiazole salt. Infect. Immun. 8: 544–548.

110. Renoux, G., and Renoux, M. 1974. Modulation of immune reactivity by phenylimidothiazole salts in mice immunized by sheep red blood cells. J. Immunol. 113: 779–790.

111. Renoux, G., Renoux, M., and Aycardi, D. 1976. Levamisole promotes the killing of Listeria monocytogenes by macrophages. Fed. Proc. 35: 335.

112. Renoux, G., Renoux, M., and Pabst, A. Influences of levamisole on T-cell reactivity and on survival of untractable cancer patients. Second Conference on Modulation of Host Immune Resistance in the Prevention or Treatment of Induced Neoplasias, 1975. Fogarty International Center Proceedings No. 28. U.S. Govt. Printing Office, Washington, D.C. (in press).

113. Rockdeschel, J. C., Stephen, B. S., Codish, S. D., Stronahan, A., and McKneally, M. F. 1972. Postoperative empyema improves survival in lung cancer. N. Engl. J. Med. 287: 1013–1017.

114. Rojas, A. F., Feierstein, J. N., Mickiewicz, E., Glait, H., and Olivari, A. J. 1976. Levamisole advanced human breast cancer. Lancet 1: 211–215.

115. Rosenthal, M., Trabert, U., and Muller, W. 1976. Leucocytotoxic effect of levamisole. Lancet 1: 369.

116. Russell, R. J., Wilkinson, P. C., Sless, F., and Parrott, D. M. V. 1975. Chemotaxis of lymphoblasts. Nature 256: 646.

117. Ruuskanen, O., Remes, M., Makela, A., Isomaki, H., and Toivanen, A. 1976. Levamisole and agranulocytosis. Lancet, October 30.

118. Sadowski, J. M., and Rapp, F. 1975. Inhibition by levamisole of metastases by cells transformed by herpes simplex virus type 1 (38776). Proc. Soc. Exp. Biol. Med. 149: 219–222.

119. Sampson, D., and Lui, A. 1976. The effect of levamisole on cell-mediated immunity and suppressor cell function. Cancer Res. 36: 952–955.

120. Schmidt, M. E., and Douglas, S. D. 1976. Effects of levamisole on human monocyte function and immunoprotein receptors. Clin. Immunol. Immunopath. 6: 299–305.

121. Schreiber, A. D., Parsons, J., and Cooper, R. A. 1975. Effect of levamisole on the human monocyte IgE receptor. Blood 46: 1018.

122. Schuermans, Y. 1975. Levamisole in rheumatoid arthritis. *Lancet* 1: 111.

123. Sensenig, D. M., Rossi, N. P., and Ehre-haft, J. L. 1963. Results of the surgical treatment of bronchogenic carcinoma. *Surg. Gynecol. Obstet.* 116: 279–384.

124. Shibata, H. R., Jerry, L. M., Lewis, M. G., Mansell, P. W. A., Capek, A., and Marquis, G. 1976. Immunotherapy of human malignant melanoma with irradiated tumor cells, oral bacillus Calmette-Guerin, and levamisole. *Ann. N.Y. Acad. Sci.*

125. Silverman, N. A., Alexander, J. C. Hollinshead, A. C., and Chretieu, P. B. 1976. Correlation of tumor burden with *in vitro* lymphocyte reactivity and antibodies to herpes virus tumor-associated antigens in squamous cell carcinoma of the head and neck. *Cancer* 37: 135–140.

126. Snyderman, R., Daniels, C. A., and Pike, M. C. Levamisole and human monocyte chemotaxis: Reversal of an influenzal induced chemotactic defect, *in* Proceedings of the Third Converence on Modulation of Host Immune Resistance in the Prevention or Treatment of Adrenal Neoplasias, 1976 (in press).

127. Sokal, J. E., and Firat, D. 1965. Varacella-Zoster infection in Hodgkin's disease. *Amer. J. Med.* 39: 452–463.

128. Sokal, J. E., Aungst, C. W., and Snyderman, M. 1974. Delay in progression of malignant lymphoma after BCG vaccination. *N. Engl. J. Med.* 291: 1226–1230.

129. Sparks, F. C., Silverstein, M. J., Hunt, J. S., Hasken, C. M., Pilch, J. H., and Morton, D. L. 1973. Complications of BCG immunotherapy in patients with cancer. *N. Engl. J. Med.* 289: 827.

130. Sparks, F. C., Wile, A. G., Ramming, K. P., Silver, H. K. B., Wold, R. W., Morton, D. L. 1976. Immunology and adjuvant chemoimmunotherapy of breast cancer. *Arch. Surg.* 111: 1057–1062.

131. Stecker, V. J., Liauw, L., and Chinea, G. 1976. Effect of levamisole on adherence and chemotaxia of leukocytes. *Fed. Proc.* 35: 531.

132. Stein, J. A., Adler, A., Efraim, S. B., and Maor, M. 1976. Immunocompetence, immunosuppression, and human breast cancer. *Cancer* 38: 1171–1187.

133. Stjernsward, J., Vanky, F., Jondal, M., Wigzell, H., and Sealy, R. 1972. Lymphopenia and change in distribution of human B and T-lymphocytes in peripheral blood induced by irradiation for mammary carcinoma. *Lancet*, pp. 1352–1356.

134. Strom, T. B., Deisserath, A., Mongonroth, J., Carptenter, C. B., and Merrill, J. P. 1972. Alteration of the cytotoxic action of sensitized lymphocytes by cholinergic agents and activations of adenylatecyclose. *Proc. Natl. Acad. Sci. U.S.A.* 69: 2995–2999.

134a. Sumner, W. C., and Foraker, A. G. 1960. Spontaneous regression of human melanoma, clinical and experimental studies. *J. Cancer* 13: 79.

135. Sutherland, E. W., and Robinson, G. A. 1966. The role of cyclic 3′,5′-AMP in the response to catecholamines and other hormones. *Pharmacol. Rev.* 18: 145–160.

136. Sutherland, E. W., Robinson, G. A., and Butcher, R. W. 1968. Some aspects of the biological role of adenosine 3′,5′-monophosphate (cyclic AMP). *Circulation* 37: 279–404.

137. Symoens, J. 1975. Levamisole: An anti-anergic chemotherapeutic agent. An overview. Janssen Pharmaceutica, Research Laboratoria B-2340 Beerse, Belgium.

138. Thienpont, D., Vanparijs, O. F. S., Raeymaekens, A. H. M., Vandenferk, J., Demoen, P. J. A., Allewijn, F. T. N., Marsboom, R. P. H., Niemegeers, C. J. E., Schellekens, K. H. L., and Janssen, P. A. J. 1966. Tetramis-le (R8299), a new patent broad spectrum antihelminthic. Nature 209: 1084–1086.

139. Thrasher, S. G., Yashida, J., Von Oss, C. J., Cohen, S., and Rose, N. R. 1973. Alteration of macrophage interfacial tension by supernatnats of antigen-activated lymphocyte cultures. J. Immunol. 110: 321–326.

140. Tripodi, D., Parks, L. C., and Brugmons, J. 1973. Drug-induced restoration of cutaneous delayed hypersensitivity in anergic patients with cancer. N. Engl. J. Med. 289: 354–357.

141. Twomey, P. L., Catalona, W. G., and Chretieu, P. S. 1974. Cellular immunity in cured cancer patients. Cancer 3: 435–440.

142. Verhaegen, H., DeCree, J., DeCock, W., and Verbruggen, F. 1973. Levamisole and the immune response. N. Engl. J. Med. 289: 1148–1149.

143. Verhaegen, H., DeCock, W., DeCree, J., Verbruggen, F., Verhaegen-Declerq, M., and Brugmas, J. 1975. In vitro restoration by levamisole of thymus-derived lymphocyte function in Hodgkin's disease. Lancet 1: 978.

144. Versijp, G., von Zwet, T. L., and von Furth, R. 1975. Levamisole and functions of peritoneal macrophages. Lancet 1: 798.

145. Wanebo, H. J., Jeeu, M. Y., Strong, E. W., and Oettgen, H. 1975. T-cell deficiency in patients with squamous cell cancer of the head and neck. Amer. J. Surg. 130: 445–451.

146. Wanebo, H. J., Rosen, P. D., Thaler, T., Urban, J. A., and Oettgen, H. F. 1976. Immunobiology of operable breast cancer. Ann. Surg. 184: 258–267.

147. Ward, H. W. C. 1976. Levamisole in the treatment of cancer. Lancet, March 13, pp. 594–595.

148. Watson, R. D., Smith, A. G., and Levy, J. G. 1974. The use of immunoabsorbent columns for the isolation of antibodies specific for antigens associated with human bronchogenic carcinoma. Brit. J. Cancer 29: 183–188.

149. Webster, D. J. T., and Hughes, L. E. 1975. Levamisole. Lancet 1: 389.

150. Wells, S. A., Burdick, J. F., Joseph, W. L., et al. 1973. Delayed cutaneous hypersensitivity reactions to tumor cell antigens and to nonspecific antigens. Prognostic significance in patients with lung cancer. J. Thorac. & Cardiovasc. Surg. 66: 557–562.

151. Whittaker, M. G., and Clark, C. G. 1971. Depressed lymphocyte function in carcinoma of the breast. Brit. J. Surg. 58: 717–720.

152. Wilson, J. F., Marsa, G. W., and Johnson, R. E. 1972. Herpes Zonter in Hodgkin's disease, clinical, histologic, and immunologic correlations. Cancer 29: 461–465.

153. Woodruff, M. F. A. 1975. Tumor inhibitory properties of anaerobic corynebacteria. Transplant. Proc. 7: 229–232.

154. Woods, W. A., Fliegelman, M. J., and Chirigos, M. A. 1975. Effect of levamisole (NSC-177023) on DNA synthesis by lymphocytes from immunosuppressed C57BL mice. Cancer Chemotherapy Rep. 59: 531–536.

155. Woods, W. A., Fliegelman, M. J., and Chirigos, M. A. 1975. Effect of levamisole on the in vitro immune response of spleen lymphocytes. Proc. Soc. Exp. Biol. Med. 148: 1048–1050.

156. Wynants, J., Woestenborghs, R., and Heykants, J. 1975. The gas chromotographic determination of levamisole in body fluids and tissues. Unpublished Biological Research Report, Janssen Research Products Information Service, October.

157. Yaron, M., Yaron, I., and Herzberg, M. 1976. Levamisole in rheumatoid arthritis. Lancet 1: 369.

158. Yeoh, T. S., Yap, E. H., Singh, M., and Ho, B. C. 1975. Drug inhibition of anophytoctin histamine release from peritoneal cells of rats infected with Toxocara conis. Int. Arch. Allergy Appl. Immun. 49: 371–380.

159. Young, R. C., Conder, M. P., Haynes, H. A., and DeVita, V. T. 1972. Delayed hypersensitivity in Hodgkin's disease. Amer. J. Med. 52: 63–72.

160. Ziegler, J. L., and Magrath, I. T. 1973. BCG immunotherapy in Burkitt's lymphoma: Preliminary results of a randomized clinical trial. Natl. Cancer Inst. Monogr. 39: 199–202.

CHAPTER 8

CLINICAL ACTION OF LEVAMISOLE IN CANCER PATIENTS

Alejandro F. Rojas*
Julio N. Feierstein*
Américo J. Olivari
Horacio M. Glait

*Members of
Argentine Foundation of
Oncological Studies
Moreno, Argentina

INTRODUCTION

Deeper knowledge of the levamisole effect on the immune system is extremely necessary and mandatory before associating it with other anticancer therapy because of the possibility of obtaining opposite results. LMS therapy is not a definitive solution for cancer diseases, but it was clearly shown that immune factors need to be controlled, possibly improving them. It is also possible to augment immune recognition to tumor cells or to ameliorate general defenses of the host. Both could give positive results. According to our experience, this was true in cancer patients rendered free of disease by conventional therapies and using LMS as adjuvant.

Since conventional "radical" therapies are not capable of eradicating the totality of tumor cells in the host, certain cancer patients receive little help from localized treatments because distant metastases appear shortly after (58); then, the search for new adjuvant therapies is one of the more important objectives of modern oncology.

Chemotherapy has proved to be capable of destroying tumor cells thereby reducing tumor burden, but until now has been unable to "cure" widespread cancer disease. Last year's intensive chemotherapy has rendered very important results—a good and deep knowledge for controlling toxicity has been obtained. Prophylactic regimens with chemotherapeutic agents have been successful in controlling residual cancer disease after radical treatments (4, 6, 15, 16).

On the other hand, normal and cancer cells have antigenic differences; hence the possibility of recognizing abnormal cells as "non-self" and controlling their growth through the immune machinery also exists (3, 19, 24, 56). The success of immunotherapy in cancer could be dependent on the presence of recognizable tumor antigens in such cells. Spontaneous regression of cancer disease in human cases has frequently supported such concepts, but it appears to be an uncommon phenomenon. There are concrete evidences that cancer patients have a diminution of the immune defenses when compared to normal people, and probably the possibliity of rejecting cancer cells is also impaired (1, 9, 10). It has been repeatedly shown that a relationship between the general immune status of the host and the clinical course of cancer exists (8, 20, 25); the normalization of such functions of the host could be used as another adjuvant to manage cancer's evolution. Since the last century there have been antecedents of cancer immunotherapy (38, 39). More recently, using immuno-stimulants in cancer patients, favorable results have been obtained (34, 35, 36, 57). But these results are dependent on variations of the quality of bacterial strains, and some hazardous side effects appeared in immunodepressive hosts (48). Immunotherapy has yet to prove its potential for controlling cancer diseases.

According to the concepts just mentioned, adjuvant therapies could be planned for killing resting cells, using chemotherapy, or through the normalization of the immune functions of the host (without discarding possible management of the hormonal behavior). Choice of chemical or immune therapies to be used in prophylactic regimens will depend on previous concepts or experience. Since 1972, we have been using immunotherapy in patients rendered free of disease by conventional therapies, comparing them to patients receiving placebo or no further treatments after radical therapies. Only one variable could influence the modification of the clinical course in such patients—immunotherapy. Levamisole was selected as the drug with a probable effect upon the immune system, bearing in mind its possible inefficacy. The choice was made because this is a synthetic compound; its quality is easy to control, it showed low toxicity in previous clinical experiences as antihelmic, and it is easily administrable orally.

Levamisole (LMS) is a phenyl-imidazo thiazole derivative well known as a "dewormer." First reports on the possible effects of LMS on the immune system were made in 1971 (43). After a pilot experience, our first clinical trial on cancer patients began in 1972. Several attempts, with positive results, have been made using LMS, during the last few years (11, 23, 28, 29, 52, 53, 54), but discordant results were also obtained (21, 44); reasons for that probably are that its effects on the immune machinery are not well known yet. LMS seems to have a different mechanism of action compared to other immunostimulators (2, 52).

This chapter describes clinical trials using LMS and placebos on cancer patients after radical therapies, with no evidence of disease progression. We used LMS for this type of patient, instead of advanced or terminal cases, because we wished to prove the effectiveness of the drug in prolonging the disease-free interval.

Obtaining a result in this period is very important because it greatly influences the future clinical course.

Simple techniques were applied for controlling immune status. In this way it was possible to control a great number of patients under protocolized treatments. It could be argued that the information obtained is not conclusive about immune effects of the drug, but our thinking gave more importance to clinical results than to mechanistic ones.

METHODOLOGY

PATIENTS. Five hundred and fifty-two patients were considered in the present study, 228 levamisole (LMS) treated, 48 dextromisole (DMS) treated, 206 under placebo treatment or with no further therapy, and 70 as the "historical control group." One hundred and seventy-nine had breast cancer, 165 head and neck cancer, 133 urogenital malignant diseases, 35 lymphomas, 13 more than one primary tumor (multiples), and 27 other malignant diagnoses (stomach, colon, lung, soft-tissue sarcoma, melanomas).

All were treated and observed after radical therapies. An assessment of having "no evidence of progressing disease" (N.E.D.) was made; they had histological demonstration of their diseases.

Forty-five benign-disease patients were also included for DNCB reactivity comparison. Such patients were reviewed every 3 months, and received no further treatment.

TREATMENTS. LMS is chemically L-2,3,5,6 tetrahydrophenyl-imidazo (2, 1b) thiazole hydrochloride (Fig. 1), and the dextroisomer is named dextromisole (DMS). Both were administered orally, 150 mg once a day. LMS treatments have two schedules:

a.   trial 2 = 150 mg/day, *three consecutive days, every other week*
b.   trial 4 = 150 mg/day, *six consecutive days, every other week*

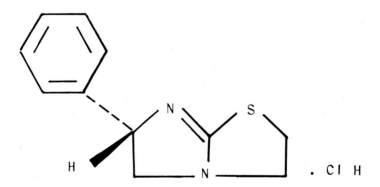

(-) 2,3,5,6, tetrahydro 6 phenylimidazo (2,1b)
thiazole hydrochloride

Fig. 1.   Chemical structure of levamisole.

DMS treatment consisted in only one scheme: 150 mg/day, 3 consecutive days, every other week. Both treatments were maintained until evidence of progressing disease. Daily dose was not changed. Out of protocol, some patients (with advanced diseases) received higher daily doses of up to 600 mg/day.

Skin Tests.   DNCB sensitization was performed with 2000 μg, dissolved in 0.1 ml of acetone. It was applied to the upper arm within the confines of a plastic ring. The acetone was allowed to evaporate; the site was kept dry with a dressing for 5 days; challenge doses of 25 and 100 μg were applied 14 days later to the right forearm and covered for 48 hours. After 48 hours, reactions were read according to the following scale:

Negative response		0 :	No response
		1 :	Erythema
Positive response	*weak*	2 :	Erythema and induration (+ 5 mm)
	strong	3 :	Induration and vesicles
		4 :	Induration and bulla

Patients were also tested for preexisting delayed hypersensitivity to common antigens, *Candida* antigen (1: 1,000 Rivero Lab., Argentina) and SK:SD (40:10 units, Lederle Lab., Pearl River, N.Y.). These antigens were injected intradermally (0.1 ml) in the left forearm. Reactions were read at 48 hours and considered "weak" positive if induration was 5 to 14 mm in diameter or "strong" when exceeding 14 mm, or having central necrosis.

Lymphocyte Culture.   In vitro lymphocyte reactivity to PHA-P (Difco Lab.) was determined using a modification of Park and Good microtechnique. Cultures were performed using three different concentrations: 50, 100, and 150 μg/ml of PHA-P. All cultures (stimulated and controls) were made in triplicates (twelve cultures per patient). Each individual culture contained 50 ml of blood and 50 ml of medium RPMI 1640 (with or without mitogen). After incubation at 37°C for 24 hours, 0.5 μCi of methyl-thymidine (20 Ci/mM, Amersham-Searle) was added in 50 ml of RPMI 1640. After a second incubation at 37°C for 24 hours, cultures were harvested with an automatic multiple harvester (Otto-Hiller Co.) through glass fiber paper (Reeve-Angel) and incorporated labeled-thymidine quantified in a scintillation counter with automatic quench correction by external standardization. The results were expressed as dpm per 50 ml of blood. Values under 9000 dpm were considered abnormal. Noncancer control (n = 40) patients have values over 9000 dpm.

Statistics.   Chi-square test with Yates' correction or Fischer's exact test was used. The McNemar test was used when a before-after comparison was necessary. Generalized Wilcoxon test with Gehan modification was employed to analyze life table results. Student's t test was also used. All P values were obtained for two side tail (18).

RESULTS

DNCB Reactivity

A positive change of DNCB reactivity was observed. Results obtained with challenge doses of 25 and 100 μg have been broken in total positive, weak, and strong positive responses. The most important increment was seen on strong reactivity (Figs. 2 and 3).

DNCB reactivity increased rapidly. The maximum percentage was obtained after 9 months of LMS treatment; at that time 91.0% of treated patients had positive response to $DNCB_{100}$ (70% strong positive) and 73% had similar reactivity to $DNCB_{25}$. After 12 months, 50% of strong reactiv-

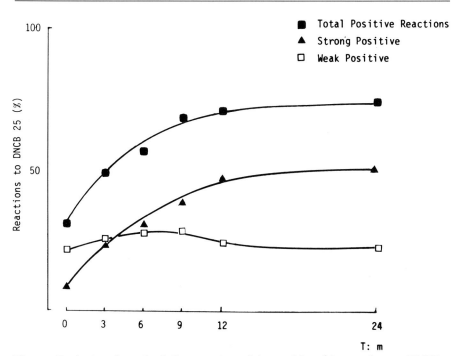

Fig. 2. Evolution along the follow-up time of the positive skin reactions to $DNCB_{25}$ in levamisole-treated patients.

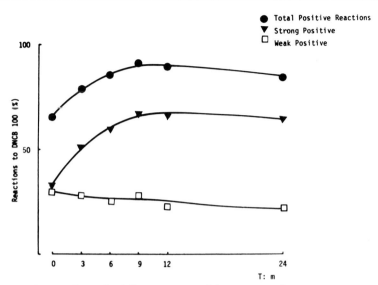

Fig. 3. Evolution along the follow-up time of the positive skin reactions to DNCB$_{100}$ in levamisole-treated patients.

ity to DNCB$_{25}$ was found. The similiarity of the percentage can be seen between strong positive response to DNCB$_{100}$ and total positive to DNCB$_{25}$. After one year of treatment, this relationship is slightly broken because of a stabilization of strong reactivity to DNCB$_{100}$ and an increase of total positive responses to DNCB$_{25}$. This relationship has been found in a majority of the 1,283 cancer patients studied.

An increase in strong reactivity caused the increment on DNCB reactivity. In 1283 cancer patients we demonstrated a total positive response to DNCB of 67.0%; and only 28.7% had strong reactivity. Cancer patients, after LMS treatment, were shown to have a different DNCB reactivity in comparison to the nontreated group. A closed relationship between the DNCB response and the clinical course was demonstrated (Fig. 4). This figure was obtained from a general study of 125 cancer patients followed up with no further treatment after radical therapies. The median disease-free interval was related to DNCB reactivity. There are differences between negative, weak positive, or strong positive responders to DNCB and their clinical course.

Based on these data, the effect of LMS treatment on DNCB reactivity could be relevant to its clinical evolution. It could be argued that DNCB repetitive challenge doses can produce a "resensitization" to DNCB, especially in patients followed up *repeatedly*, and the observed results

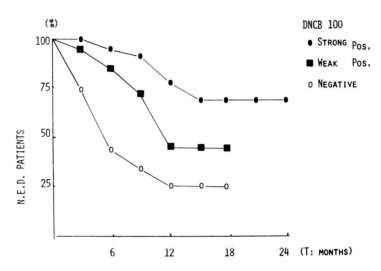

CLINICAL EVOLUTION ACCORDING DNCB RESPONSE IN CA. PATIENTS (125)

Fig. 4. Disease-free interval duration according to $DNCB_{100}$ skin reactivity in cancer patients followed with no further therapy after radical procedures.

could reflect that phenomena. Because of that, we considered the increment, no change, or descent of DNCB reactivity in each patient with time.

DNCB reactions were classified in five grades (see "Methodology"). Any positive change (0–1 or 3–4 or any other) was considered as "an increment" and any change in the other, "a descent."

Analysis of LMS and placebo-treated patients showing an increase in their DNCB reactivity is shown in Figure 5. Resensitization occurred in LMS and placebo groups, but in a different proportion. The higher increase was shown in patients under LMS therapy. Statistical differences appear at 3 months—the LMS group increasing continuously up to 12 months and the placebo group increasing DNCB reactivity up to six months. After that a lowering was observed. On the other hand, the placebo group only reached an increment of 40% and the LMS group reached 80% at 12 months ($P < 0.001$). Both groups had similar clinical conditions, the same follow-up, and received no further treatment, after radical ones, except LMS or placebo therapy.

Obviously, LMS induced a different rate of DNCB resensitization. This phenomenon gives another parameter to be measured: the rate of DNCB increase. From the general study of cancer patients, we obtained information on this aspect in benign disease patients and cancer patients

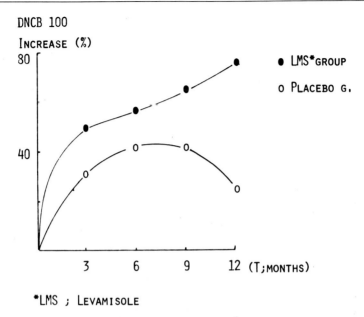

DNCB 100
INCREASE (%)

LMS*GROUP

o PLACEBO G.

(T;MONTHS)

*LMS ; LEVAMISOLE

Fig. 5. Increase of $DNCB_{100}$ skin reactivity along the follow-up time in levamisole- or placebo-treated patients after finishing radical therapies.

(Fig. 6). Skin tumors and lymphomas were also analyzed. The first group had a localized disease and showed no statistical immune depression; the second had a poor prognosis and DNCB response (Fig. 7) and was frequently associated with immuno deficiencies. A clear difference could be established between the benign disease and the cancer group by means of DNCB increment ($P < 0.0005$). A similar trend exists between skin tumors and lymphomas. There is a relationship between normal immune status and DNCB resensitization phenomena. Poor responders have a lower rate of DNCB increment and good responders have a higher one. According to these concepts, LMS reestablished resensitization capacity, i.e., "normalized" DNCB response in cancer patients. It could be postulated that LMS ameliorated either recognition of new antigens or the efficiency of the afferent limb of the immune mechanism. Table 1 shows $DNCB_{100}$ responses in placebo and LMS groups before and after starting treatments. Figure 8 shows LMS and placebo effects on DNCB response; LMS clearly demonstrated a decrease of negative responses and an increase of the strong ones ($P < 0.0005$). The rate of descent of DNCB reactivity was also different; placebo-treated patients showed a 8.2% rate of decreasing reactivity compared to 4.3% in LMS patients.

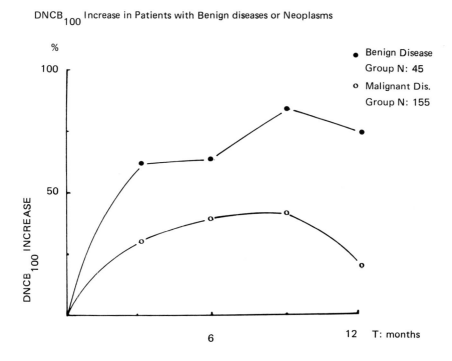

DNCB$_{100}$ Increase in Patients with Benign diseases or Neoplasms

%

- Benign Disease
  Group N: 45
o Malignant Dis.
  Group N: 155

Fig. 6.   Increase of DNCB$_{100}$ skin reactivity along the follow-up time in cancer patients or those having benign diseases after finishing radical therapies. Both groups received no further treatment after such procedures.

It can be assumed that LMS treatment improved DNCB response and "normalized" immune conditions in cancer patients as a comparison between Figures 5 and 6 clearly shows. On the other hand, it was not uncommon that skin reactions to DNCB had a "reactivation," several days after challenge doses in patients receiving LMS.

Preexisting Delayed Hypersensitivity

A different picture has been seen when response to recall antigens (*Candida*, SK SD) was analyzed. Figures 9 and 10 show a small increase of positive responses to SK SD and *Candida* after 3 and 6 months treatment, respectively. After that, a decrease of recall antigens reactivity can be seen. Neither weak nor strong reactions showed any positive change with time.

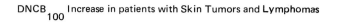

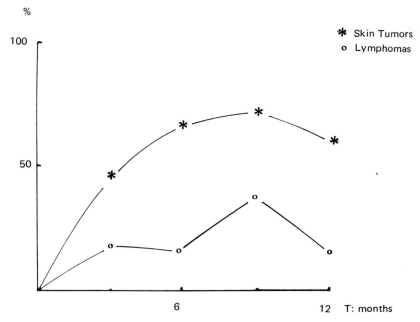

Fig. 7. Increase of $DNCB_{100}$ skin reactivity along the follow-up time after NED assessment in patients having lymphomas or skin tumors and receiving no further treatment.

Table 1. $DNCB_{100}$ response in treated patients

	Before Treatment		After Treatment	
	Total Positives	Strong Positives	Total Positives	Strong Positives
Levamisole-treated (N=219)	65.8%	30.6%	88.1%	63.4%
Placebo-treated (N=200)	70.0%	39.5%	75.0%	50.0%

P value: $0.1 < P < 0.2$ (n.s.) $P < 0.005$

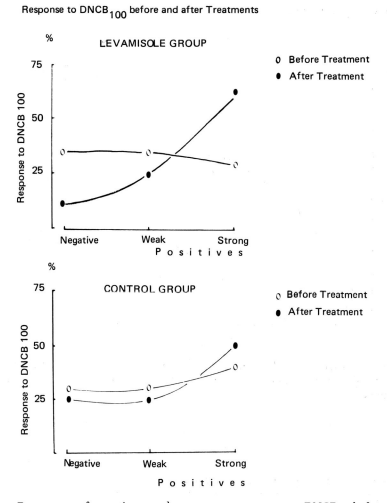

Fig. 8. Percentage of negative, weak, or strong responses to $DNCB_{100}$ before and after levamisole or placebo treatment. Skin reactivity was assessed after radical therapies in cancer patients.

LMS treatment was not associated with an increase of preexisting delayed hypersensitivity, but a decrease trend was observed. In our study of cancer patient evolution and immune reactivity, no relationship was found to *Candida* responses and clinical course, and a slight one was found with SK SD positive response.

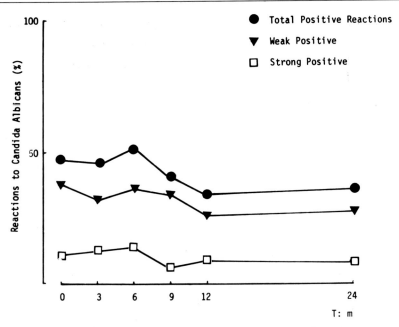

Fig. 9. Evolution of the positive skin reactions to *Candida Albicans* antigen along the follow-up time in levamisole-treated patients.

An increase of lymphocyte count and PHA-P reactivity was observed after three months treatment (Fig. 11). At 6 months, similar values of lymphocyte count were found in relation to previous treatment levels. Lower values of PHA-P reactivity than pretreatment ones have been observed from 6 to 12 months. High PHA-P reactivity and an increase in lymphocyte count have been seen in patients after 24 months of LMS treatment. Lymphocyte count and PHA-P reactivity showed similar variation during the first year, but a higher reactivity per cell was found after 2 years of treatment.

Before LMS therapy, there was an average of 453,000 dpm/10^5 cells; similar values were found up to 12 months (381,000 dpm/10^5 cells); at 24 months, activity was 774,000 dpm/10^5 cells. A relationship between PHA-P lymphocytes reactivity and intradermal weak response to SK SD was seen (Figs. 10 and 11). Great variations have been found, day to day, in PHA-P reactivity in healthy donors under LMS treatment, using whole blood cultures. A different response was found when their purified lymphocytes were cultured.

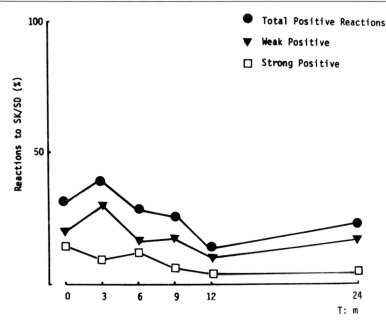

Fig. 10. Evolution of the positive skin reactions to Streptokinase-Streptodornase (SK:SD) along the follow-up time in levamisole-treated patients.

Differences in the time between last drug intake and blood sample withdrawal make it difficult to interpret such results in cancer patients.

Dose Response

Studies were performed using two dosages per week (450 mg/week or 900 mg/week) in trials 2 and 4 (see "Methodology"). Preliminary data showed that patients who were capable of increasing DNCB in a short time had, in general, the best clinical evolution. Some patients needed a long time to increase their reactions or did not increase their DNCB responses; they had the worst clinical course. It was postulated that a higher dosage than was used initially could improve DNCB response and ameliorate clinical course more effectively. Based on our previous experience, we decided to prolong the administration from 3 to 6 days per week. Basically, we did not increase daily doses (similar side effects were expected), and intermittent treatment (every other week) was maintained.

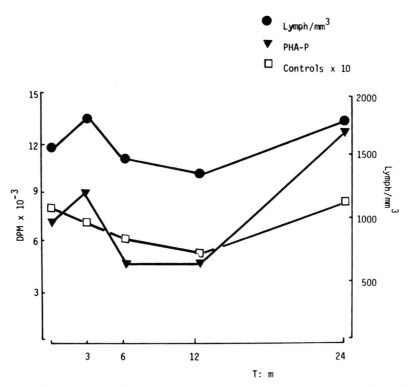

Fig. 11. Average of lymphocyte count, PHA-P stimulated or unstimulated lymphocyte cultures (whole blood technique) measured by H-3 Thymidine uptake in levamisole-treated patients along the follow-up time.

To evaluate the effect of both trials, the $DNCB_{100}$ response of patients under each was analyzed (Fig. 12). A better rate of DNCB increment was seen in trial 4. Under trial 2 it took 12 months to reach 80% $DNCB_{100}$ reactivity, while the same response was obtained in 6 months under trial 4 with a greater statistical difference than trial 2 relative to the control

Table 2. Levamisole side effects

	None	Mild	Severe
Trial 2 (450 mg/week every other week)	106 (89.8%)	10 (8.5%)	2 (1.7%)
Trial 4 (900 mg/week every other week)	81 (81.8%)	15 (15.2%)	3 (3.0%)

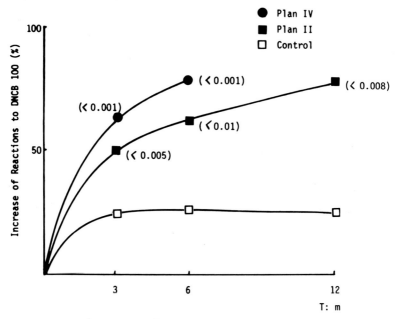

Fig. 12. Increase of $DNCB_{100}$ skin reactivity along the time in NED cancer patients with plan IV (levamisole 900 mg/week), plan II (levamisole 450 mg/week), or placebo.

group (Table 2, Fig. 12). A new scheme for LMS treatment has been adopted since these findings. Patients having strong responses to DNCB (such patients need to maintain their response) receive 450 mg/week alternatively (trial 2). Negative or weak positive responders to $DNCB_{100}$ receive trial 4 (900 mg/week) until they reach a DNCB response of a "strong level." When such reactions occur, trial 2 is used. The concepts of "induction" and "maintenance" have thus been introduced in LMS therapy.

Side Effects

A 13.8% response was observed in LMS-treated patients; they were classified in four groups (Table 3), nausea and vomiting being the most frequent. Some of them have an obvious relation to CNS (48.9%) (sickness, headache, smell, and taste alterations). Furthermore, nausea

Table 3. Type of side effects in 30
levamisole-treated patients

Nausea, vomiting	15 (40.5%)
Sickness, headache	12 (32.4%)
Smell and taste alterations	5 (13.5%)
Skin alterations	2 (5.4%)

and vomiting could be interpreted as effects on specific centers of CNS, in addition to a direct action on the gastrointestinal tract.

Anorexia, nervousness, nightmares, sleep disturbances, influenza-like syndromes and two lymphopenias were also observed. One patient related a tendency to suicide and a great depression under LMS treatment; both symptoms disappeared one day after suspension of medication. We did not find severe agranulocytosis.

A relation between the general status and side effects was also seen, but the reasons for the appearance of side effects are still unknown. We analyzed skin reactivity to DNCB in patients with and without side effects. The first group presented a lower DNCB response before treatment, but a higher increment during treatment. The most important difference has been found in strong reactivity to $DNCB_{25}$; patients who presented side effects had a 4.0% rate before and 40.0% after LMS treatment in comparison to 8.5% before and 26.5% after in patients without side effects. After LMS treatment, $DNCB_{25}$ reactivity has not shown a statistical difference between the groups ($P < 0.2$), but a trend was established. Patients having mild side effects increased their DNCB reactivity strongly and quickly.

LMS ACTION ON CLINICAL TRIALS

Locally Advanced Breast Cancer

It is well established that control of this type of tumor by radiotherapy is not sufficient to prevent the use of adjuvant therapy.

Zucali et al. (58) have reported a series showing a 10-month relapse mean time as well as a 2.5- to 3-year mean survival time. With the addition of LMS, administered by mouth, we have initially achieved, and presently confirmed, that the first period can be extended up to nearly 30 months, while keeping a survival rate of over 50% four years after the onset of "radical" therapies.

Patients

After having established radiation therapy on the chest wall, in internal and external tangential fields, in the supraclavicular area, and in the posterior axillary field (delivered by a cobalt-60 source over a mean period of 2 months), patients were reviewed until there was evidence of a first recurrence, either local or distant metastases. We can divide the study into two parts. The first one was conducted with patients under randomization. Thus, 43 patients in stage III of breast cancer (U.I.C.C. classification) were adequately treated: 23 acted as control; and 20 received LMS orally, 150 mg a day for 3 consecutive days every other week, until there was evidence of progressing disease. The second part consisted of analyzing 70 patients who had received radiation therapy, since demonstrating stage III breast cancer between late 1971 and mid-1974 (historical control group). All the diagnoses were confirmed by biopsy.

Table 4.   Control and 20 levamisole-treated patients

	Control	Levamisole
Age, menopausal status, and parity *of patients prior to radiotherapy*		
Average age	58.3	60.0
	(39–80)	(34–82)
Average age at menopause	49.1	49.5
	(41–57)	(42–56)
Number of premenopausal patients	3	2
Average number of children	2.2	1.8
	Control	Levamisole
Distribution of patients *according to TNM classification (UICC)*		
T3 N1 MO	34.8% (8)	30.0% (6)
T3 N2 MO	26.1% (6)	35.0% (7)
T3 N3 MO	13.0% (3)	10.0% (2)
T4 N1 MO	4.3% (1)	5.0% (1)
T4 N2 MO	17.4% (4)	5.0% (1)
T4 N3 MO	4.3% (1)	15.0% (3)
Total number of patients	23	20

The historical control group served to verify results obtained in the first control group; another 33 stage III breast cancer patients were studied and treated with LMS without randomization procedures. There was a follow-up of all patients, consisting of physical examination, liver-function tests, complete blood count and differential and platelet counts. Skeletal survey, bone scan, and chest X rays were repeated every 3–6 months, or earlier if warranted by the patients' symptoms. The breakdown of the randomized group—age, TNM classification, and menopausal status—appears in Tables 4 and 5.

The randomized control group and patients under treatment were sensitized after the completion of radiotherapy, using DNCB (see "Methodology"). The tables show that the groups were comparable, especially the randomized one. In the other groups (historical control vs. new LMS group) certain differences with regard to the tumor size can be appreciated; a larger number of T4s being present in the historical control

Table 5. Historical control and 33 levamisole-treated patients

	Historical Control	Levamisole
Age and Menopausal Status of Patients Prior to Radiotherapy		
Average age	59.1 (23–88)	55.8 (33–82)
Average age at menopause	49.3 (40–59)	49.2 (42–56)
Number of premenopausal patients	22	12
	Historical Control	Levamisole
Distribution of Patients According to TNM classification (UICC)		
T3 N1 MO	21.4% (15)	30.3% (10)
T3 N2 MO	32.9% (23)	36.4% (12)
T3 N3 MO	5.7% (4)	9.1% (3)
T4 N1 MO	22.9% (16)	12.1% (4)
T4 N2 MO	10.0% (7)	3.0% (1)
T4 N3 MO	7.1% (5)	9.1% (3)
Total number of patients	70	33

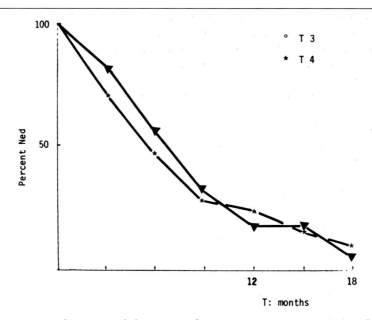

Fig. 13. Disease-free interval duration in breast cancer stage III patients (historical control group) according to their tumor size before radiation therapy.

group. This, as well as the difference in the number of N1, N2, and N3 axillary nodes, might modify the results.

The historical control showed that the mean time for T3 and T4 tumors was essentially the same, with a 6-month median time in the case of T4s, and about 7.5 months for T3s. Both groups had less than 10% disease-free patients after 18 months' time (Fig. 13).

Similar results were found for N1, N2, and N3 nodes. In those classified as N3 55% were disease-free 3 months after completion of radiotherapy, while 75% of the patients were disease-free with N1 and N2 nodes. However, median times are essentially the same and fluctuate between 6 and 7.5 months (Fig. 14).

Another important prognostic point concerns the number of those in the premenopausal period. There exists (Table 5) a high percentage of such patients in the nonrandomized group under LMS treatment—12 out of 33. Obviously, if the evolution of premenopausal patients (as it has been reported) is worse than that of postmenopausal, this could be a disadvantage to the possible effects of LMS. This will be dealt with later in more detail.

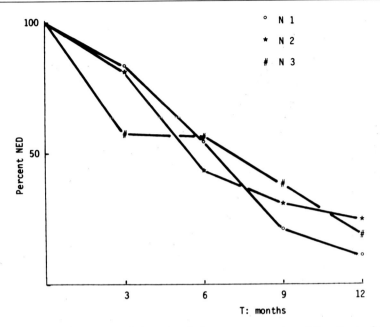

Fig. 14.   Disease-free interval duration in breast cancer stage III patients (historical control group) according to lymph node involvement before radiation therapy.

Results

CLINICAL EVALUATION.   In the randomized group, 43 patients were evaluated: 20 in the treated group and 23 in the control group. All patients have been reviewed for a period of at least 30 months. Figure 15 shows the evolution of the appearance of the progressing disease in randomized groups. The control group shows a median time of 9.2 months, while in the LMS-treated group the median time is 22 months (P < 0.01; generalized Wilcoxon test).

At 24 months after radiation therapy the untreated group is 9% disease-free, vs. 25% for the treated group.

Patients' survival data appear in Figure 16; it will be noted that the median survival time for the control group is 21 months, and up to 40 months for the LMS-treated group. More than 50% are alive in the treated group, while only 23% remain alive in the control group.

Another important fact is the type of metastasis appearing in the treated group and in that serving as the control (Table 6). It is important to

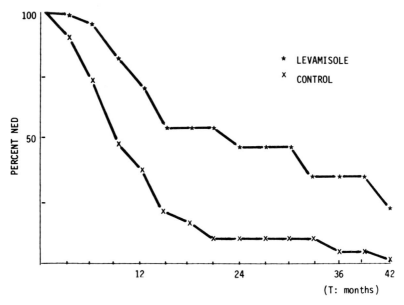

Fig. 15. Disease-free interval-duration in breast cancer stage III patients receiving levamisole or no further therapy (randomized study) after finishing radiotherapy.

Table 6. Comparison of sites of metastases in randomized group

Site of Metastasis	Control	Levamisole
Local recurrence	26.1% (6/23)	30.8% (4/13)
Skin	17.4% (4/23)	7.7% (1/13)
Nodes	21.7% (5/23)	15.4% (2/13)
Lungs	21.7% (5/23)	61.5% (8/13)[a]
Bones	39.1% (9/23)	23.1% (3/13)
Liver	17.4% (4/23)	0.0% (0/13)
Other	13.0% (3/23)	7.7% (1/13)

a. $P < 0.005$, χ^2 test.

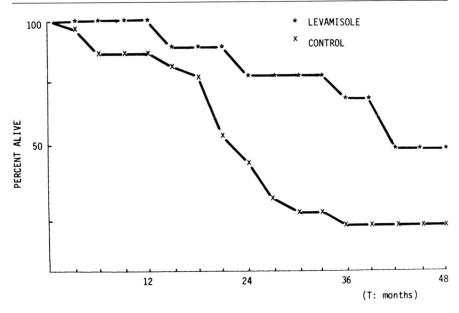

Fig. 16.   Survival in breast cancer stage III patients receiving levamisole or no further therapy (randomized study) after finishing radiation treatment.

emphasize that only patients showing a relapse have been included. In the LMS group, only 13 patients developed metastases, while all in the control group showed progressing disease.

Table 6 reveals a change in the incidence of sites of metastasis. There are no substantial differences, with the singular exception of lung and/or pleura metastases, a 61.5% in LMS-treated group vs. 21.7% for the control group ($P < 0.05$, χ^2 test, with Yates' correction).

HISTORICAL CONTROL VS. NONRANDOMIZED LMS GROUP.   In order to assure that the observed evolution in patients of the control group under randomization actually reflected the evolution of inoperable stage III breast cancer patients, 70 historical control patients were studied.

Median time for relapse onset in the historical control group was 7.5 months; it can be compared to that of the LMS-treated group, extending up to 31 months (Fig. 17). The historical control group showed a slightly shorter period, although without statistical significance, as compared with the randomized control group. At 36 months, 40% of the

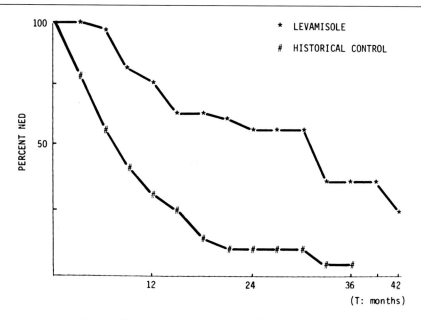

Fig. 17. Comparison of the disease-free-interval duration in stage III breast cancer patients receiving no further therapy (historical control group) or levamisole (nonrandomized group) after finishing radiotherapy.

treated patients were disease-free, while only 5% in the historical control group were.

Median survival median time for historical control was 21.8 months, while the median survival for those treated reached 39 months (P < 0.01, generalized Wilcoxon test).

Figure 18 shows recurrence times for the historical control and non-randomized LMS group. (Here only the evolution of relapsing patients has been taken into account.) Both curves are very similar. Median time for recurrence is 6 months for the historical control group and 10 months for the LMS-treated group.

Statistical analysis, however, reveals a P < 0.01 (generalized Wilcoxon test). There is a statistical increase in the interval of appearance of metastases in the treated group, but it is obvious that this is not a reflection of the clinical evolution of the total group. Patients having no evidence of disease cause a median time shift to nearly 30 months. Table 7 shows recurrence sites for historical control and LMS-treated groups. Here again, there is a marked increase in the frequency of pulmonary and pleural metastasis; the treated group shows a 47.4% increase against an

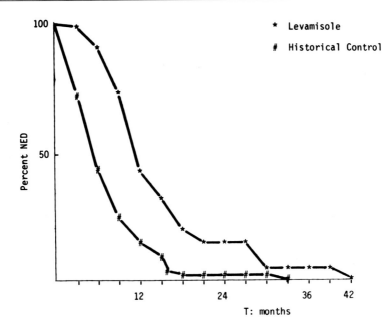

Fig. 18. Onset of relapses in those patients who presented it treated with levamisole or no further therapy after radiation treatment.

Table 7. Comparison of sites of metastases in historical control and 33 levamisole-treated patients

Site of Metastasis	Historical Control	Levamisole
Local recurrence	16.7% (9/54)	36.8% (7/19)[a]
Skin	16.7% (9/54)	5.3% (1/19)
Nodes	22.2% (12/54)	10.5% (2/19)
Lungs	18.5% (10/54)	47.4% (9/19)[b]
Bones	37.0% (20/54)	21.1% (4/19)
Liver	5.6% (3/54)	5.3% (1/19)
Other	3.7% (2/54)	5.3% (1/19)

a. $P < 0.025$, χ^2 test.
b. $P < 0.05$, χ^2 test.

18.5% for the historical control $(P < 0.05)$ $(\chi^2$ test, with Yates' correction). The LMS group has an increase in the number of local recurrences (in comparison with our first treated group) and also with the historical control group; LMS shows 36.8% against 16.7% $(P < 0.025)$ $(\chi^2$ test).

This increase had not been observed before. The reason may lie in the larger number of premenopausal patients, or in a different interval for the onset of local relapses. Only those patients with evidence of disease were studied in order to evaluate—as in the previous case—the presence of a different action by LMS on the sites of metastasis.

Although metastasis sites differ, in the case of the lungs and local recurrences, between the nonrandomized LMS group and the historical control, determining whether there is any variation in the onset time of that type of metastasis is also important, since similar numbers could be arrived at with completely different times. That is why the data were classified according to an analytical method based on Weibull distribution. Thus, a frequency breakdown could be established for each metastasis site.

The onset time in three sites for the LMS vs. historical control groups was also studied. The first data analyzed were those of bone metastases. Within the historical control the greatest frequency for the onset of bone metastasis appears at 6 months, while in the LMS group this is true at 9 months' time: the distribution is very similar. The positive reactions to DNCB in treated patients having bone metastases was zero. In the specific case of pleuropulmonary metastasis, it was noted that the historical control group showed a high incidence during the first 6 months after completion of treatment, while pulmonary metastases in the LMS-treated group appeared with a median time of 13.3 months and extended up to about 2 years.

Patients with lung metastases revealed a response of 28.6% strong reactions to $DNCB_{100}$ before and 33.3% after treatment. Therefore, it was a population with a low percentage of strong reactions to $DNCB_{100}$. The change, in spite of the treatment, was not significant.

Patients showing negative or weak reactions to $DNCB_{100}$ revealed their metastases before 13 months $(\bar{x} = 10.3$ m$)$, while those who showed strong or increased reactions had their metastases after that period $(\bar{x} = 16.5$ m$)$. The high incidence of pulmonary metastases after radiotherapy revealed an action on the pulmonary tissue which is increased by the action of LMS. It was interesting to verify the lack of correlation between the irradiated side and the site of lung metastasis.

In respect to local recurrences the situation was somewhat different. The maximum frequency of onset of local progressions appeared, for the historical control, at 9 months, while within the LMS group, two populations could be identified. There was one in which local progressions

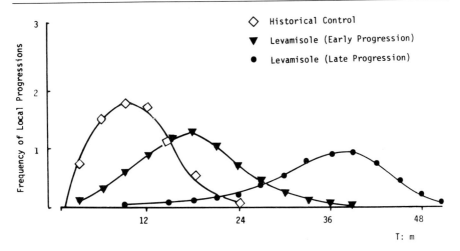

Fig. 19. Frequency of appearance of local progressions along the time in historical control patients or levamisole-treated stage III breast cancer patients (Weibull analysis).

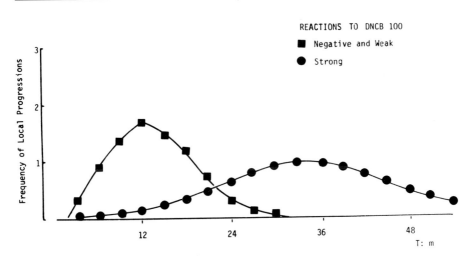

Fig. 20. Appearance of local progressions along the time in levamisole stage III breast cancer patients according to their $DNCB_{100}$ skin reactivity (Weibull analysis).

appeared with maximum frequency at 18 months and tended to disappear beyond 30 months (median time = 17.3m); while the other (median = 36.2 m) had its maximum frequency at 30 months after completion of treatment. This second type of local progression did not exist in the historical control group. LMS caused this new phenomena of the onset of a local progression with a maximum incidence at 39 months (Fig. 19).

Local progressions occurred in a population showing an incidence of 57.1% strong reactions to $DNCB_{100}$. A follow-up study of patients showing local progressions and their correlation with reactions to $DNCB_{100}$ is condensed in Figure 20. Local progressions for patients with negative or weak positive reactions showed a maximum frequency of local progression at 12 months, while the maximum frequency in patients having strong positive reactions occurred at 33 months ($\bar{x}$ = 41.6 m; median time: 36.2 m). An analysis of Figures 19 and 20 clearly shows that patients presenting the "early local progression" were treated (patients who had maintained negative or weak positive reactions from the beginning, or who digressed to that level). Those who showed a "late local progression" were those who, from lower levels, reached or maintained the strong reaction level to $DNCB_{100}$.

IMMUNE REACTIVITY. LMS augmented the rate of DNCB reactivity compared to the control group. The maximum difference was obtained after 9 months (Fig. 21). This figure shows a continuous increment of DNCB response in LMS patients, while no control patient increased over 50% and a trend toward decreased reactions at twelve months ($P < 0.05$) was noted.

Figure 22 shows the pre- and post-treatment responses in LMS patients. Before treatment, the population showed a positive reaction of 45%; after it, 83.3% of the patients showed positive reactions. The same figure clearly shows that more than half the post-treatment responses were considered strong, i.e., grades 3 and 4 (60%).

Figures 23 and 24 show the percentage of positive responses to DNCB-recall antigens and lymphocyte count in stage III breast cancer patients before, immediately, and 6–12 months after radiotherapy in control or treated groups. An important decrease in the percentage of $DNCB_{100}$ and $DNCB_{25}$ Candida positive responses and in the lymphocyte count can be appreciated immediately after radiotherapy.

In the control group, the negative trend continued up to one year. On the other hand, the LMS group showed a similar decrease in positive responses immediately after radiation, but a positive trend was finally appreciated; at twelve months the DNCB positive responses and lymphocyte counts showed a higher value than preirradiation ones. The positive response to recall antigens showed little change, but it is necessary to note

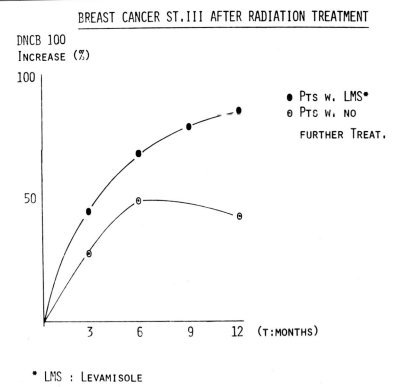

BREAST CANCER ST.III AFTER RADIATION TREATMENT

DNCB 100
INCREASE (%)

● PTS W. LMS*
Ө PTS W. NO
FURTHER TREAT.

(T:MONTHS)

* LMS : LEVAMISOLE

Fig. 21. Increase of $DNCB_{100}$ skin reactivity along the follow-up time in stage III breast cancer patients receiving levamisole or no further treatment after finishing radiotherapy.

that in the control group an important diminution of such responses was observed. The differences between both groups are highly significant ($P <$ 0.001). It was noticed that patients showing sustained negative reactions to $DNCB_{100}$, or those whose reactions became negative, revealed a median relapse time of 12 months (Fig. 25).

Patients who maintained weak positive reactions or who increased their negative reactivity to that level, showed a median relapse time of 14 months, but a stabilization after that time kept 48% of these patients disease-free up to 36 months.

Median time for strong reactions has not been determined yet, but it is estimated at close to 36 months; at 24 months there are 68% of disease-free patients when they showed positive strong reactions. The evolution of historical control patients, post- (50) and premenopausal (37), was stud-

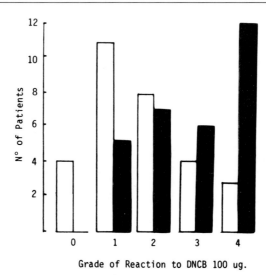

Fig. 22. Grade of skin reactivity to DNCB$_{100}$ in stage III breast cancer patients before (clear) and after (dark) levamisole therapy.

ied. Essentially, the median time for recurrence of the disease was quite similar in both groups (Fig. 26).

Historical control premenopausal disease-free patients were zero after 21 months, and 6% at 32 months in the postmenopausal group. However, these differences did not have statistical significance, according to the generalized Wilcoxon test.

Pre- and postmenopausal LMS-treated patients showed similar median relapse times (Fig. 27). However, at 42 months, the premenopausal group was 55% disease-free, and 22% in the postmenopausal. Neither curve differs statistically yet (generalized Wilcoxon test), but a favorable change has been observed in the evolution trend of premenopausal patients.

TOXICITY.   Toxicity in these patients was negligible, and in only 3 cases was there mild toxicity with 150 mg a day for 3 consecutive days every other week (Table 8). No patient in this group had to give up the treatment because of severe toxic reactions.

DISCUSSION.   As can be observed in Tables 4 and 5, treated and nontreated patient groups are comparable. LMS significantly increased the number of patients with "no evidence of disease" and notice-

BREAST CANCER ST.III - CONTROL GROUP

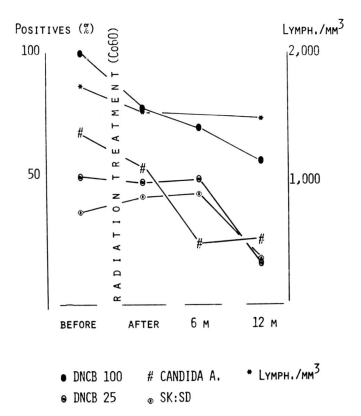

Fig. 23. Percentage of positive skin responses to DNCB$_{100}$, DNCB$_{25}$, *Candida* Antigen and SK:SD and the average lymphocyte count in stage III breast cancer patients receiving radiotherapy and no further therapy after it. Results are expressed before, immediately after and at six and twelve months after finishing such therapy.

ably extended the N. E. D. period after radiation treatment in treated groups.

Historical controls and control groups under randomization revealed similar recurrence periods. Therefore, we can discard the hypothesis that the first group studied (control under randomization) was one that did not reflect the real evolution in these patients.

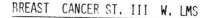

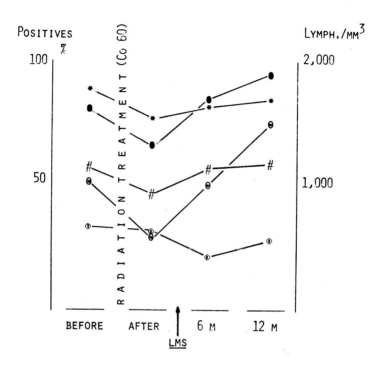

Fig. 24. Percentage of positive skin responses to DNCB$_{100}$, DNCB$_{25}$, *Candida* Antigen, SK:SD, and lymphocyte count in stage III breast cancer patients receiving radiotherapy and levamisole after it. Expressed results were obtained before radiotherapy, immediately after and at six and twelve months after finishing it.

It is confirmed that LMS shows a definitive and positive effect on the evolution of patients with inoperable breast cancer after radiation therapy.

Between pre- and postmenopausal-treated patients, there is reason to believe that there was a distinct effect on immune reactivity of the first

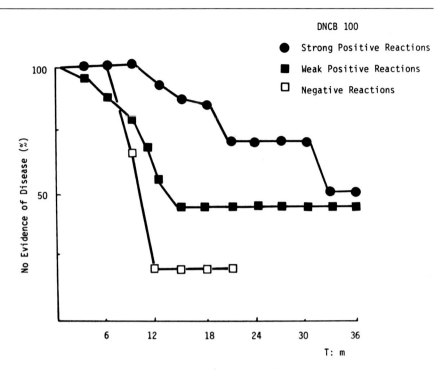

Fig. 25. Disease-free-interval duration in stage III breast cancer patients receiving levamisole after radiotherapy according to their $DNCB_{100}$ skin reactivity along the follow-up time.

population, which was younger than the second. But postmenopausal women changed more, although there were no significant differences between both groups. It is difficult to explain this effect, especially in terms of immune reactivity. We have observed certain alterations in the menstrual rhythm of treated patients.

There is suggestive evidence that LMS could have effects on the central nervous system. It may condition responses, not only immunological but of the breast cancer evolution too.

The effect of LMS on the metastasis site and local recurrence is also something to be reckoned with. As to the observed local recurrences, it is important to note their correlation with responses to DNCB. All patients who developed local recurrences beyond 36 months had strong, positive reactions from the beginning or else increased their reactions (late local progressions). The "late local recurrence" is easy to control; two patients with this progression having more than 52 months' evolution have not

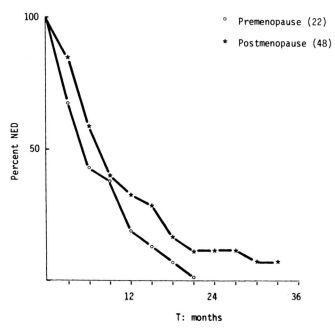

Fig. 26. Disease-free-interval duration in stage III breast cancer patients receiving no further therapy after finishing radiation treatment according to their menopausal status (historical control group).

Table 8. Breast cancer stage III under levamisole treatment

	Number in trial	Side Effects		
		None	Mild	Severe
Trial 2 (450 mg/week)	36	33	3 (8.3%)	—
Trial 4 (900 mg/week)	17	17	—	—

Type of Side Effects

Vomiting	1
Headache—smell alterations	1
Skin rash	1
Other	1
Total	4

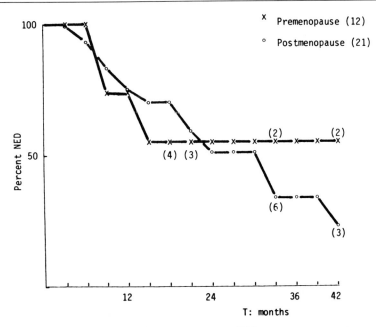

Fig. 27. Disease-free-interval duration in stage III breast cancer patients receiving levamisole after finishing radiotherapy according to their menopausal status.

had another distant evidence of the disease, and a new local therapy reestablished the disease-free status.

Operable Breast Cancer

Patients. A pilot study was done using LMS as prophylactic treatment in breast cancer stage II after surgery and radiation therapy and compared to a placebo group (Table 9). Twenty patients received placebo; the average age in this group was 51.9 years. Seven were in premenopausal status and 30% had positive axillary nodes; twenty-six received LMS (150 mg/day, alternate weeks, 3 or 6 days according to DNCB response); the average age was 50.7 years. Twelve were in premenopausal status and 46.2% had positive axillary nodes. The average follow-up period was 9.3 months in placebo and 11 months in the LMS group. Strong positive responders received trial 2, and negative or weak positive responders received trial 4; 73.1% of the treated patients received the latter.

Table 9. Breast cancer stage II

	Placebo		Levamisole	
	Before	After	Before	After
DNCB$_{25}$				
Total positives	11/20	11/20	10/26	19/26
	(55.0)	(55.0)	(38.5)	(73.1)
Strong positives	1/20	3/20	1/26	10/26
	(5.0)	(15.0)	(3.8)	(38.5)
DNCB$_{100}$				
Total positives	14/20	16/20	18/26	24/26
	(70.0)	(80.0)	(69.2)	(92.3)
Strong positives	9/20	8/20	7/26	15/26
	(45.0)	(40.0)	(26.9)	(57.7)

Immune Reactivity. Results of the DNCB$_{100}$ increase, rate of LMS, and placebo groups are shown in Figure 28. A positive increment was observed after three months of LMS therapy ($P < 0.05$, McNemar). The placebo group showed a negative trend of DNCB increasing rate; this is very important at 12 months. A different trend occurred in the LMS group; a little increase after 3 months but a strong one at 12 months was seen. LMS was able to prevent a decrease of the DNCB reactivity observed in the control group. Before treatment there were 70% positive and 45% strong positive responders to DNCB$_{100}$ in the placebo group; after that 80% and 40%, respectively, were obtained.

In the LMS group 69.2% had a positive response and 26.9% a strong one before treatment; after LMS they became 92.3% and 57.7%. More important differences were obtained when DNCB$_{25}$ reactivity was analyzed. An increment from 3.8% to 38.5% in strong reactivity was found under LMS therapy, while changes from 5% to 15% occurred in placebo-treated patients.

LMS did produce a change in DNCB reactivity with statistical value ($P > 0.005$, McNemar test) while the placebo did not (P = n.s.). Recall antigen responses show lower values during both treatments than without pretreatment (Table 10). After treatment, low lymphocyte count was found in placebo-treated patients, while the LMS group had similar values.

PHA-P lymphocyte reactivity showed similar changes in both groups. Seven patients presented side effects (26.9%), two (7.7%) had severe reac-

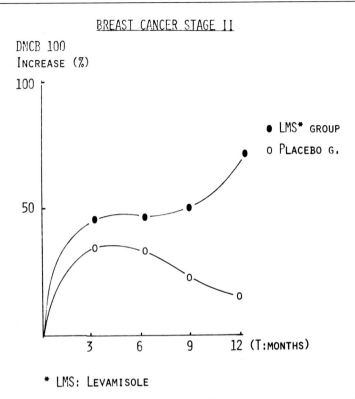

Fig. 28.   Increase of $DNCB_{100}$ reactivity along the follow-up time in stage II breast cancer patients receiving levamisole or placebo after radical procedures.

Table 10.   Breast cancer stage II

	Placebo		Levamisole	
	Before	After	Before	After
Candida antigen Positives	10/19 (52.6)	7/19 (36.8)	9/25 (36.0)	5/25 (20.0)
SK:SD (40:10) Positives	13/20 (65.0)	9/20 (45.0)	12/25 (48.0)	8/25 (32.0)
Lymph count χ/mm³	1,720 (1020–2312)	1,629 (1200–2352)	1,706 (1260–2664)	1,741 (1500–2403)
PHA-P response χ DPM	10,205	18,465	8,344	11,379

Table 11.   Side effects—breast cancer stage II

None	19 (73.1%)	Sickness, headache	4 (57.1%)
Mild	5 (19.2%)	Nausea	1 (14.3%)
Severe	2 (7.7%)	Malaise, intolerance	2 (28.6%)
Total	26	Total	7

tions and the treatment was stopped (Table 11). Median follow-up time is too short to obtain definitive conclusions. There are also some other differences between the groups; for example, a higher frequency of premenopausal patients and the number of axillary positive nodes in the LMS group. Keeping these concepts in mind, it is possible to observe that 3 patients (15.0%) in the placebo group and 2 (7.7%) in the LMS group showed evidence of progressing disease ($P = 0.1$, Fisher's exact test). Their recurrence rate is low in both groups at this time; more observation time is needed. The trend indicates the possibility of obtaining a statistical difference in a shorter time. Prophylactic regimens comparing LMS and chemotherapeutic schemes are necessary in breast cancer stage II to evaluate the kind of side effects and response rates in both arms.

Head and Neck Cancer Patients

Patients.   Head and neck cancer patients were treated with LMS or placebo after radical therapies and disease assessment. A total of 165 patients were studied; 88 in the LMS group and 77 in the placebo one.

There were several subgroups in this group: 22 skin tumors; 17 lip; 34 larynx; 24 tongue; 22 floor of mouth; 16 oropharynx; 30 nasopharynx; and other pathologies. It is a very complicated group about which to recommend clinical action because of the complexity of the staging and prognosis of each subgroup.

Immune Reactivity.   Tables 12 and 13 provide results on $DNCB_{100}$ reactivity in each group. Before placebo or LMS treatment, patients showed similar results: 62.3% vs. 67.1% of total positive responders and 24.7% vs. 31.8% of strong positive responders, respectively (P = n.s.).

DNCB reactivity increased continuously in the LMS group up to 12 months, where 75% of the treated patients increased their DNCB response. The placebo group increased up to 46% at six months and main-

Table 12.   Levamisole-treated head and neck cancer patients: response to $DNCB_{100}$ (percent)

	Before		After	
	Total Positives	Strong Positives	Total Positives	Strong Positives
Lips (9)	88.9	33.3	100	88.9
Skin (10)	67.4	31.8	94.3	71.6
Larynx (21)	71.4	28.6	100	85.7
Tongue (12)	50.0	25.0	100	50.0
Floor of mouth (11)	45.5	18.2	72.7	45.5
Oropharynx (17)	58.8	29.4	94.1	64.7
Total (88)	67.1	31.8	94.3	71.6

Table 13.   Head and neck control cancer patients: response to $DNCB_{100}$ (percent)

	Before		After	
	Total Positives	Strong Positives	Total Positives	Strong Positives
Lips (8)	100	37.5	100	62.5
Skin (12)	75	16.7	83.3	58.3
Larynx (13)	61.5	30.8	84.6	53.8
Tongue (12)	50.0	33.3	66.7	50.0
Floor of mouth (11)	90.9	18.2	90.9	45.5
Oropharynx (8)	25	12.5	50	25.0
Nasopharynx (13)	46.2	23.1	38.5	38.5
Total (77)	62.3	24.7	71.4	48.1

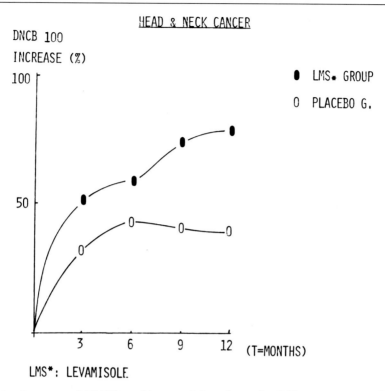

Fig. 29. Increase of $DNCB_{100}$ skin reactivity along the follow-up time in head and neck cancer patients receiving levamisole or placebo after radical procedures and NED assessment.

tained the same value at 12 months (Fig. 29). Statistical differences were found between the groups ($P < 0.01$).

Posttreatment differences were also found in percentage of the total and strong positive responders between LMS and placebo: 94.3% vs. 71.4% and 71.6% vs. 48.1%, respectively ($P < 0.001$). Results in head and neck cancer patients, after LMS treatment, differ greatly from those obtained in a general group of such cancer patients, especially in the percent of strong responders to $DNCB_{100}$. A clear relationship was observed in the clinical course according to the negative, weak positive, or strong positive responses to DNCB. It is important to maintain or increase DNCB reactions up to the "strong level" because of their relationship with further clinical evolution.

The evolution of 143 patients (excluding those having skin tumors) showed: 57 with negative nodes or small-sized tumors (accordingly, TNM classifications were stage I or II); and 86 patients with the extension of the disease to the lymph nodes or large-sized tumors (stages III or IV). There were 36 different subgroups. Median follow-up was 12 months. The overall recurrence rate showed the benefit of LMS treatment: 11/73 (15.1%) over the placebo at 21/70 (30%) ($P < 0.05$).

The median follow-up time is still short and there are also many subgroups to give valid conclusions on each. But the benefit of LMS therapy has been confirmed in the general evolution.

Other Groups Treated With LMS

Patients.   Cancer patient groups, other than those previously mentioned, have been entered in clinical trials using LMS. They include: 27 melanomas; 37 lymphomas; 13 patients with more than one primary tumor; 21 bladder carcinomas; 21 prostrate adenocarcinomas; 18 testicle and kidney tumors. A total of 146 were studied; 61 under LMS therapy and 85 corresponding to the control group.

Immune Reactivity.   This group of patients showed a high DNCB reactivity before treatment. This was probably because the group included melanomas and prostate adenocarcinomas, which are well known as good responders to DNCB. The LMS group had 72.1% of positive responders and 37.7% strong responders to $DNCB_{100}$; the placebo group had 73.3% and 51.2%, respectively. After treatment similar reactivities were found in the last group, but the LMS one showed 83.6% and 62.3% respectively.

Statistical differences were observed in the $DNCB_{100}$ rate increment (Fig. 30). The LMS group increased continuously up to 12 months, while the placebo one showed a first increment up to 43.3% and a decrease up to 25% at 12 months. At the same time, the LMS group reached 64.7% ($P < 0.05$).

Recurrence Rate.   There were 11/61 (18%) patients who had evidence of progressing disease in the LMS group and 17/85 (20%) in the control group (P = n.s.). All the subgroups showed better clinical results in LMS patients with the exception of lymphomas and those including stomach and colon carcinomas. But all groups had too few numbers to reach a definite conclusion. In this heterogenous group there also were little differences in DNCB reactivity.

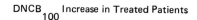

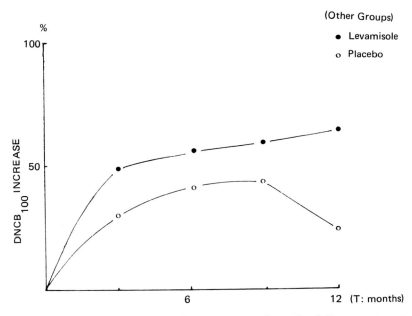

Fig. 30. Increase of DNCB$_{100}$ skin reactivity along the follow-up time in cancer patients (excluding breast and head and neck cancer patients) receiving levamisole or placebo after radical procedures.

General Results on Duration of Disease-Free Interval

Analysis of the whole data (excluding breast cancer stage III) makes it possible to observe the NED interval of LMS (174) or placebo (184) patients (Fig. 31). The placebo group has a median disease-free interval of 22.5 months while the LMS group has a 70.6% of disease-free patients at two years from the beginning of treatment ($P = 0.06$, generalized Wilcoxon test).

The recurrence rate is 13.8% in LMS with an average follow-up of 9.8 months, and 23.9% in the placebo group with 9.3 months of follow-up ($P < 0.001$). In the LMS group, trial 4 was administered to 46.6% of the treated patients.

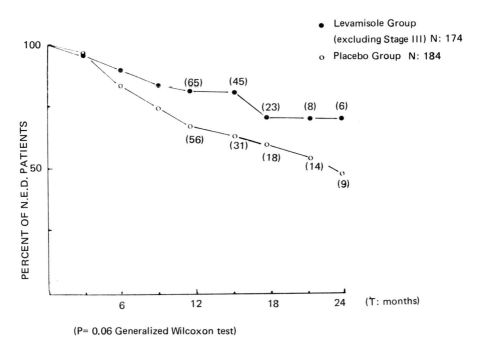

Disease-free-interval in Levamisole & Placebo Groups

(P= 0.06 Generalized Wilcoxon test)

Fig. 31. Disease-free-interval duration in cancer patients (excluding stage III breast cancer patients) treated with levamisole or placebo after radical therapies and NED assessment.

Dextromisole—Levamisole

Forty-eight patients have been treated using the dextroisomer (Dextromisole). All had urogenital tumors; 11 were women; 59 received a placebo or no further therapy after radical treatment. A positive increment in $DNCB_{100}$ reactivity was also seen in DMS-treated patients against control group (Fig. 32). At 6 months the placebo group showed 54.7% reaction increase and the DMS 70.6%. After 12 months, 82.8% of the treated patients had increased DNCB response; 50.0% of the placebo patients showed a similar event. The whole group had a high spontaneous increment. Women having cervix uteri tumors have spontaneously increased their DNCB responses greatly. A nonstatistical difference was observed

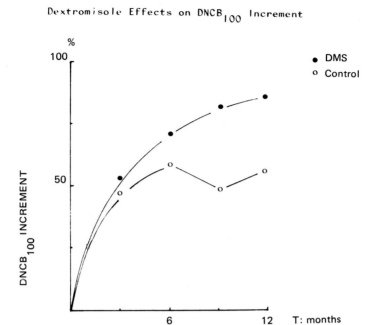

Fig. 32. Increase of $DNCB_{100}$ skin reactivity along the follow-up time in cancer patients receiving dextromisole or placebo after radical therapies and NED assessment.

Table 14. Dextromisole side effects

	GYN	Bladder	Prostate	Testicle	Kidney	Total (%)
None	3	8	5	6	4	26 (54.2)
Mild	5	4	3	2	2	16 (33.3)
Severe	3	2	1	0	0	6 (12.5)
Total	11	14	9	8	6	48

Type of Side Effects (DMS)

Sickness—irritability	
Insommia—anorexia	15 (38.5%)
Nausea—vomiting	15 (38.5%)
Malaise	6 (15.4%)
Other	3 (7.7%)
Total	39

between the DMS (10.9%) and placebo groups (15.3%) in relation to recurrence rate. DMS treatment showed a high percentage of side effects (45.8%) (Table 14). A number of patients (12.5%) had severe reactions causing termination of the treatment.

Side effects in relation to CNS and nausea or vomiting had the higher frequency.

To do a comparison between LMS and DMS effectiveness on $DNCB_{100}$ increment rate, an analysis was made of patients having bladder, prostate, testicle, or penis tumors treated with each drug and placebo; 17 were treated with LMS, 37 with DMS, and 29 using placebo.

Both treatments showed a similar activity in DNCB response in comparison to the placebo group (Fig. 33), but it is important to point out that LMS-treated patients received 11.03 gr per patient (because of trial 4) and DMS patients 9.2 gr per patient. DMS showed a slightly positive dif-

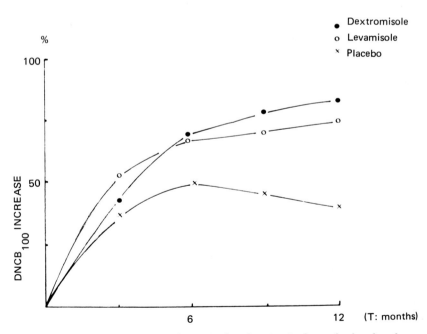

Effects of LMS,DMS or Placebo on DNCB 100 Increase

Fig. 33. Comparison among levamisole, dextromisole and placebo therapy on $DNCB_{100}$ skin reactivity along the follow-up time in cancer patients after receiving radical therapies and NED assessment.

Table 15.   Comparison of the side effects of LMS and DMS

A. Number of Side Effects

	None	Mild	Severe
Levamisole			
Trial II	106 (89.8%)	10 (5.5%)	2 (1.7%)
Trial IV	81 (81.8%)	15 (15.2%)	3 (3.0%)
Total	187 (86.2%)	25 (11.5%)	5 (2.3%)
Dextramisole	26 (54.2%)	16 (33.3%)	6 (12.5%)

B. Type of Side Effects

	Levamisole	Dextramisole
Sickness—irritability	17 (50.0%)	15 (38.5%)
Insomnia—anorexia		
Nausea–vomiting	15 (40.5%)	15 (38.5%)
Malaise	—	6 (15.4%)
Other	2 (5.4%)	3 (7.7%)
Total	34	39

C.	Patients with Side Effects	Number of Manifestation/ Patients with Side Effects
LMS	30/217 (13.8%)	34/30 : 1.13
DMS	22/48 (45.8%)	39/22 : 1.77

ference at twelve months which is without statistical value. A comparison of the side effects of both drugs (Table 15) showed a higher percentage in DMS treatment ($P < 0.0005$).

GENERAL DISCUSSION

The positive action of LMS therapy on DNCB reactivity has been shown by comparison with the placebo. DNCB response of treated patients increased at a high rate. The "$DNCB_{100}$ increase rate" as one parameter in measuring LMS or placebo effects upon immune reactivation has also been considered. It was clearly shown that benign disease patients and localized skin tumors are capable of spontaneously increasing DNCB response (probably because of rechallenges), while malignant diseases and lymphoma patients show only a slight change. There are statistical differences between the first groups and later ones. LMS was able to improve responsiveness to DNCB which could imply an activation of the recognizing capacity.

According to these results, an increase in DNCB response is not dependent on spontaneous increment alone because of retesting; there is a specific effect of LMS on "resensitization capacity." The same capacity was seen in patients with an excellent prognosis because of having localized tumors or benign diseases; DNCB resensitization phenomena have been associated with a normalization of immune status.

However, a spontaneous DNCB increase has also been observed in placebo groups. Forty percent of such patients increased $DNCB_{100}$ response during the first 6 months, but after that time a decrease was demonstrated. The LMS group did not show this kind of decrease. According to these results, LMS produced an increasing rate in treated cancer patients similar to those having benign diseases. In this way, LMS "normalized" DNCB response.

In our experience, LMS therapy did not improve preexisting immunity to *Candida* antigen or SK:SD; instead, it produced a decreasing trend of such responses. Conflicting results were obtained from PHA-P lymphocyte reactivity. It had variations depending on administration time; an improvement was seen at 3 and 24 months from the beginning of therapy, while a depression was observed at 6 to 12 months. Day to day variations in PHA lymphocyte reactivity were obtained when a study on treated healthy donors was carried out.

Depressions and stimulations were found using a whole blood microtechnique, but only an increasing response was noted using purified lymphocytes. Both microtechniques were performed using blood from the same donors.

Serum activity, differential action on pure lymphocyte, or differential activity on whole blood cells were postulated to interpret such results (41). In this way, a different methodology could show very different results according to laboratory conditions. Obviously interpretations of the data would depend on the methodology used.

Of all the immunological data obtained, the most important are those derived from DNCB reactivity. In our experience, a close relationship was established between variations in DNCB response and the duration of the disease-free interval. It was inferred from a general study done on immune factors in the progression of cancers (Fig. 4).

Negative responders and strong positive responders have a different probability to continue in NED conditions. Unfortunately, it was only a probability of the whole group of patients more than any one patient considered alone. There are negative responders who are NED up to 2 years and strong positive responders to DNCB who have a relapse in a few months after the immune study, but there is a highly statistical difference between both groups. At 12 months, negative responders had 25% NED patients, while strong positive responders had 80% in similar conditions.

Total reliability has not been determined using such methodologies, but we are convinced that positive changes in DNCB reactivity are generally followed by a better clinical course, while a negative change reflects the opposite: concordances are greater than exceptions.

The previous concept points out the importance of LMS action on DNCB reactivity.

LMS therapy positively modified the clinical course in locally advanced breast cancer patients and DNCB response (45, 46).

Clinical results could be interpreted as an action mediated through the immune system. LMS clearly has prevented the immune depression after localized radiotherapy; similar events did not occur in the control group. Figure 24 shows a normalization to similar or higher values than preradiation ones in the LMS-treated group, while lower values were seen in the control group (Fig. 23).

Premenopausal breast-cancer treated patients showed a more dramatic change in their clinical course than did postmenopausal patients when they were compared to the evolution of similar cases in the historical control group. This modification in the clinical course has no correlation with a more important change or strong response of the immunological profile. It could be assumed that because premenopausal patients are younger women, immune status could be modified more effectively than in older women (in postmenopause). However, this was not confirmed.

Differences in the clinical course are not yet significant ($P < 0.1$), but the tendency is very strong to conclude that both groups are different. In reference to the historical control group, results were analyzed after the first pilot trial in such a way as to confirm previous ones. The data were obtained from patients in radiation treatment, during the same period of performance as our clinical trials, and who did not receive further treatment after radiotherapy until presenting evidence of progressing disease. Differences can be ruled out in radiation therapy or diagnosis with the exception of the immune follow-up.

Some observations indicate possible LMS actions on hormonal behavior. Suppression of menstrual rhythm has been observed in a 13-year-old girl under LMS treatment: normal rhythm appeared under placebo administration and a further inhibition occurred when LMS was reestablished.

These concepts could have special importance for the evolution breast cancer patients.

We have postulated on the possible action of LMS on CNS and

through it the possible modulation of the immune system. The previously mentioned alteration of menstrual rhythm could be related to these concepts.

To support this postulation, more suggestive evidence was found: animal studies of LMS distribution showed high brain concentrations. We demonstrated it using S35 and ^{3}H-labeled LMS; other authors have obtained similar results (17).

Furthermore, there are several authors who have established a relationship between the immune system and CNS (13, 26, 27, 33, 49). LMS-treated groups have a dose-related response upon DNCB reactivity; high weekly dosages produced an earlier DNCB increment than classical schemes. A regimen of 450 mg/week, in alternating weeks, was established as a maintenance policy in patients having strong reactivity to $DNCB_{100}$. Higher doses (900 mg/week, alternate weeks) were used as "induction" therapy in negative or weak positive responders; those patients who showed a strong level from a lower dosage received lower weekly doses to maintain this kind of response. Some observed differences among clinical trials could be explained in this way. Fifty-eight percent of our patients received a higher weekly dosage than the classical one. Head and neck cancer patients were treated in Memorial Sloan-Kettering Cancer Center using the classical scheme; clinical results appeared after one year of treatment. It could be possible to obtain an earlier clinical result if higher weekly dosages are used, especially if negative or weak responders to DNCB receive this kind of therapy. On the other hand, it was observed that lung cancer patients weighing over 70 kg need longer dosages to receive benefits similar to patients with a lower weight (50).

We have considered the response to DNCB more important than the patients' weight in adopting weekly dosages.

In the head and neck group, an unusual response to $DNCB_{100}$ was obtained after LMS therapy (94.3% positive and 71.6% strong responders) when comparing it to a general study done on 360 non-treated head and neck cancer patients. The latter group had a 63.1% total positive and 26.2% strong positive responses. In the same group a clear relationship was found between the duration of a disease-free interval and the DNCB response. Negative responders had a median disease-free interval time of 5 months, weak positive responders of one year, and strong responders had 80% of disease-free patients up to 15 months.

According to a previous relationship between DNCB and the disease-free interval found in head and neck non-treated cancer patients after radical treatments, a positive effect in the clinical course is expected in LMS patients.

Nonstatistically as yet, positive results were observed in breast cancer stage II patients and in a heterogeneous group of malignant diseases. The duration of the disease-free interval from the whole clinical data (excluding stage III breast cancer patients) showed a positive effect in LMS-treated groups compared to placebo ones ($P \cong 0.06$). Necessary statistical value has not been reached yet, but considerable differences have been observed between both treatments.

LMS therapy has a tendency to be more effective in advanced stages (2). Our own results in stage III breast cancer patients could be related to this. Debois obtained positive results in breast cancer patients stage IV and no results in other stages (48). Analysis of these data makes it possible to observe that the stage III reference group has 80% of the patients alive at 25 months. Our control groups have a median survival time of 24 months. Then it is possible to assume that our stage III breast cancer patients had more advanced diseases. Stage III breast cancer is the most heterogenous group in the UICC classification. Debois has shown statistical differences in stage IV; we have similar ones, but in stage III breast cancer patients. Local rules for localized treatment or different clinical considerations could be responsible for the observed differences. Amery et al. have demonstrated the benefit of LMS therapy in lung cancer patients having a large-sized tumor instead of a small one (50).

The reasons for that are still unknown, especially because the tumoral load had an opposite effect on clinical results when other immunostimulant treatments were used. A possible explanation could be found if a high tumor load implies a strong recognition of tumor antigens. LMS therapy improves recognition of new antigens. In this way the most important benefit would be seen in patients who have their tumor antigens recognized; probably it is those patients who are bearing a high tumor burden.

It is also possible that activation of general immune defense of the host has a more important effect on advanced diseases.

Low incidence of side effects and acute or chronic toxicity have induced the use of LMS in a wide range of diseases and it is used indiscriminately in cancer patients.

From our breast cancer experience and from other reports (14, 32, 42) we have the concept that it is possible to induce a differential effect on the site of distant metastases. There was in this group, a high frequency of lung metastases in treated rather than in control patients. The time of appearance of such metastases was longer in treated group, and there was no significant correlation between irradiated breast and lung metastases sites. Such patients showed no significant change of DNCB reactivity, in spite of LMS therapy.

The appearance of local recurrences in breast cancer was also modified. The LMS group had two different subpopulations according to the time of appearance, the first having local relapses of between one and two years after radiotherapy, and the second in which local relapses were seen from 3 to 4 years after that therapy. In the later group, not having other distant metastases, a new local therapy was done. Now those patients are NED again. It has all been closely correlated to the DNCB response.

The reasons for these phenomena are still unknown. On the other hand, a pilot experiment done in mice receiving an LD_{70} of radiotherapy and LMS showed a shorter survival time than the control group receiving irradiation and saline solution.

Moreover, a melanoma patient showed a torpid evolution when receiving LMS (900 mg/week) after intensive chemotherapy. There were positive reactions before LMS therapy and negative ones (grade 0) after that.

Bearing in mind that LMS breakdown produces more than fifty metabolites, the clinical effectiveness could be mediated by one or more of these (5, 7, 22).

Patients showing no positive response to LMS therapy could have the incapacity to produce the active metabolite. On the other hand, there is another imidothiazole derivative, niridazole, which has potent long-acting inhibitor capacity on T cell function (12, 30, 31, 40, 55). This fact leads to the possibility that LMS breakdown could produce a metabolite having inhibitory properties. Furthermore, metabolism of chemotherapeutic drugs could be modified by immunostimulant treatments (47).

Before planning combination schemes with LMS it is necessary to have a deep knowledge of all the effects of LMS (and the other therapies) on immune system. Patients with NED under LMS therapy need a close immunological check-up and clinical follow-up to control any possible immune depression. Combination schemes need further and deep considerations; especially to administration time after immune depressive treatments.

The DMS pilot experiment gave us an unexpected slant on immune reactivity. DMS was considered an inactive drug (2), but clinical results using this drug are scarce. Our data showed the positive effect of the purified dextroisomer on DNCB reactivity; it was compared to LMS in the same group of patients, and both drugs had similar effectiveness.

In vitro studies of LMS have shown direct action which could be considered an immunostimulating action at the peripheral level. DMS has not shown such action.

Thus, a possible explanation could be that a similar breakdown of both drugs could produce a common "active metabolite" in vivo, in this way producing similar observable results in cancer patients.

It is also possible that LMS and DMS actions on immune system could be mediated through an action on the CNS.

Studies involving tetramisole (the racemic salt) could not be interpreted as the effects of LMS alone.

CONCLUDING REMARKS

LMS has produced an effective change in DNCB reactivity and in the duration of the disease-free interval in cancer patients under therapy. LMS therapy showed a close relationship to the DNCB increase rate according to dosages. Some suggestive evidence was found on the possible action of LMS on hormonal behavior or modulation of the immune system through CNS. A definite evaluation regarding the direct immune action is impossible since the modification of the immune reactivity.

Results in patients having a high tumor load and the observed differential effect on certain metastases sites have not, until now, had a clear explanation.

ACKNOWLEDGMENTS

We thank Dr. O. R. Burrone and J. M. De Gregorio for their inestimable help; Ms. Raquel Baldrich and Ms. Magdalena Racedo for technical assistance; Ms. Cecilia Nan for help in the preparation of this manuscript. We also wish to thank Ms. Helen C. Nauts for the economic aid given by the Cancer Research Institute, Inc., New York, since 1974.

REFERENCES

1. Alexander, P., Currie, G. A., and Thomson, D. M. P. 1975. In *Immunological Aspects of Neoplasia*. Williams and Wilkins Co., Baltimore.

2. Amery, W. K., Spreafico. F., Rojas, A. F., Denissen, E., and Chirigos, M. A. Adjuvant treatment with LMS in Cancer. *Cancer Treatment Review* (in press).

3. Bansal, S. C., and Sjögren, H. O. 1974. *Israel J. Med. Sci.* 10: 939.

4. Bonnadona, G., Brusamolino, E., Valagussa, et al. 1976. *N. Engl. J. Med.* 294: 405.

5. Boyd, J. E., Bullock, M. W., Champagne, D. A., Gatterdam, P. E., Morici, I. J., Plaisted, P. H., Spicer, L. D., Wayne, R. S., Zulalian, J. 1960. Lecture given at the 158th National Meeting of the American Chemical Society, New York.

6. Carbone, P. O. 1975. *Cancer* 36: 633.

7. Champagne, D. A., Gatterdam, P. E., Plaisted, P. M., Zulalian, J., Boyd, J. E. 1969. Lecture given at the 158th National Meeting of the American Chemical Society New York.

8. Cochram, A. J., Mackie, R. M., Ross, C. E., Ogg, L. J., and Jackson, A. M. 1976. In J. Wybran and M. Staquet (eds.), *Clinical Tumor Immunology*, Pergamon Press, Oxford and New York.

9. Cooperband, S. R., Numberg, R., Schmid, K., Marmick, J. A. 1976. *Transplant Proc.* 8: 225.

10. Cooperband, S. R., Badger, A. M., and Marmick, J. A. 1976. In J. J. Op-

penheim and D. L. Rosenstreich (eds.), *Mitogens in Immunobiology*. Academic Press, New York, San Francisco and London.

11. Debois, J. Am. 1977. *In* M. A. Chrigos (ed.), *Control of Neoplasia by Modulation of the Immune System*, Vol. 2. Raven Press, New York.

12. Deodhar, S. D., Lee, V. W., Chiang, T., Mahmoud, A. A. F., Warren, K. S. 1976. *Cancer Res.* 36: 3147.

13. Fesell, N. J., Forsyth, R. P. 1963. *Arthritis Rheum.* 6: 770.

14. Fidler, I. J., and Spitler, L. E. 1975. *J. Natl. Cancer Inst.* 55: 1107.

15. Fisher, B. F., Slack, N., Katrych, D., Wolmark, N. 1975. *Surg. Gynec. Obstet.* 140: 528.

16. Fisher, B. F., Carbone, P. P., Economou, S. *et al.* 1975. *N. Engl. J. Med.* 292: 117.

17. Fisher, B. F. 1976. Lecture given at Third Conference of Modulation of Host Defence, Bethesda, Maryland, December.

18. Gehan, E. A. 1965. *Biometrika* 52: 203.

19. Hellström, K. E., and Hellström, I. 1974. *In* F. H. Bach and R. A. Good (eds.), *Clinical Immunobiology*, Vol. 2. Academic Press, New York.

20. Hersh, E. M., Gutterman, J. U., Mavligit, G. M., Mountain, C. W., McBride, C. M., and Burgers, M. A. 1976. *Ann. N.Y. Acad. Sci.* (in press).

21. Hirshaut, Y., Pinsky, C., Fried, J., and Oettgen, E. 1974. *Proc. Amer. Assoc. Cancer Res.* 15: 126.

22. Holbrock, A., and Scales, B. 1967. *Anal. Biochem.* 18: 46.

23. Holmes, E. C., and Golub, S. H. 1976. *J. Thorac. Cardiovasc. Surg.* 71: 161.

24. Howell, S. B., Dean, J. H., and Law, L. W. 1975. *Int. J. Cancer* 15: 152.

25. Kaiser, D. W., and Reif, A. E. 1975. *In* A. E. Reif (ed.), *Immunity and Cancer in Man*. Marcel Dekker, New York.

26. Korneva, E. A. 1967. *Fiziol. ZH. SSSR Sechenov* 53: 42.

27. Korneva, E. A., and Khay, L. M. 1963. *Fiziol. ZH. SSSR Sechenov* 49: 42.

28. Levo, Y., Rotter, V., and Ramot, B. 1975. *Biomedicine* 23: 198.

29. Lewinski, U. H., Mavligit, G. M., Gutterman, J. V., and Hersh, E. M. 1977. *In* M. A. Chirigos (ed.), *Control of Neoplasia by Modulation of the Immune System*, Vol. 2. Raven Press, New York.

30. Lucas, S. V., Daniels, J. C., Schubert,R. D., Simpson, J. M., Mahmoud, A. A. F., Warren, K. S., David, J. R., Webster, L. T., Jr. 1977. *J. Immunol.* 118:418.

31. Mahmoud, A. A. F., Mandel, M. A., Warren, K. S., Webster, L. T., Jr. 1975. *J. Immunol.* 114: 279.

32. Mantovani, A., and Spreafico, F. 1975. *Eur. J. Cancer* 11: 537.

33. Macris, N. T., Schiavi, R. C., Camerino, M. S., Stein, M. 1970. *Amer. J. Physiol.* 219: 1205.

34. Mathé, G. 1969. *Brit. Med. J.* iv: 7.

35. Mathé, G. 1970. *Brit. Med. J.* iv: 487.

36. Mathé, G., Amiel, J., Schwarzenberg, L., Schneider, M., Cattan, A., Schlumberger, J. R., Havat, M., Vassal, F. 1973. *Revue fr. Etud. clin. biol.* 13: 454.

37. Mathé, G. 1973. *Ciba Foundation Symp.* 18: 305.

38. Nauts, H. C. 1975. *Cancer Res. Inst. Monogr.* 16.

39. Nauts, H. C. 1976. *Cancer Res. Inst. Monogr.* 4, 2nd edition.

40. Pelley, R. P., Pelley, R. J., Stavitsky, A. B., Mahmoud, A. A. F., and Warrent, K. S. 1975. *J. Immunol.* 115: 1477.

41. Peña de de, N. C., Lustig de, E. S., Rojas, A. F., Olivari, A., and Canónico, A. 1975. Presented at the Antivirals with Clinical Potential Symposium, Stanford, Calif.

42. Potter, C. W., Carr, I., Jennings, R., Rees, R. C., McGinty, F., and Richardson, V. M. 1974. *Nature* 249: 567.

43. Renoux, G., and Renoux, M. 1971. *C.R. Acad. Sci. (Paris)* 272: 349.

44. Renoux, G. 1972. *Nature New Biol.* 240: 217.

45. Rojas, A. F., Mickiewicz, E., Feierstein, J. N., Glait, H. M., and Olivari, A. J. 1976. *Lancet* 1: 7953.

46. Rojas, A. F., Feierstein, J. N., Glait, H. M., Varela, O. A., Pradier, R., and Olivari, A. J. 1977. *In* M. A. Chirigos (ed.), *Control of Neoplasia by Modulation of the Immune System,* Vol. 2. Raven Press, New York.

47. Soyka, L. F., Hunt, W., Knight, S., Foster, R., Jr. 1976. *Cancer Res.* 36(12): 4425.

48. Sparks, F. C., Silverstein, M. J., Hunt, J. S., Haskell, C. M., Pilch, Y. H., Morton, D. L. 1973. *N. Engl. J. Med.* 289: 827.

49. Stein, M., Schiavi, R. C., and Camerino, M. 1976. *Science* 191: 435.

50. Study Group for Bronchogenic carcinoma. 1975. *Brit. Med. J.* 3: 461.

51. Symoens, J. 1977. *In* M. A. Chirigos (ed.), *Control of Neoplasia by Modulation of the Immune System,* Vol. 2. Raven Press, New York.

52. Tripodi, D., Parks, L. C., and Brugmans, J. 1973. *N. Engl. J. Med.* 289: 354.

53. Verhaegen, H., De Cree, J., De Cock, W., and Verbruggen, F. 1973. *N. Engl. J. Med.* 289: 1148.

54. Verhaegen, H., De Cock, W., De Cree, J. Verbruggen, F., Verhaegen-Declerq, M., and Brugmans, J. 1975. *Lancet* 1: 978.

55. Webster, L. T., Jr., Butterworth, A. E., Mahmoud, A. A. F., Mngola, E. N., Warren, K. S. 1975. *New Engl. J. Med.* 292: 1144.

56. Whitney, R. B., Levy, J. G., and Smith, A. G. 1974. *J. Natl. Cancer Inst.* 53: 111.

57. Wybran, I., and Staquet, M. 1976. *In Clinical Tumor Immunology.* Pergamon Press, Oxford and New York.

58. Zucali, R., Uslenghi, C., Kenda, R., and Bonnadona, G. 1976. *Cancer* 37: 1422.

CHAPTER 9

IMMUNOLOGICAL PROPERTIES OF SYNGENEIC AND XENOGENEIC IMMUNE RNA TO A MURINE TUMOR

Matthew C. Dodd
Stephen B. Evans

Department of Microbiology
Ohio State University
Columbus, Ohio 43210

Syngeneic and xenogeneic IRNA were shown to be specifically cytotoxic for C3H mouse fibrosarcoma. Xenogeneic IRNA had no effect on normal cell lines derived from C3H mice and acted more like syngeneic IRNA than like the guinea pig lymphocytes which were the RNA donors. Xenogeneic RNA was shown to protect mice against tumor challenge. IRNA and RNA from lymphocytes of tumor-bearing mice (TLRNA) were both shown to produce antibody (ADCC) to the tumor, whereas the latter also produced "blocking" factors.

Introduction

The first attempts in this laboratory to transfer immunity using immune RNA began in the late 1960s (28). In 1973, we reported that a variety of humoral and cellular factors, including antibody to sheep red blood cells, antibody and MIF to tuberculin, and specific lymphocyte cytotoxicity to a murine fibrosarcoma, could be transferred to normal lymphocytes in vitro by either syngeneic or xenogeneic immune RNA derived from spleens or lymph nodes of mouse or guinea pig donors (8). The antitumor effects of xenogeneic immune RNA suggested the approach to the immunotherapy of human tumors. This simply proposed that, if a specific antihuman tumor RNA could be created in a xenogeneic system, such as a guinea pig, without accompanying reactions to normal human antigens, such human IRNA could be used in the immunotherapy of cancer. This report also emphasized that the antitumor effect was specific, RNA-dependent, and that this immunologic activity was associated only with RNA preparations in which the ratio of the 8–18 S peak to the 0–8 S peak on sucrose gradients was 2.0 or more, and finally the active principle was separated by Sephadex filtration and shown to lie in the range 6–12 S with a molecular weight of approximately 135,000.

Such findings prompted a further and extensive examination of the use of xenogeneic guinea pig IRNA as an antitumor agent in this mouse fibrosarcoma which might serve as a model for the use of xenogeneic guinea pig IRNA in the treatment of human tumors. Syngeneic IRNA to the same tumor was used in comparison of the specificity and to monitor any reactions which might occur to normal tissue antigens.

Subsequently, extensive work involved the examination of both kinds of IRNA to the mouse fibrosarcoma for their capacity to transfer in vitro manifestations of cellular immunity such as cytotoxicity, MIF, and lymphoblastogenesis, but also the capacity of xenogeneic IRNA to protect mice from tumor challenge. In the process, hundreds of milligrams of xenogeneic IRNA have been made which will routinely transfer specific cytotoxicity to mouse lymphocytes for tumor cells but none for normal mouse cells. The various factors in the preparation and extraction of tissue which insure successful production of immunologically active RNA containing not more than 5% contamination with DNA or protein have been demonstrated. Since specifically cytotoxic lymphocytes and so-called "blocking" factors have been found in animals and humans with tumors, RNA from lymphocytes of mice bearing the sarcoma (TLRNA) was compared with ILRNA from immunized mice and the two were shown to have distinct immunological properties, both transferring antibody which was cytotoxic for tumor cells, but whereas TLRNA also transferred a blocking antibody and a suppressor factor that directly blocked the cytotoxicity of specifically sensitized anti-tumor lymphocytes, ILRNA did not.

Review of Previous Work

The most consistent results in transferring a cell-mediated tumor response have been obtained in vitro and include a wide variety of tumors and assays. The tumor systems studied include mouse (8), rat (26), guinea pig (35), and human (4). The techniques used to measure cell-mediated response have mainly been cytotoxicity assays, but migration inhibition (8, 35) and lymphocyte blastogenic assays have also been used (7, 10).

Using an in vitro cytotoxicity assay which measures the direct effect of treated lymphocytes on plated target cells, work in this laboratory has consistently demonstrated transfer of cytotoxicity to a murine fibrosarcoma tumor to normal nonimmunized lymphocytes. The transfer has been shown to be specific and inhibited by prior treatment of the RNA with RNAse but not pronase, or DNAse (9). Similarly, Pilch and his colleagues, using a target cell label-release assay, have demonstrated the in vitro transfer of cytotoxicity to tumor cells to a variety of lymphocyte species including mouse (16), rat (16), and human (27). Likewise, Schlager et al. (35), working in a guinea pig tumor system, have used a migration inhibition assay to demonstrate the transfer of the cell-mediated response to the guinea pig tumor, to lymphocytes of other species via "immune" RNA. All three laboratories have shown that the transfer of the cell-mediated response can be accomplished by using either syngeneic or xenogeneic RNA (10, 25, 35).

Two separate observations have possibly been the foundation for the current study of "immune" RNA and its involvement in the retardation or rejection of tumor growth in vivo. The first was the finding by Alexander et al. (1) that thoracic duct lymphocytes from specifically immunized rats could adoptively transfer a degree of immunity to tumor-bearing rats. The response was tumor-specific and, while complete cures were rarely seen, temporary regressions were relatively common.

The second observation was that of Mannich and Egdahl (21), who demonstrated the transfer of immunity to skin allografts in rabbits. After incubation of autologous spleen cells in vitro with RNA extracted from spleens and regional lymph nodes of specifically immunized rabbits, the treated cells were then reinfused. The transfer of the skin graft rejection was found to be RNA-dependent and ineffective if the RNA was injected directly, without prior incubation *in vitro,* with lymphoid cells.

Following the two previous observations, Alexander *et al.* (2) found that they could achieve a temporary regression of a primary rat sarcoma after the injection of RNA from lymphocytes of sheep and allogeneic rats which had been immunized with the tumor to be treated. The crude RNA extract used was found to contain variable amounts of DNA and to a much lesser extent, protein. Subsequent work in a variety of systems has served to confirm Alexander's preliminary findings.

Rigby (33) has prolonged the survival of mice bearing Ehrlich ascites tumors by administering syngeneic spleen cells that had previously been incubated with RNA from the spleens of mice immunized with this tumor. Londner *et al.* (17) reported slower growth of transplants of a spontaneously arising sarcoma in rats treated with the intraperitoneal injection of RNA extracted from the spleens of rats immunized with the tumor being treated.

Kennedy *et al.* (15) described the protection of C3H mice against transplants of a benzpyrene-induced sarcoma by foot pad injections of RNA extracted from the lymph nodes and spleens of C57 Bl mice immunized with this tumor. Complete protection was afforded in only 4 out of 45 mice treated, but a significant prolongation of mean survival time was obtained in the 41 mice which succumbed to the tumor. The protection was RNA-dependent, and displayed a very critical dose response.

Ramming and Pilch (32) showed that the growth of isographs of a chemically induced murine sarcoma was inhibited by the injection of syngeneic spleen cells incubated with RNA extracted from guinea pigs immunized with the same mouse tumor. The inhibitory effect was, at least partially, tumor-specific and did not cross-react with another chemically induced sarcoma. Following their success in the murine sarcoma system, Pilch and colleagues (26) expanded to a rat system in which they employed xenogeneic RNA of guinea pig origin and directly injected the RNA into the footpads. Once again, they were able to demonstrate a significant reduction of tumor incidence in the "immune" RNA treated animals.

Transfer of Antitumor Cytotoxicity by Syngeneic "Immune" RNA

The research using syngeneic IRNA to transfer an antitumor response was based on previous studies (9) with the 4198 V fibrosarcoma in C_3H mice which demonstrated lymphocyte-mediated cytotoxicity to the tumor cell, by lymphocytes from either immunized or tumor-bearing animals. The cytotoxicity was detected by an *in vitro* cytotoxicity assay, which was an adaptation of the Takasugi and Klein microcytotoxicity assay (37). Although the ultimate goal was the transfer of tumor immunity by xenogeneic IRNA, which would be necessary for human tumor immunotherapy, the original experiments involved the production of evidence that normal C3H mouse lymphocytes could be endowed with specific antitumor cytotoxicity by treatment with syngeneic IRNA derived from spleen cells of C3H mice either immunized to or actually carrying the previously mentioned fibrosarcoma tumor.

RNA was extracted from the spleens of three different groups of mice. The first group consisted of animals immunized by a series of intraperitoneal injections with tumor cells. These animals were proved to be resistant to tumor challenge. The second group consisted of animals with obvious tumors. The third group consisted of untreated, or normal mice. The cytotoxicity results obtained using the syngeneic RNA-treated lymphocytes are reported in Table 1. The target cells were the 4198V tumor cell and the syngeneic but non-tumorigenic LM cell, which was used as a control of specificity. The lymphocytes were incubated with 100 μg quantities of the different RNA preparations prior to addition to the target cells.

As can be seen in the table, cytotoxicity of cells treated with RNA derived from immunized animals, designated as SIRNA, ranged from 20%

Table 1.   Cell-mediated cytotoxicity by syngeneic RNA-treated lymphocytes for the 4198 V and LM cell lines

Lymphocytes[a] Tested	Cytotoxicity[b] (%, S.E.)	Number of Tests
NL	0[c]	
SIRNA	34.1 (4.0)	5
STRNA	31.2 (6.3)	4
SNRNA	2.0 (1.7)	3

a. NL, lymphocytes from normal mice; SIRNA, lymphocytes treated with syngeneic "immune" RNA; STRNA, lymphocytes treated with RNA from tumor-bearing mice; SNRNA, lymphocytes treated with RNA from syngeneic, non-immune mice.

b. Percent cytotoxicity with standard error, percent reduction of target cells by test lymphocytes as compared to target cell survival with normal lymphocytes.

c. Percent cytotoxicity against the LM cell with these populations was negligible, ranging from −2% to 8%.

to 45% for the five different RNA preparations tested. The average cytotoxicity for the five groups was 34%. Percent cytotoxicity produced by cells treated with RNA from tumor-bearing animals, designated by cells treated with RNA from tumor-bearing animals, designated by STRNA, ranged from 20.3% to 48%. The average for these four RNA's was 31.3%. The RNA derived from the untreated animals, designated as SNRNA, did not confer significant cytotoxicity. Tests with NRNA in subsequent experiments to be referred to later did show cytotoxicity which was not specific. None of the RNA preparations tested displayed significant cytotoxicity for the LM cell. In each case cytotoxicity was calculated using normal lymphocytes as the control, showing no cytotoxicity. This was necessary since due to some undefined reason the target cells grow slightly better in the presence of lymphocyte preparations. It is quite obvious, however, that IRNA as well as RNA from tumor-bearing animals are capable of transferring specific cytotoxicity to normal syngeneic lymphocytes.

In the process of producing the previous data on IRNA, it became obvious that maximal specific cytotoxicity is dose dependent. As can be seen in Figure 1, a wide range of RNA concentrations from 10 to 500 μg was effective in transferring the cytotoxicity. In fact, the only dose not shown to transfer significant cytotoxicity was the 1000 μg quantity. It was found that after treating the lymphocyte populations with this high dose of RNA, the lymphocyte viability was decreased. This could possibly account for the lack of cytotoxicity by these treated lymphocytes. Nevertheless, it can be deduced from Figure 1 that doses of 10 to 500 μg of IRNA produced significant cytotoxicity in normal lymphocytes and it is also quite possible that loss of cytotoxicity by cells treated with the larger dose could be the result of RNA from lymphocytes with suppressor effects but present in smaller amounts. Since cytotoxicity was maximally transferred by 100 μg of IRNA (although the quantitative aspects of this test are not necessarily significant) this concentration was used routinely in further studies unless otherwise noted.

As noted in the final biochemical analysis of IRNA, it does contain minimal contamination by DNA and less than 5% protein. In order to eliminate any role of these factors in the transfer of immunocompetence by IRNA, each preparation used was treated with RNAse, DNAse, and pronase. The treated extracts were analyzed spectrophotometrically by absorbance at 260nm on sucrose density gradients, and also by the in vitro microcytotoxicity assay.

Previous work in our laboratory has shown it critical that the RNA extracts have a characteristic three peak appearance. The three peaks have sedimentation coefficients of 30S, 18S and 4S. As can be seen in Figure 2, effective "immune" RNA displays a typical three peak appearance.

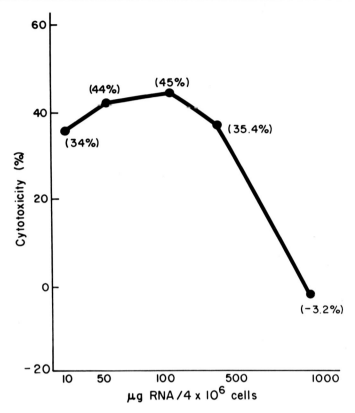

Fig. 1.   Dose effect of syngeneic "immune" RNA's ability to mediate tumor cell (4198 V) cytotoxicity. "% Cytotoxicity" represents the percent reduction of target cells by test lymphocytes as compared to normal lymphocyte controls.

Treatment of the RNA with RNAse resulted in degradation of the RNA with the majority of the resulting RNA residing in the 4S region. Treatment with either DNAse or pronase has no effect on the RNA density profile.

These same RNA preparations were then tested for their ability to transfer *in vitro* cytotoxicity to tumor cells. Similar procedures were followed as previously described with the only difference an enzymatic pretreatment of the RNA prior to incubating it with the lymphocytes. Figure 3 depicts the results obtained. RNAse treatment effectively abrogated the transfer of cytotoxicity. Treatment with either DNAse or pronase did not significantly reduce the transfer of cytotoxicity. These results certainly demonstrate the necessity of RNA in achieving the transfer of

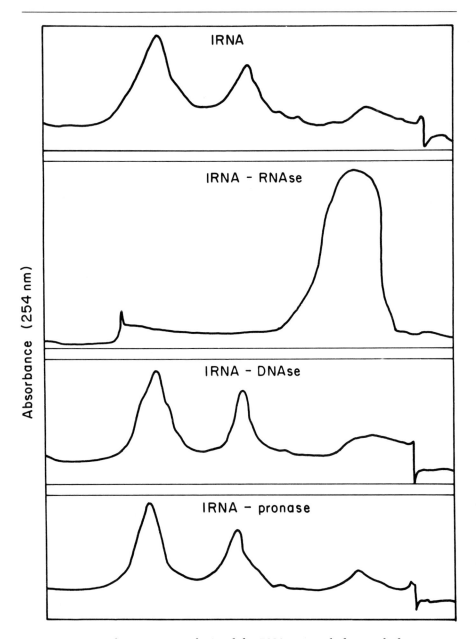

Fig. 2. Spectrophotometric analysis of the RNA extract before and after enzyme treatment.

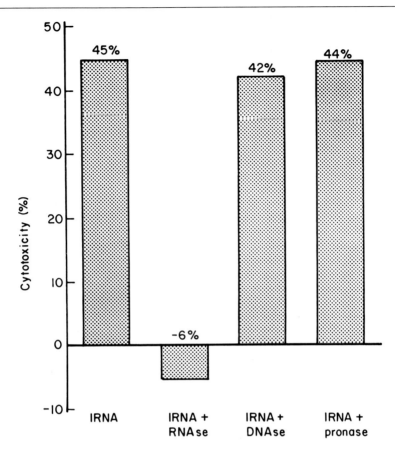

Fig. 3.   Cytotoxicity mediated by IRNA after treatment with RNAse, DNAse, and pronase. "% Cytotoxicity" represents the percent reduction of target cells by test lymphocytes as compared to normal lymphocyte controls.

cytotoxicity and at least suggests that both contaminating DNA and protein are not involved.

Under the conditions of the above controlled tests, it is clear that IRNA has the capacity to transfer specific anti-tumor cytotoxicity which is relatively dose dependent. It was completely unexpected, therefore, that while varying the doses of the RNA extracted from cells of untreated animals, it was found that this RNA was capable of mediating a nonspecific cytotoxicity for plated target cells.

Table 2 depicts the results obtained. The cytotoxicity was found to be optimally mediated by an RNA concentration of 50 μg. Cytotoxicity was

Table 2. Normal RNA-dependent lymphocyte-mediated cytotoxicity

Lymphocytes[a]	% Cytotoxicity[b] of Target Cells			
	V	LM	D$_2$	HeLa
SNRNA + RNAse	79	51	87	18
	23	2	nt[c]	5
XNRNA	83	61	50	16

a. SNRNA, lymphocytes treated with 50 μg of RNA from untreated mice before and after RNAse treatment; XNRNA, lymphocytes treated with RNA derived from untreated guinea pigs.

b. % Cytotoxicity: percent reduction of target cells by test lymphocytes as compared to normal lymphocyte controls.

c. Not tested.

obtained against all target cells tested including the 4198V tumor cell, the LM cell, the D$_2$ cell, and to a lesser extent, the Hela cell. The phenomenon was observed over a very limited dose range, and was not apparent at either higher or lower doses. Both syngeneic and xenogeneic (guinea pig) RNA species were found capable of mediating the cytotoxicity. Treatment of the RNA preparations with RNAse significantly reduced the amount of cytotoxicity indicating a requirement for intact RNA. The reason for this non-specific cytotoxicity by low doses of "normal" RNA is not completely clear, but possible explanations will be discussed later.

Transfer of Antitumor Cytotoxicity by Xenogeneic "Immune" RNA (IRNA)

Having established the fact that syngeneic RNA transferred cytotoxicity to mouse lymphocytes, the next step was to demonstrate transfer by xenogeneic RNA to mouse lymphocytes. If RNA transfer of responsiveness is to be of value in the human tumor situation, xenogeneic RNA will have to be effective. The RNA tested was derived from the spleens of untreated and immunized guinea pigs. The guinea pigs were immunized by a series of injections with the target cells, with or without Freunds' incomplete adjuvant. After immunization, the guinea pigs were skin tested with the appropriate cells, and if a skin test of greater than 10 mm was obtained after 48 hours, then the animals were sacrificed, and the RNA extracted from their spleens.

Three different xenogeneic RNA preparations were tested by the *in vitro* microcytotoxicity assay. The first was from animals immunized with the 4198V tumor cell, and designated XIRNA. The second was from animals immunized to the LM cell, depicted by XLMIRNA. The third was from untreated animals, and is signified by XNRNA. Table 3 displays the results obtained. Mouse lymphocytes treated with RNA derived from the tumor-immunized animals averaged 25.3% cytotoxicity of the tumor cells. The cytotoxicity was found to be specific by a lack of cytotoxicity by the same RNA preparations for the LM cell. RNA derived from LM cell immunized animals was shown to confer cytotoxicity to the LM cell, but not to the 4198V tumor cell. Again, RNA from untreated animals did not mediate significant cytotoxicity for either the 4198V or LM cells, at the doses tested. Untreated lymphocytes were used as the 0% cytotoxicity level.

As noted previously with syngeneic RNA, tumor cell cytotoxicity with xenogeneic RNA was also dose dependent. The results, as depicted in Figure 4, are quite similar to those obtained with the syngeneic RNA, in which a wide range of activity was found. Doses of xenogeneic RNA of 50, 100, and 500 μg transferred significant cytotoxicity for the tumor cells. As with syngeneic RNA 1,000 μg did not, possibly due to the same reasons

Table 3. Cell-mediated cytotoxicity to 4198 V and LM cell lines by lymphocytes treated with xenogeneic RNA

Lymphocytes Tested[a]	Cytotoxicity (%)[b]	
	4198 V	LM
NL	0	0
XIRNA	25.3[c]	−1.0[c]
XLMRNA	0	16
XNRNA	−4.7[d]	−8.3[d]

a. NL, normal lymphocytes; XIRNA, lymphocytes treated with RNA from 4198 V immunized guinea pigs; XLMRNA, lymphocytes treated with RNA from LM immunized guinea pigs; XNRNA, lymphocytes treated with RNA from normal guinea pigs.

b. Cytotoxicity: percent reduction of target cells by test lymphocytes as compared to target cell survival with normal lymphocytes.

c. Mean of three values.

d. Mean of two values.

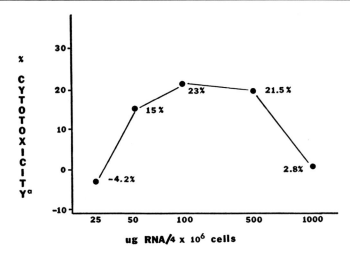

Fig. 4.   Dose effect of xenogeneic "immune" RNA's ability to mediate tumor cell (4198 V) cytotoxicity. "% Cytotoxicity" represents the percent reduction of tumor cells by "immune" RNA-treated lymphocytes as compared to normal lymphocyte controls.

suggested previously. Unlike the syngeneic RNA, however, the lowest dose of xenogeneic RNA tested (25 us) did not transfer cytotoxicity. This again emphasizes the dose dependency of the transfer of tumor cytotoxicity.

Another example of the specific cytotoxicity of IRNA for the fibrosarcoma was performed by Dr. John C. Rees, using a different method of measuring killing and making a comparison with another C3H normal mouse cell line 4094 as well as the LM cells. At the same time, extensive analysis of the procedure for production of this kind of immunologically active RNA and its application was carried out by Ms. Sherry Flinchum.

Albino, outbred guinea pigs were immunized with cell lines obtained from monolayer cultures. The animals were given three injections one week apart with 1×10^7 viable cells. The initial injection was given in Freund's incomplete adjuvant into footpads. The second injection was given in phosphate buffered saline intraperitoneally, the final injection was given subcutaneously. One week following the final injection each animal was skin tested with 1×10^7 viable cells in 0.1 ml. Those animals showing indurations of greater than 10-mm diameter were chosen as donors of RNA.

Lymphoid tissue was removed from immunized animals within one week of skin testing. The animals were exsanguinated by cardiac puncture. The spleen was chosen most frequently for extraction since it could be removed quickly and cleaned of extraneous material. The spleens were placed into oven sterilized beakers containing acetone at −70°C. The beakers were held in an insulated flask containing acetone and dry ice. Care was taken to exsanguinate the animals and place the spleen into the acetone within five minutes. The excess acetone was drained and the tissue stored at −70C until RNA extraction.

Ethanol and distilled liquid phenol were stored at −20C. All buffers were prepared in triple distilled water which had been treated with 50 μl/L diethylpyrocarbonate (Sigma Chemical Co., St. Louis, Mo.) and autoclaved. Buffer A contained 0.01 M sodium acetate, 0.1% 8-hydroxyquinoline, 0.5% sodium dodecyl sulfate, 0.004% polyvinyl sulfate, pH 5.0. Buffer B contained 2.5 M sodium acetate, pH 5.0. Buffer C contained 0.3 M sodium acetate, 0.005% polyvinyl sulfate, pH 5.1. Sucrose density buffer contained 0.01 M Tris(Hydroxymethyl)Aminomethane (Sigma Chemical Co., St. Louis, Mo.) 0.001 M EDTA, 0.05 M NaCl, pH 7.0. Bentonite was prepared according to Fraenkel-Conrat et al. (11).

A biphasic system of hot phenol and water was employed for RNA isolation with some modifications (19, 34, 38). One part tissue was homogenized in 30 parts (w/v) 90% freshly distilled phenol saturated with buffer A for 15 min. at 450 rpm using a VirTis Model 45 homogenizer (VirTis Co., Gardiner, N. Y.). An equal volume of buffer A containing 2 mg of bentonite was added and the mixture homogenized 10 min. more. The homogenate was extracted 10 min. at 60C with gentle agitation, bringing the mixture gradually to 55C. The extraction mixture was chilled to 10C and centrifuted 3 min. at 4C, 18,000 rpm in a Sorvall RC 2-B centrifuge (Ivan Sorvall Inc., Newtown, Conn.). The aqueous layer was withdrawn and the phenol layer re-extracted with one-half volume of buffer A containing bentonite. The mixture was chilled and centrifuged as before. The second aqueous layer was pooled with the first. One-half volume of chilled 90% phenol was added to the combined aqueous phases along with 2 mg of bentonite. The mixture was extracted, chilled, and centrifuged as before. The aqueous phase was removed and the procedure repeated once again. This final aqueous phase was brought to 0.3 M acetate with buffer B and added to 3 parts chilled ethanol at −20C overnight to precipitate the RNA. RNA was recovered by centrifuging 15 min. at 18,000 rpm at −20C and drying the pellet under a stream of nitrogen. The pellet was resuspended in 7 ml of buffer C and precipitated a second time with three parts ethanol at −20C. RNA was recovered as before, resuspended in buffer C and stored at −70C until lyophilization.

RNA was estimated spectrophotometrically at 260 nm, assuming $A_2^{1\%}{}_{60}$ = 240. The relative concentrations of RNA to protein were estimated by the ratios at 260 nm/230 nm and 260 nm/280 nm. DNA contamination was determined by the diphenylamine assay of Burton (5). Protein was estimated by the method of Lowry et al. (18).

The extent of degradation of isolated RNA was determined by centrifugation in linear sucrose gradients of 6 to 21% in sucrose density gradient buffer layered with 75 to 100 μg of RNA. The gradients, prepared in cellulose nitrate tubes, were centrifuged in a Spinco SW-27 rotor for 18 hr at 4C at 25,000 rpm using a Beckman L-2 Ultracentrifuge (Beckman Instruments Inc., Palo Alto, Calif.). The gradients were analyzed with an ISCO Model 184 uv monitor at 254 nm.

Biological activity of the IRNA was assessed by lymphocyte mediated cytotoxicity of C3H lymphocytes against two non-tumorigenic and one tumorigenic cell lines all of C3H origin. The non-tumorigenic cell lines were the 4094, originating from the parotid gland of C3H mice and spontaneously transformed (40) and the LM fibroblast derived from normal C3H mice (13). The tumor cell-line was the 4198V, a high tumor antigen variant derived from polyoma transformed 4094 cells (39). All cells were maintained in RPMI-1640 containing 2 mM L-glutamine and 10% heat inactivated fetal calf serum. The tumorigenicity of the 4198V cell line was periodically checked by injecting 1×10^6 to 1×10^7 viable cells intramuscularly into 5 week old C3H mice. Such treatment resulted in tumors in 100% of the mice by 14 days.

Cytotoxicity of RNA-treated C3H lymphocytes was determined using a tritium-labeled target cell assay. Target cells were plated at a concentration of 1×10^4/ml onto microtiter plates (Falcon Plastics #3040, Oxnard, Calif.) in 0.1 ml aliquots. The cells were labeled with 1.0 μC of methyltritiated thymidine, specific activity 6.7 Ci/mM (New England Nuclear, Boston, Mass.), overnight at 37C at 5% CO_2. The incorporation was stopped by the addition of 0.1 ml of medium containing 7.2 μg/ml unlabeled thymidine. Lymphocytes, either treated with IRNA, or untreated, were added to the labeled target cells at a ratio of 200 lymphocytes per target cell. Cultures were prepared as six replicates in each experimental group. The cultures were incubated for 72 hr, at which time the lymphocytes were decanted and the remaining attached target cells washed twice with 0.1 ml of medium. The remaining cells were scraped from the plate and aspirated onto glass fiber filter paper using a multiple analysis sample harvester (Otto Hiller, Inc., Madison, Wisc.). The strips were dried and the individual spots placed in a toluene-based scintillation cocktail. Radioactivity was estimated using a Packard Tri-Carb liquid scintillation spectrophotometer. The mean and standard error for the six replicate cultures were calculated. Cytotoxicity was calculated by dividing the cpm of wells receiving untreated lymphocytes minus the cpm of wells receiving IRNA-treated cells by the cpm of the wells receiving the untreated cells. This figure was then multiplied by 100 for the percent cytotoxicity.

Lymphocytes from 5-to-6-week old C3H mice were isolated from minced spleens using Ficoll/Hypaque gradients according to a modification of the procedure of Boyum (3). These normal lymphocytes were resuspended to 2×10^6/ml in 2.0 ml aliquots in RPMI-1640 without serum. Each aliquot received 25 μg of DEAE-dextran (Sigma Chemical Co., St. Louis, Mo.) per ml of medium immediately before the addition of the IRNA. The IRNA was added to the cultures in concentrations ranging from 25 μg/4 $\times$ 10^6 cells to 1000 μg/4 $\times$ 10^6 cells. The cultures were incubated at 37C on a 2 rpm rotator for 30 min. Following this the cells were concentrated at 400 $\times$ g for 10 min., washed once in RPMI-1640 containing 10% fetal calf serum and 100 μg Gentamicin (Schering Corp., Kenilworth, N.J.) and resuspended to the original concentration. Each experimental group contained lymphocytes treated with DEAE-dextran alone as the controls.

The immune status of several guinea pigs immunized with 4198V cells were assessed using the cytotoxicity assay. Lymphocytes from these donor animals were capable of significant killing of both the 4198V (35.1%) as well as the two antigenically similar, nontumorigenic controls, the 4094 (33.4%) and the LM (62.8%). Skin testing data confirmed these findings.

It was of singular importance to determine whether the IRNA extracted from the spleens of these animals would transfer this broad specificity of responses to normal C3H lymphocytes. In a series of experiments IRNA from 4198V immunized guinea pigs extracted individually were used to treat normal splenic lymphocytes from C3H mice at concentrations from 25 μg to 1000 μg. These treated cells were then tested for cytotoxic response against the tumor and the LM cell as compared to responses with lymphocytes treated with DEAE-dextran alone. The mean cytotoxicity results of this series of experiments are presented in Figure 5. Normal lymphocytes incubated with IRNA meeting the physiochemical conditions of intactness and purity demonstrated increased cytotoxicity against the 4198V cells in contrast to the lack of cytotoxicity against the syngeneic control cell. Cytotoxicity against the 4198V seen with 25 and 500 μg differ significantly from that seen toward the LM (p 0.05; p 0.001). The transfer of specific cytotoxicity is apparent with IRNA treated cells in spite of the fact that the IRNA came from guinea pigs showing immune responses to both cell types. Another important aspect of these data concerns the complex dose-response relationship. It is apparent that the dose of IRNA used to treat 4 $\times$ 10^6 lymphocytes is critical; variation from this narrow range can result in failure to detect transfer.

Further experiments were then performed with IRNA from guinea pigs immunized with the 4094 cell. Normal C3H lymphocytes were incubated with doses of this IRNA as previously described. These cells were

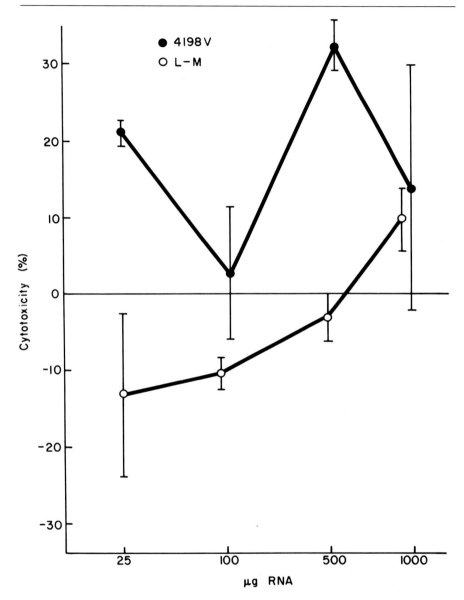

Fig. 5. Cytotoxicity with C3H treatment with IRNA from 4198 V immunized guinea pigs.

Table 4. Cytotoxicity of normal mouse lymphocytes treated with 4094/IRNA

Target Cell	Dose[a] IRNA	CPM (±S.E.)	Cytotoxicity[b] (%)
LM	25	48,176 (1691)[c]	28.1[d]
	100	64,084 (2593)	4.4
	500	61,777 (2141)	7.0
	1000	64,775 (2344)	3.4
	NRNA[e]	66,977 (1910)	0.1
	none[f]	67,027 (2109)	—
4198 V	25	16,893 (811)	<0
	100	11,788 (892)	6.9
	500	12,758 (1619)	<0
	1000	17,904 (1015)	<0
	NRNA	15,400 (657)	<0
	none	12,665 (1597)	—

a. μg IRNA per 4×10^6 lymphocytes.
b. Cytotoxicity calculated as follows: (cpm with untreated cells) minus (cpm with IRNA-treated cells) divided by (cpm with untreated cells) multiplied by 100.
c. Mean of six replicate determinations.
d. p value < 0.001.
e. RNA from unimmunized guinea pigs.
f. Cells treated with 25 μg of DEAE-dextran.

then tested for their ability to induce cytotoxicity against the tumor cells and the syngeneic LM cells. These data are presented in Table 4. No cytotoxicity against the 4198V was expressed by lymphocytes treated with 4094/IRNA. Resultant cytotoxicity against the LM was minimal at doses greater than 100 μg. Significant cytotoxicity against the LM was apparent with lymphocytes treated with 25 μg (28.1%; $p = 0.001$). Lymphocytes treated with RNA from unimmunized animals were not cytotoxic for either the LM or the 4198V. Lymphocytes treated with 4198V/IRNA showed significant cytotoxicity against the 4198V target cells (26.6%).

Various factors encountered in the extraction and purification process are citical. Among these is that maximal yield of IRNA is relative to the amount of tissue homogenized. With both guinea pig and mouse spleens larger amounts of tissue appear to increase the percent yield of IRNA. These increases must be viewed with caution, however, since consistently unacceptable levels of DNA are present. The results of 15 representative extractions from guinea pig spleens are presented in Table 5. Examination

Table 5.   IRNA extractions from guinea pig spleens

Immunizing Agent	Grams of Tissue	mg IRNA Recovered	Yield (mg/g)
None	1.20	4.36	3.63
None[a]	2.10	10.50	5.00[b]
None	1.21	3.33	2.75
4198 V	0.71	2.95	4.16
4198 V[a]	2.43	24.75	10.19[c]
4198 V	0.87	2.89	3.32
4198 V	1.40	6.79	4.85
4198 V	1.30	4.95	3.81
4198 V	1.83	7.95	4.35
4198 V	1.41	5.40	3.83
SRBC	0.80	3.00	3.75
SRBC	1.19	5.50	4.62
SRBC	1.56	9.30	3.75
Mean	1.38	7.04	4.63
(±S.E.)	(0.14)	(1.62)	(0.52)

a. IRNA extracted from two pooled spleens.
b. DNA contamination was 27%.
c. DNA contamination was 65%.

of these data indicate that the mean yield of IRNA per gram of tissue extracted was 4.63 mg. When 2.43 grams of splenic tissue were extracted, the yield was apparently greater (10.19 mg/gram); however, in this instance and another shown (2.10 grams) the amount of DNA in the final product was unacceptable (65% and 27%) and interfered with accurate quantitation. Successful transfer of cytotoxicity is closely dependent upon dosage (Figure 5). Inaccurate quantitation due to large amounts of DNA may, in effect, decrease the amount of RNA employed for in vitro transfer. In addition, little is known concerning the effects of DNA on RNA uptake or upon expression of biological parameters following treatment. The immune status of the donor has, apparently, little effect upon yields.

To obtain IRNA with demonstrable biological activity various factors were found to be critical during 15 separate extractions of guinea pig spleens. Most investigators of the immunological aspects of IRNA agree that biological activity is lost upon degradation. When all factors during the isolation were controlled to present degradation and maximize yield, it was shown that immunologically active IRNA invariably presented a

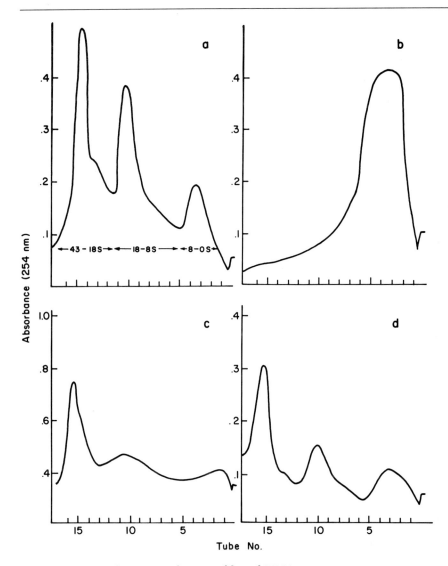

Fig. 6.   Sucrose density-gradient profiles of IRNA.

sucrose density gradient profile as shown in Figure 6a for guinea pig IRNA. Using successful transfer of specific cytotoxicity to normal C3H mouse lymphocytes as a criterion, it was shown that such activity depended upon a gradient pattern in which the ratio of the height of the 18–8 S peak to the 8–0 S peak was 2.0 or greater. Figure 6b shows inactive

IRNA resulting from degradation with RNAse. Figure 6c represents an RNA sample containing 25% contamination with DNA. The RNA in this sample was found to be undergraded when analyzed at a higher attenuation (Figure 6d). The presence of large amounts of DNA has not been shown to materially affect immunological activity per se, but since dosage of RNA is a critical factor such contamination may affect accurate quantitation and may lead to ineffective transfer due only to lowered amounts of IRNA.

Extraction of 230.86 mg of IRNA from 36 guinea pig spleens either normal, immune to murine fibrosarcoma cells, immune to non-tumorigenic C3H cells, sheep red blood cell immune, or BCG immunized animals has indicated that 6 mg of IRNA in a useable undegraded form can be expected from a single guinea pig spleen, if the conditions outlined in this report are adhered to strictly. In addition, further research has indicated that 0.7 to 0.8 mg of IRNA can be isolated from C3H mouse spleens if the amount of tissue extracted is limited to at least 10 but not more than 15 spleens (1.4 to 1.8 grams). If the requirements of less than 5% contamination with DNA, less than 5% protein, and a ratio of 18–8 S to 8–0 S is at least 2.0 or more are met, the material will transfer immunological responses which, to date, include lymphocyte mediated cytotoxicity, localized hemolysis in gel (8), antibody dependent cellular cytotoxicity (24), and MIF production (22).

The following statements may be made concerning the IRNA isolation procedure. The tissue must be removed from the animal within 5 min. after exsanguination. The tissue chosen must be frozen quickly. Our experience has indicated that rapid freezing before extraction results in consistently satisfactory products. Extractions of fresh, as opposed to frozen, tissue results in lower yields and greater degradation. Our most efficient yields of IRNA were obtained with 2 grams of tissue, extraction of larger amounts frequently resulted in preparations containing unacceptable amounts of DNA. In light of the critical relationship between RNA, cell numbers, and perhaps antigen, the presence of high amounts of DNA may affect quantitation; since all nucleic acids absorb at 260 nm (20), the presence of DNA would essentially mean that the final product would contain less IRNA than that actually measured.

IRNA extracted and characterized according to the procedures discussed here was capable of transferring to normal mouse lymphocytes the ability to induce cytotoxicity against murine fibrosarcoma cells. Although cytotoxicity and skin test results indicate that the donor animals possessed lymphocytes capable of response to the tumor cell and to the antigenically similar LM and 4094 cells, the IRNA from these animals transferred only the ability to kill the tumor cell. The transfer of the cytotoxic response was dose dependent. This complex dose/response relationship has been observed in this laboratory using other *in vitro* correlates of cellular immunity. Treatment of normal lymphocytes with 4198V/IRNA enables some cells within the population to express cytotoxicity against the tumor cell (32.8%) but no apparent response to normal (non-tumor) antigens (−3.3%). The cytotoxic response expressed by these lymphocytes following treatment with a precise dose of IRNA is apparently directed at tumor specific antigens on the 4198V cells. If responses against normal antigens are transferred, their expression is suppressed by cells or cell products within the treated population.

This is again emphasized by the fact that lymphocytes treated with similar doses of IRNA from 4094 immunized guinea pigs did not show cytotoxicity for the 4198V cells. However, some killing of LM cells (28.1%) was observed following treatment with 25 μg. It can be assumed that any cytotoxicity for normal mouse cells was somehow shut off by the cells treated with IRNA from tumor immunized animals. It is curious, therefore, that 4094/IRNA caused mouse lymphocytes to kill LM cells since the only known difference in the 4094 and the LM is the presence of a non-tumor associated antigen not shared by the 4094. This would indicate that killing was directed toward a shared, therefore normal, antigen involved in the LM cell transformation. This indicates that capacity for cytotoxicity for normal mouse cells was perhaps present in the guinea pig IRNA but expressed only in the presence of the non-tumorigenic variant (LM). Again, since significant killing was evident only with the lowest dose tested, it may involve a different, non-specific effect of IRNA-treated lymphocytes. Quite obviously, the 4198V/IRNA is quite specific since it transferred no recognition of this shared antigen nor the LM specificity.

It seems pertinent to note also that evidently mouse lymphocytes sensitized by xenogeneic IRNA to this mouse tumor express a highly specific antitumor cytotoxicity, quite in contrast from the cytotoxicity for this tumor shown by sensitized guinea pig splenic lymphocytes directly. The latter would appear to be a dual recognition process involving both species and tumor antigens. Thus, IRNA treated mouse lymphocytes are different from sensitized guinea pig lymphocytes and appear much as syngeneic tumor sensitized lymphocytes. In fact, syngeneic C3H tumor sensitized lymphocytes, C3H lymphocytes treated with syngeneic IRNA, and C3H lymphocytes treated with xenogeneic IRNA show similar patterns of cytotoxic responses.

One aspect of syngeneic or xenogeneic IRNA treated lymphocytes can be seen in Figure 5. The dose dependency of activity seen here has been observed using MIF and antibody production to tumor antigen, tuberculin, and to sheep red blood cells. In turn, a given dose of IRNA may be shown to cause treated cells to behave differently with different doses of antigen. Both phenomena seem related to the production or transfer of suppressive factors. It may be surmised that the lack of response following treatment with some doses of IRNA may be due to the transfer of "suppressor" factors or information.

Immuno-Prophylaxis of Tumor with Xenogeneic IRNA

Preliminary data indicate that guinea pig splenic lymphocyte IRNA to this mouse fibrosarcoma is effective in preventing tumor growth in mice injected with a 100% tumor dose. This work was carried out by the authors with the invaluable aid of Drs. John C. Rees and Kenneth J. Pennline, who are continuing studies on both prophylaxis and immunotherapy.

The IRNA used was prepared by immunizing guinea pigs with cultured cells of the C3H mouse fibrosarcoma as previously described. After skin testing with tumor cells indicated sensitization, spleens were removed, and IRNA extracted from the cells. C3H mice were sacrificed, spleens removed, and their lymphocytes were separated and treated with the xenogeneic IRNA. These treated lymphocytes were shown to be cytotoxic for the tumor as already described. Such treated cells which are not cytotoxic but do not affect normal mouse cells were injected into normal mice. The mice thus received syngeneic "tumor-immune" to protect the IRNA from degradation by enzymes in the body. Each animal received 2×10^7 treated lymphocytes injected intraperitoneally one day prior to tumor challenge (day 0), the latter consisting of a 100% challenge dose of tumor cells given the next day, and the same dose of treated lymphocytes repeated two days later (day 3). Controls consisted of mice injected with the same numbers of normal lymphocytes and mice receiv-

Table 6.   Summary of tumor challenge data

Group[a]	Tumor[b] Formation	Percent Tumor Formation
Normal mice	8/8	100
Mice injected with untreated cells	7/7	100
Mice injected with IRNA-treated lymphocytes	6/15	40

a. The data presented is a summation of results of separate experiments.
b. The number of mice which had tumors divided by the total number of mice challenged with a tumor-forming dose of 4198 tumor cells.

ing only tumor cells. Each dose of 2×10^7 lymphocytes was the equivalent of cells treated with 500 μg of IRNA.

As noted in Table 6, all 15 control mice developed tumors by day 24, while only 6 of 15 animals receiving IRNA-treated cells did so. The 60% of mice which were protected remained tumor-free for three more months, at which time control animals were dead of the tumor. The protected animals were also immune to subsequent tumor challenge several months later, but were not immune to another tumor for C3H mice.

Distinct Immunologic Properties of RNA from Lymphocytes of Tumor Immune and Tumor Bearing Mice

In vitro examination of the immune response in tumor-bearing animals usually reveals the same humoral factors as found in immune animals such as cytolytic antibody, antibody-dependent cell cytotoxicity (ADCC), as well as specifically cytotoxic lymphocytes (12, 14, 29, 30). However, the response in the former animals also includes "blocking" or "enhancing" factors variously described as antibody (37), tumor antigen (6), or a soluble complex of both (36), which effectively abolishes the cytotoxic action of specifically sensitized lymphocytes. Recently Nelson et al. demonstrated that supernates obtained from cultured lymphocytes of tumor-bearing animals (TL) as opposed to similar supernates from immune lymphocytes (IL) abolished the cytotoxicity of sensitized lymphocytes (23).

This report describes the production of specific "blocking" factors by normal lymphocytes treated in vitro with RNA from lymphocytes of tumor-bearing animals (TLRNA) which are not produced by normal lymphocytes treated with RNA from immunized animals (ILRNA). Both TLRNA and ILRNA were found to stimulate the production of ADCC. Since, antibody and blocking factors were produced by cultured lymphocytes in an antigen-free system, it is clear that "immune" lymphocyte RNA and RNA from tumor-bearing animals are different, and that the immune response includes "blocking" or "enhancing" factors only when tumor antigen is constantly provided from the growing tumor, but not as artificially supplied by injections of living tumor cells.

C3H mice were injected with 5×10^5 cells of a polyoma induced fibrosarcoma in one rear leg. Tumors appeared in all mice within 14 days. These mice were sacrificed seven days later and their spleens were used as the source of lymphocytes for the extraction of TLRNA. ILRNA was obtained from splenic lymphocytes of C3H mice immunized by three intraperitoneal injections of 4×10^6 viable tumor cells every six days, three to five days after the last injection. RNA extracted from splenic lymphocytes of normal mice is indicated as NLRNA. Each type of RNA was extracted from spleen cells of the appropriate mice by the use of hot phenol as previously described.

Lymphocytes used for treatment with the various RNAs were obtained from normal C3H mouse spleens which were removed aseptically and placed in a petri dish with 7 ml of RPMI-1640 medium containing 1% gentamicin. Spleen cells were teased free and lymphocytes separated by Hypaque-Ficoll gradient, and adjusted to a final concentration of 2×10^6 cells per ml in the same medium. Cell treatment consisted of the addition of 100 μg of the appropriate RNA (TLRNA, ILRNA, or NLRNA) and 50 μg of DEAE-dextran to 2 ml of the lymphocyte suspension containing 4×10^6 lymphocytes and then incubated for 30 minutes at 37C in the presence of 5% of CO_2. Triplicate treatments with each RNA were performed. All suspensions were centrifuged at 250 G for 10 minutes, residual medium and RNA aspirated, each cell suspension resuspended and washed three times in the same medium and were finally suspended in 5 ml of RPMI containing 20% fetal calf serum, 1% gentamicin and 1% L-glutamine in 25 ml Erlenmeyer flasks and incubated at 37C and 5% CO_2. Supernatants from each cell suspension were obtained at 42 hour periods by transferring the suspensions to sterile test tubes and centrifuging at 250 G for 6 minutes. The supernatants were filtered, heat inactivated at 56C for 30 min and stored at $-20C$. The cell pellets were resuspended in medium, a sample removed for testing viability, and re-incubated. Lymphocytes from spleens of normal (NL), tumor-bearing (TL), and tumor-immune (IL) C_3H mice were maintained in the same manner except for RNA treatment.

Supernatants were tested for blocking or ADCC activity on tumor cells suspended in RPMI with 10% fetal calf serum which were added to wells of 3034 Falcon microcytotoxicity plates, 100 cells per well in 0.01 ml quantities, allowed to attach for 12 hours, at this time the medium was decanted from the plates and the various supernatants added to the cells in the various wells. The supernatants remained in contact with the tumor cells for 30 minutes, were decanted, and the appropriate lymphocytes added at an effector cell to target cell ratio of 100:1. For blocking, actively tumor immune C3H mouse splenic lymphocytes were used, while for demonstration of ADCC, normal C3H mouse splenic lymphocytes were employed. Supernatants from NL and NLRNA treated lymphocytes were used as controls for the calculation of percent blocking and ADCC as previously described (23).

It was realized initially the viability of RNA-treated cells in an antigen-free culture would be a limiting factor in the time span of the experiment, since it was known, as shown in Table 1, that whereas 90% of

Table 7. Percent viability of untreated and RNA-treated lymphocytes at various intervals during culturing time

Lymphocytes	Culturing Time (hr)					
	24	48	57	72	93	100
NL treated with 50 μg TLRNA:	90	75	48	—[a]	18	—
NL treated with 100 μg TLRNA:	93	84	68	—	27	—
NL treated with 100 μg ILRNA:	81	63	40	—	15	—
NL treated with 100 μg NLRNA:	70	39	23	—	8	—
TL	99	97	95	95	—	95
IL	99	94	94	90	90	—
NL	57	38	21	10	—	—

a. — not tested.

splenic IL and TL remain viable for 4 to 5 days, less than 50% of NL survive for 48 hours under the same conditions. Table 7 also shows that treatment of NL with either TLRNA or ILRNA in 100 or 50 μg quantities increased the 50% viability of NL to at least 57 hours, whereas an equal amount of NLRNA had no detectable effect on lymphocyte viability. Evidently, RNA from sensitized lymphocytes provides some of the information responsible for the more vigorous metabolism of these cells under these conditions.

Figure 7 shows that supernatants from normal mouse lymphocytes treated with TLRNA but not after treatment with ILRNA, contained a blocking factor which prevented cytotoxicity of tumor cells by specifically sensitized lymphocytes. TL, but not IL, also produced this blocking effect, which has been previously reported by Nelson et al. (23). It is interesting to note that TLRNA-treated lymphocytes produced blocking factor earlier and in greater amounts than TL cells, although production by the latter cells was more sustained, undoubtedly due to their superior survival capacity. The last detectable blocking factor by TLRNA-treated cells coincides fairly well with the time of 50% loss of viability seen in Table 7. No blocking factor was produced by NL- or NLRNA-treated lymphocytes when cultured similarly.

Figure 8 demonstrates that all four types of lymphocytes, TLRNA- and ILRNA-treated, TL and IL, produced ADCC antibody in supernatants of their culture fluids which allowed normal lymphocytes to kill tumor cells treated with these supernatants. Antibody was produced earlier by

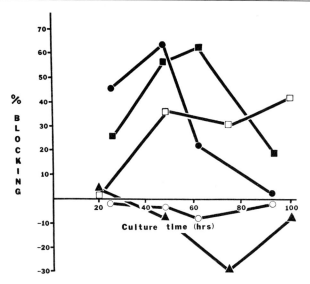

Fig. 7. Blocking activity of culture supernatants collected from untreated and RNA-treated lymphocytes: IL (▲———▲), TL (□———□), and NL treated with 100 μg of ILRNA (○———○), 50 μg of TLRNA (●———●) and 100 μg of TLRNA (●———●).

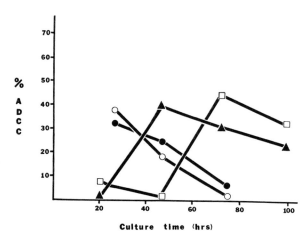

Fig. 8. ADCC activity of culture supernatants collected from untreated and RNA-treated lymphocytes: IL (▲———▲), TL (□———□) and NL treated with 100 μg of ILRNA (○———○) and 100 μg of TLRNA (●———●).

TLRNA- and ILRNA-treated lymphocytes, and as with blocking, the more rapid decrease in production is associated with decreased viability of these cells.

The blocking effect of supernatants from TLRNA-treated lymphocytes shown in Figure 8 resulted from treatment of normal lymphocytes from 100 μg of TLRNA. Absorption of the supernatants with a suspension of tumor cells (Figure 9) removed most blocking activity indicating the effect to be due to specific antibody as previously reported for supernatants of TL (23). However, supernatants from normal lymphocytes treated with 50 μg of TLRNA contained not only the tumor cell absorbable antibody, but in addition, such supernatants contained a dose-dependent blocking factor demonstrable by the lack of cytotoxicity by tumor sensitized lymphocytes exposed to such supernatants after 48 hours in culture (Figure 9). In the absence of tumor antigen in these experiments with TLRNA-treated lymphocytes, the argument in favor of tumor antigen as the explanation for the paradoxical presence of in vitro cytotoxic lymphocytes which are inactive in the in vivo tumor situation does not apply. Rather, the situation is two RNA species, one highly dose-dependent, that directs normal lymphocytes to produce not only blocking antibody but a factor, perhaps lymphokine, which directly blocks cytotoxic lymphocytes. These RNA preparations contain less than 5% protein. Even supposing all of this existed as "super" antigen-RNA complex, it would provide very little for

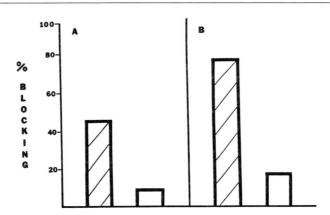

Fig. 9. A. Blocking activity of supernatants from NL treated with 50 μg (▨▨▨) and 100 μg (▭) of TLRNA which were collected after 48 hrs in culture and absorbed with 1×10^7 tumor cells. **B.** Blocking exhibited by treating tumor-immune lymphocytes with 48 hr culture supernatants from NL treated with 50 μg (▨▨▨) and 100 μg (▭) of TLRNA.

four million cells to continue to reproduce for 50–60 hours, and it should have been even more in evidence from 100 μg doses.

The presence of these blocking factors generated in the culture fluid of only lymphocytes treated with TLRNA provides evidence in favor of the point made by Prehn (31) that the original immunologic event in the tumor situation results in enhancement. Such enhancing RNA species apparently do not occur following artificial immunization with living tumor cells. Since complete tumor removal is followed by the disappearance of blocking and the establishment of tumor immunity, blocking is reversible and the situation imposed by the ILRNA can be established. The reason for the divergent RNA content of lymphocytes following the two immunization procedures is not clear. Lymphocytes treated with either ILRNA or TLRNA are capable of producing the immune factors generated by the particular RNA donor sensitized lymphocytes. On the basis of viability they survive intermediately between sensitized and normal lymphocytes suggesting some metabolic activity of the RNA donor cells is not transferred.

ACKNOWLEDGMENTS

This study was supported in part by Grant CA-16867 from the National Cancer Institute, National Institutes of Health, Bethesda, Maryland.

REFERENCES

1. Alexander, P., Delorme, E. J., and Hall, J. G. 1966. The effect of lymphoid cells from the lymph of specifically immunized sheep on the growth of primary rat sarcomata in rats. *Lancet* 1: 1186.

2. Alexander, P., Delorme, E. J., Hamilton, L. D. G., and Hall, J. G. 1967. Effect of nucleic acids from immune lymphocytes on rat sarcomata. *Nature* 213: 569.

3. Boyum, A. 1968. Isolation of mononuclear cells and granulocytes from human blood. *Scand. J. Clin. Invest.* 97: 77.

4. Brower, P. A., Ramming, K. P., and deKernion, J. B. 1975. Immune cytolysis of human neoplasms mediated by RNA. *Surg. Forum* 26: 156.

5. Burton, K. 1956. A study of the conditions and mechanisms of the diphenylamine reaction for the colorimetric estimation of deoxyribonucleic acid. *Biochem. J.* 62: 315.

6. Currie, G. A., and Basham, C. 1972. Serum mediated inhibition of the immunological reactions of the patient to his own tumor: A possible role for circulating antigen. *Brit. J. Cancer* 26: 427.

7. Deckers, P. J., Wang, B. S., Stuart, P. A., and Mannick, J. A. 1975. The augmentation of tumor specific immunity with immune RNA. *Transplant. Proc.* 7: 259.

8. Dodd, M. C., Scheetz, M. E., II, and Rossio, J. L. 1973. Immunogenic RNA in the immunotherapy of cancer. N. Y. Academy of Sciences International Conference on RNA in the Immune Response. Ann. N. Y. Acad. Sci. 207: 454.

9. Evans, S. B., Miller, L. S., Pennline, K. J., and Dodd, M. C. 1976. RNA-mediated lymphocyte responsiveness to a murine fibrosarcoma tumor, as measured by microcytotoxicity and lymphoblastogenesis. Abstract. Seventy-sixth Ann. Meeting American Society for Microbiology.

10. Evans, S. D., Pennline, K. J., and Dodd, M. C. 1975. RNA induced lymphocyte-mediated cytotoxicity to a murine fibrosarcoma tumor. J. Reticuloendothelial Soc. 18: 17b.

11. Fraenkel-Conrat, H., Singer, B., and Tsugita, A. 1961. Purification of viral RNA by means of bentonite. Virology 14: 54.

12. Friedman, H. 1964. Antibody plaque formation by normal mouse spleen cell cultures exposed in vitro to RNA from immune mice. Science 146: 934.

13. Giles, R. R., Merchant, D. J., and Masselink, E. 1966. Chromosomes of LM cells and variants. J. Natl. Cancer Inst. 37: 663.

14. Hellström, I., and Hellström, K. E. 1969. Studies on cellular immunity and its serum mediated inhibition in Moloney-virus-induced mouse sarcomas. Int. J. Cancer 4: 587.

15. Kennedy, C. T. C., Cater, D. B., and Hartveit, F. 1969. Protection of C3H mice against B P-8 tumor by RNA extracted from lymph nodes and spleens of specifically sensitized mice. Acta. Pathol. Microbiol. Scand. 77: 796.

16. Kern, D. H., and Pilch, Y. H. 1974. Immune cytolysis of murine tumor cells mediated by xenogeneic "immune" RNA. Int. J. Cancer 13: 679.

17. Londner, M. V., Morini, J. C., Font, M. T., and Rabasa, S. L. 1968. RNA-induced immunity against a rat sarcoma. Experimentia 24: 598.

18. Lowry, O. H., Rosenberg, N. J., Farr, A. L., and Randall, R. J. 1951. Protein measurement with the Folin Phenol Reagent. J. Biol. Chem. 193: 265.

19. Mach, B., and Vassalli, P. 1965. Template activity of RNA from antibody-producing tissues. Science 150: 622.

20. Mahler, H. R., and Cordes, E. H. 1971. Biological Chemistry, 2nd ed., p. 224. Harper & Row, New York.

21. Mannick, J. A., and Egdahl, R. H. 1964. Transfer of heightened immunity to skin homografts by lymphoid RNA. J. Clin. Invest. 43: 2166.

22. Nawrocki, J. F., and Dodd, M. C. 1975. In vitro transfer of tuberculin sensitivity by immune Ribonucleic Acid (iRNA). J. Reticuloendothel. Soc. 18: 51b.

23. Nelson, K., Pollack, S. B., and Hellström, K. E. 1975a. Specific anti-tumor responses by cultured immune spleen cells. I. In vitro culture method and initial characterization of factors which block immune cell-mediated cytotoxicity in vitro. Int. J. Cancer 15: 806.

24. Pennline, K. J., Evans, S. B., Minton, J. P., and Dodd, M. C. 1976. Distinctive immunological properties of RNA extracted from tumor-immune and tumor-bearing mice (unpublished results).

25. Pilch, Y. H. 1972. Immune RNA: New model for the immunotherapy of cancer. Ann. Int. Med. 77: 431.

26. Pilch, Y. H., Ramming, K. P., and Deckers, P. J. 1973. Induction of anti-cancer immunity with RNA. Ann. N. Y. Acad. Sci. 207: 409.

27. Pilch, Y. H., Veltman, L. L., and Kern, D. H. 1974. Immune cytolysis of human tumor cells by xenogeneic "immune" RNA: implications for immunotherapy. *Surgery* 76: 23.

28. Pollock, H. M. 1970. RNA transfer of immunity between inbred strains of mice. Ph.D. Dissertation. The Ohio State University, Columbus, Ohio.

29. Pollock, S., Heppner, G., and Brown, R. 1972. Specific killing of tumor cells *in vitro* in the presence of normal lymphoid cells and sera from hosts immune to the tumor antigens. *Int. J. Cancer* 9: 316.

30. Pollock, S. 1973. Specific "arming" of normal lymph node cells by sera from tumor-bearing mice. *Int. J. Cancer* 11: 138.

31. Prehn, R. T. 1971. Perspectives on oncogenesis: Does immunity stimulate or inhibit neoplasia? *J. Reticuloendothel. Soc.* 10: 1.

32. Ramming, K. P., and Pilch, Y. H. 1970. Mediation of immunity to tumor isografts in mice by heterologous ribonucleic acids. *Science* 168: 492.

33. Rigby, P. G. 1969. Prolongation of survival of tumor-bearing animals by transfer of "immune" RNA with DEAE-dextran. *Nature* 221: 968.

34. Scherrer, K. 1969. Isolation and sucrose gradient analysis of RNA, *in* K. Habel and K. P. Salzman (eds.), *Fundamental Techniques in Virology*, p. 413. Academic Press, New York.

35. Schlager, S. I., Paque, R. E., and Dray, S. 1975. Complete and apparently specific local tumor regression using syngeneic or xenogeneic "tumor immune" RNA extracts. *Cancer Res.* 35: 1907.

36. Sjögren, H. O., Hellström, I., Bansal, S. C., and Hellström, K. E. 1971. Suggestive evidence that the "blocking antibodies" of tumor-bearing individuals may be antigen-antibody complexes. *Proc. Natl. Acad. Sci.* 68: 1372.

37. Takasugi, M., and Klein, E. 1970. A microassay for cell-mediated immunity. *Transplantation* 9: 219.

38. Thor, D. E. 1971. Conversion of nonsensitive lymph node cell populations to sensitive cells with an RNA extract, *in* B. R. Bloom and P. R. Glade (eds.), *In Vitro Methods in Cell-Mediated Immunity*, p. 547. Academic Press, New York.

39. Ting, R. C., and Law, L. W. 1965. The role of thymus in transplantation resistance induced by polyoma virus. *J. Natl. Canc. Inst.* 34: 521.

40. Ting, C. C., Lavrin, D. H., Takemoto, K. K., Ting, R. C., and Herberman, R. B. 1972. Expression of various tumor-specific antigens in polyoma virus-induced tumors. *Cancer Res.* 32: 1.

CHAPTER 10

IMMUNOTHERAPY OF CANCER WITH IMMUNE RNA: CURRENT STATUS

Kenneth P. Ramming
Jean B. deKernion
Yosef H. Pilch

Department of Surgery
UCLA School of Medicine
Los Angeles, California 90509
Department of Surgery
School of Medicine
University of California at San Diego
La Jolla, California 92093

Immune RNA (I-RNA) is an RNA-rich nucleic acid preparation extracted from lymphoid cells or tissues following exposure to specific antigens in vitro or sensitization to specific antigens in vivo. It induces normal, non-immune lymphoid cells to mediate specific cellular and humoral immune responses. Previous studies have demonstrated that I-RNA preparations extracted from the lymphoid organs of animals immunized with tumor cells mediate specific immune responses against tumor-associated antigens in both animal models and human tumor systems. Cancer patients were treated with I-RNA extracted from the lymphoid organs of sheep immunized with either autologous tumor cells or allogeneic tumor cells of the same histologic type. The results of these preliminary trials suggest increased survival in patients with metastatic hypernephroma and possible benefit (decreased recurrence rate) in the adjuvant immunotherapy of patients with malignant melanoma.

Introduction

Passive and/or adoptive immunotherapy of cancer involves the transfer of immunologically active cells or cell products from a specifically immunized donor(s) to a cancer patient in an attempt to transfer either humoral or cellular immune reactivity to the recipient. Sera from cured cancer patients have occasionally been administered and at least one documented instance of tumor regression in a recipient of serum from a patient who had experienced a spontaneous regression of a similar tumor has been recorded (58). However, the demonstration of complex circulating blocking and unblocking serum factors and the limited number of appropriate donors make this form of passive immunotherapy both rare and potentially hazardous until the role of these factors is further delineated (20). McKhann et al. cultured lymphocytes from cancer patients with autologous tumor cells in an attempt to sensitize the lymphocytes to tumor antigens, in vitro, prior to reinfusion (34). Other investigators have infused autologous lymphocytes following in vitro stimulation with various mitogens (6), or infused large numbers of autologous or allogeneic lymphocytes cultured in vitro (37). Morton has suggested transfusing lymphocytes from family members (39). Like McKhann, Seigler (55) and Moore (38) have advocated sensitizing cancer patients' lymphocytes to autochthonous tumor cells by cocultivation in vitro, followed by reinfusion.

Isolated instances of transfusion of allogeneic lymphocytes from a cured cancer patient to one with a growing tumor have been reported (41). This method of adoptively transferring tumor immunity is potentially hazardous since the patient's immune system may rapidly destroy the donor lymphocytes which contain foreign H-LA antigens, graft versus host reactions may occur in immunosuppressed recipients, and severe hypersensitivity reactions may ensue. Cross-immunization with tumor cells of patients with similar tumor types who are identical with respect to ABO and RH types, followed by cross-transfusion of white blood cells or plasma, has occasionally been accompanied by small tumor regressions, but has also resulted in significant complications due to incompatible H-LA antigens. Furthermore, results are difficult to interpret since immunization to H-LA as well as to tumor-associated antigens results (22). The complications associated with passive and adoptive immunotherapy schemes, difficulty in obtaining adequate amounts of serum or cells, and the modest results obtained, have hampered progress in this potentially useful method of immune therapy (7).

The use of lymphoid extracts, that is active subcellular fractions of immune lymphocytes capable of mediating specific immune responses after injection into non-immune or immunosuppressed subject, has long intrigued investigators and therapists alike. Two such immunologically active lymphoid extracts have been studied fairly extensively. They are transfer factor and Immune RNA (I-RNA).

Transfer of delayed cutaneous hypersensitivity responses to tuberculin and other antigens in man with a dialyzable extract of human peripheral blood leukocytes was initially reported by Lawrence and co-workers (30). This substance, called "transfer factor," has since been shown by other authors to transfer delayed cutaneous hypersensitivity reactions to other antigens in man (5, 21, 31, 32, 33). Transfer factor has also been shown to be effective in the treatment of certain immunodeficiency diseases, and in certain disseminated intracellular infections (56, 57). Occasional regressions of human tumors have been reported after infusion of transfer factor (17), but its role in the treatment of malignancies has yet to be defined.

The term Immune RNA (I-RNA) refers to RNA-rich extracts of immune lymphoid cells which have been shown to mediate immune responses to a variety of antigens in vitro and in vivo. It has also been shown to mediate anti-tumor immune responses in a number of animal tumor models, effecting immunoprophylaxis against otherwise lethal tumor innocula (50) in vivo, preventing or delaying the occurrence of metastatic lesions (44), and rarely, inducing partial regressions of established tumors (1, 10). It is significant that in most of the in vivo animal experiments xenogeneic I-RNA, that is I-RNA extracted from the lymphoid tissues of a donor species different from the I-RNA recipient, was able to induce an antitumor response without any associated toxicity, secondary syndromes or allergic reactions (46). It is our observations on the use of xenogeneic Immune RNA in the treatment of human neoplasms, preceded by a presentation of the laboratory investigations which inclined us to initiate human trials, which form the basis of this report.

Immune RNA differs from transfer factor in several respects. Although transfer factor probably is a complex of a polypeptide and a ribonucleotide, it is, unlike I-RNA, insensitive to inactivation by ribonuclease treatment. It is a smaller molecule than I-RNA (4000–8000 m.w. versus 100,000–200,000 m.w.) and does not contain antigen fragments (45). Transfer factor must contain a peptide moiety to be active. Immune RNA contains negligible protein, and is unaffected by pronase treatment.

Two types of Immune RNA have been identified. One is an RNA-antigen complex and may simply behave as an extremely potent antigen or "super antigen" (2). The second type does not appear to contain antigen moieties. Although this active I-RNA has not been proven to be a "messenger RNA," it may be a true informational RNA. The exact chemical nature of I-RNA has not been established. Kern et al. fractionated antitumor Immune RNA and identified an active fraction with sedimentation values between 8S and 16S (25). This active fraction comprised only 5%–7% of the total RNA present.

Mediation of Antitumor Immune Responses with I-RNA: Animal Studies

The initial interest in Immune RNA was stimulated by the observation that RNA extracted from lymphoid cells which had been exposed to specific antigens, in vitro, or extracted from lymphoid tissues of animals immunized in vivo, could convert normal, non-immune lymphoid cells to specific immunologic activity (15, 16). As demonstrated in various systems, accelerated rejection of skin allografts in vivo (36, 53) and specific immune cytolysis of target cells in vitro (3) mediated by RNA from specifically sensitized donors, confirmed the mediation of immune responses to histocompatability antigens by Immune RNA. Alexander et al. first reported the induction of antitumor immunity with I-RNA (1). They administered xenogeneic I-RNA extracted from lymphoid cells of sheep which had been immunized against primary benzpyrene-induced rat sarcomas to sarcoma-bearing rats. This treatment often inhibited the growth of the specific sarcoma used to immunize the I-RNA donor and occasionally resulted in regression of growing tumors. Subsequently, Ramming and Pilch reported the mediation of immune responses against transplants of chemically-induced murine sarcomas by xenogeneic Immune RNA (49). Guinea pigs were immunized with a benzpyrene-induced sarcoma of C3H mice after which RNA was extracted from the guinea pig lymphoid tissues. Spleen cells from normal, non-immune C3H mice were incubated with the guinea pig I-RNA in vitro and then injected intraperitoneally into normal syngeneic mice. These immunized animals rejected transplants of the same tumor which had been used to immunize the guinea pigs. RNA preparations extracted from the lymphoid organs of guinea pigs which had been immunized with normal C3H mouse tissues, Freund's adjuvant, or with a different benzpyrene-induced sarcoma did not affect the growth of tumor transplants. In these, as in subsequent experiments, the activity of the I-RNA preparations was abrogated by treatment with ribonuclease but not by treatment with pronase or deoxyribonuclease, indicating that the active moeity(ies) was one or more species of RNA (51). Deckers, Ramming, and Pilch (8, 9, 10) later reported the induction of specific resistance to transplants of the same benzpyrene-induced C3H sarcomas, when xenogeneic I-RNA derived from the lymphoid organs of immunized guinea pigs was injected systemically in medium containing the ribonuclease inhibitor, sodium dextran sulfate. Numerous other studies using a number of different tumors in several rodent species have confirmed the induction of specific tumor immunity in vivo by syngeneic, allogeneic or xenogeneic Immune RNA preparations, either by the administration of syngeneic lymphocytes treated with I-RNA, in vitro, or by the direct systemic administration of I-RNA (11, 18, 19, 24, 42, 52, 54).

Immune cytolysis of tumor cells, in vitro, mediated by Immune RNA was then demonstrated by Ramming and Pilch in a totally syngeneic animal system (50). Normal syngeneic spleen cells pre-incubated with syngeneic I-RNA extracted from spleens of inbred strain 2 guinea pigs which had been immunized by excision of growing tumor transplants produced areas of cytolysis in a monolayer of the same tumor cells. This suggested that the immune response was directed against tumor-associated antigens. In another syngeneic system, Kern et al., using a quantitative microcytotoxicity assay, reported the mediation of immune cytolysis of cells from a methylcholanthrene-induced sarcoma of Fischer 344/N rats by syngeneic lymphocytes pre-incubated with syngeneic I-RNA extracted from spleens of Fischer rats bearing growing transplants of the same tumor (26).

We have recently reported the intracellular localization of I-RNA in the lymphoid cells of RNA donor animals (12). RNA was extracted separately from homogenates of whole intact spleen cells, from nuclei-free cytoplasmic fractions of spleen cells, and from purified spleen cell nuclei. It was found that immunological activity was confined to RNA from the cytoplasmic fractions. Nuclear RNA did not mediate anti-tumor immune reactions.

Kern et al. (25) described the kinetics of synthesis of I-RNA in the lymphoid organs of immunized animals. They found that I-RNA activity was maximal 21–28 days following immunization of animals with syngeneic tumor cells and 14–21 days following immunization with xenogeneic tumor cells. Mannick and Deckers (35) reported that I-RNA extracted from guinea pig peritoneal exudate cells 30–35 days following immunization with bovine gamma globulin (BGG) mediated immune responses to BGG when incubated with normal guinea pig peritoneal exudate cells. It therefore appears that the optimal time for extraction of I-RNA from the lymphoid tissues of immunized animals varies and is dependent upon several factors including the nature and route of administration of the immunogen, the presence or absence of adjuvants, the schedule of immunization of the donor, and the specific immunologic response which is measured.

T lymphocytes were found to be intimately involved in cellular antitumor immune reactions mediated by both syngeneic and xenogeneic

Immune RNA. The cell of origin of syngeneic I-RNA was determined by extracting I-RNA separately from unfractionated spleen cell suspensions and from various subpopulations of cells obtained from spleens of inbred rats bearing growing transplants of a chemically-induced sarcoma. Each I-RNA preparation was incubated with normal, non-immune syngeneic spleen cells and their cytotoxicity for tumor target cells was measured. I-RNA-mediating cellular antitumor immune reactions were extracted from populations of lymphoid cells enriched in T lymphocytes. The activity of these I-RNAs was the same as I-RNA from unseparated spleen cells. By contrast, RNA from cells adherent to EA monolayers (B cells) was inactive. The effector cell population which was acted upon by syngeneic I-RNA was also determined in this system and appeared to be T cells. Following incubation with I-RNA, lymphoid cells which formed EA rosettes (most B cells) showed no increase in cytotoxicity for tumor target cells. Cells not forming EA rosettes or non-adherent to nylon fiber (mostly T cells) became more cytotoxic after exposure to I-RNA. The lymphoid cell type affecting cellular cytotoxic antitumor reactions after incubation with xenogeneic I-RNA was determined in a murine model. Suspensions of normal, non-immune spleens were separated by several techniques into subpopulations of cells. The cytotoxicities of these various subpopulations for tumor target cells were measured before and after incubation with xenogeneic I-RNA. Following incubation with xenogeneic I-RNA, extracted from the lymphoid organs of specifically immunized guinea pigs, the cytotoxicity of unfractionated, normal spleen cells for tumor target cells was increased. Removal of cells adherent to petri dishes did not change the cytotoxicity. However, non-adherent cells, themselves, were inactive. Lymphocytes eluted from nylon fiber columns increased in cytotoxicity following exposure to I-RNA. When these cells were treated with anti-serum and complement, their cytotoxicity, following incubation with I-RNA, was abrogated. Therefore, it appeared that the effector cells which mediated cytotoxic antitumor reactions after incubation with xenogeneic I-RNA were T-lymphocytes (D. H. Kern and Y. H. Pilch, unpublished data).

I-RNA has recently been shown to induce humoral as well as cellular immune responses to tumor-associated antigens. Globulins derived from culture medium and cell lysates that had been prepared from normal, non-immune mouse spleen cells, following incubation with xenogeneic Immune RNA were shown to contain complement-dependent cytotoxic antitumor antibody activity. Globulins derived from spleen cells incubated with I-RNA extracted from the lymphoid organs of guinea pigs that had been immunized with either of two cross-reacting chemically induced murine sarcomas reacted against target cells of both tumors, but not against target cells derived from a spontaneously arising syngeneic osteosarcoma. Globulins obtained from spleen cells that had been incubated with I-RNA from guinea pigs immunized either with osteosarcoma tumor cells or cells from a spontaneous, syngeneic mammary tumor were not cytotoxic for target cells from either of the two chemically induced sarcomas, although globulins from spleen cells that had been incubated with anti-osteosarcoma I-RNA were cytotoxic for osteosarcoma target cells. Globulins derived from spleen cells incubated with I-RNA extracted from guinea pigs that had been immunized with either complete Freund's adjuvant only or with a pool of syngeneic normal tissues exhibited no cytotoxic activity against any of the three target cells tested. The antitumor antibodies whose synthesis was induced by xenogeneic I-RNA were apparently specific for the tumor-associated antigens of the particular tumor used to immunize the I-RNA donor (D. H. Kern and Y. H. Pilch, unpublished data).

Mediation of Immune Responses to Human Tumor Cells In Vitro

The mediation of cytotoxic cellular immune responses to human tumor cells by Immune RNA was first reported by Veltman et al. (59) using a quantitative microcytotoxicity test. Peripheral blood lymphocytes were shown to become markedly cytotoxic for human tumor cells in vitro following incubation with I-RNA extracted from the lymphoid organs of guinea pigs or sheep which had been specifically immunized with human tumor cells of the same histologic type. These results were obtained with gastric carcinoma cells, breast carcinoma cells, and several different melanoma cell lines. Lymphocytes incubated with RNA from animals immunized with complete Freund's adjuvant only evidenced no increased cytotoxic activity. As before, treatment of the I-RNA preparations with deoxyribonuclease or pronase did not alter the responses while treatment with ribonuclease abrogated all responses indicating that one or more species of RNA was the active moiety.

However, when allogeneic lymphocytes are used as effector cells, the antitumor immune reactions detected following incubation with I-RNA are directed against normal, histocompatibility antigens (H-LA antigens) on the surface of the tumor cells as well as against tumor-associated antigens. This was demonstrated by the fact that RNA extracted from lymphoid organs of animals immunized with normal skin fibroblasts, when incubated with normal, allogeneic lymphocytes, also mediated cytotoxic immune reactions against tumor target cells.

Kern et al. (27) then demonstrated mediation of specific immune responses to human tumor-associated antigens in vitro with Immune RNA.

Two autologous systems were studied in which lymphocytes from two melanoma patients from whom tumor cell lines had been derived were incubated with I-RNA extracted from animals which had been immunized with autologous tumor tissue from each particular patient and tested on autologous tumor cells *in vitro*. The effector cells were then autologous with respect to both the tumor cells used to immunize the RNA donor and the tumor target cells against which the lymphocytes were tested *in vitro*. In these systems, malignant melanoma target cell cultures, matching normal fibroblastic target cells, lymphocyte effector cells, and melanoma and normal skin tissue used to immunize I-RNA donor animals were derived from the same autochthonous hosts. The results of experiments performed with material from one of these two melanoma patients are depicted in Figures 1–4. In Figures 1 and 2, reactions against melanoma target cells are presented, while in Figures 3 and 4, reactions against autologous normal fibroblasts are depicted. Note that when allogeneic lymphocytes were incubated with I-RNA and used as effector cells, both I-RNA to normal skin and I-RNA to melanoma tissue mediated increased

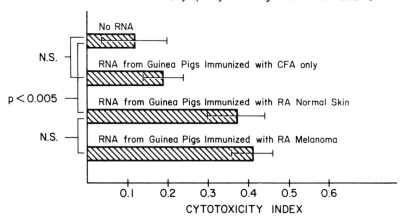

IMMUNITY AGAINST RA-H MELANOMA CELLS MEDIATED BY XENOGENEIC IMMUNE RNA

Normal Allogeneic Lymphocytes

(Lymphocyte to target cell ratio = 200:1)

Fig. 1. Cytotoxicity indices obtained when normal allogeneic lymphocytes, following incubation with no RNA or with indicated RNA preparations, were tested for cytotoxic activity *in vitro* against *melanoma cells* from patient RA. (CFA = complete Freund's Adjuvant)

IMMUNITY AGAINST RA-H MELANOMA CELLS MEDIATED BY XENOGENEIC IMMUNE RNA

Autologous Lymphocytes from Patient RA

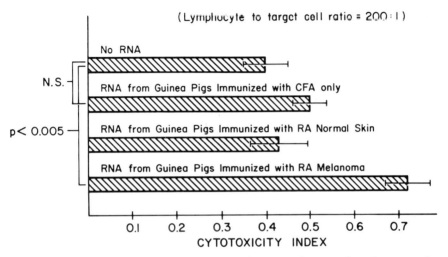

Fig. 2. Cytotoxicity indices obtained when autologous lymphocytes from melanoma patient RA, following incubation with no RNA or with indicated RNA preparations, were tested for cytotoxic activity against RA's own *melanoma cells, in vitro*. (CFA = complete Freund's Adjuvant)

cytotoxic activity against both melanoma cells and fibroblasts—reactions against HLA differences. However, when the same RNA preparations were incubated with autologous lymphocytes, only I-RNA to melanoma cells mediated cytotoxic immune responses against autologous melanoma cells and none of the RNA preparations mediated cytotoxic responses against autologous normal fibroblasts. These experiments demonstrated that, while xenogeneic anti-tumor I-RNA mediated immune reactions against normal cell surface antigens upon incubation with allogeneic lymphocytes, only immune reactions against tumor-associated antigens were detected when antitumor I-RNA was incubated with autologous lymphocytes. When incubated with autologous lymphocytes, I-RNA extracted from the lymphoid organs of donor animals immunized with melanoma tissue mediated immune reactions against autologous melanoma target cells, *in vitro*. I-RNA from animals immunized with normal skin tissue from the autochthonous host was ineffective. By con-

IMMUNITY AGAINST RA-F SKIN FIBROBLAST
CELLS MEDIATED BY XENOGENEIC IMMUNE RNA

Normal Allogeneic Lymphocytes

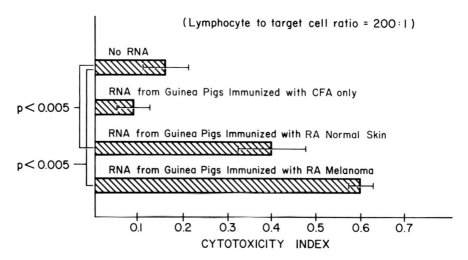

Fig. 3. Cytotoxicity indices obtained when normal allogeneic lymphocytes, following incubation with no RNA or with indicated RNA preparations, were tested for cytotoxic activity against RA's normal *fibroblasts, in vitro.* (CFA = complete Freund's Adjuvant)

trast, when allogeneic lymphocytes were used as effector cells, RNA extracted from animals immunized either with melanoma tissue or normal skin mediated cytotoxic immune reactions against both melanoma target cells and normal fibroblast target cells derived from the same patient. These data suggest that lymphocytes recognize Immune RNAs against "non-self" antigens, as tumor-associated antigens, and are induced to effect an immune response. This phenomenon may explain why the administration of xenogeneic Immune RNA *in vivo* does not result in autoimmune phenomena or graft versus host reactions.

Immune cytolysis of human renal, bladder, and lung carcinoma cells *in vitro* by xenogeneic I-RNA has also been reported by Brower et al. (4). No autologous systems were included in these studies. Furthermore, the degree of cytotoxicity seemed to depend upon several variable factors including the origin of the allogeneic effector cells, the immunizing tumor, and the animal source of the RNA.

IMMUNITY AGAINST RA-F SKIN FIBROBLAST CELLS MEDIATED BY XENOGENEIC IMMUNE RNA

Autologous Lymphocytes from Patient RA

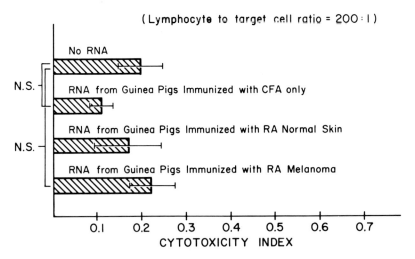

Fig. 4. Cytotoxicity index obtained when autologous lymphocytes from melanoma patient RA, following incubation with no RNA or with indicated RNA preparations, were tested for cytotoxic activity against CA's own normal *fibroblasts, in vitro*. (CFA = complete Freund's Adjuvant)

Recent experience has demonstrated effective mediation of cytotoxic immune reactions against human cancer cells *in vitro* by allogeneic Immune RNA extracted from the peripheral blood lymphocytes of putatively cured cancer patients. Kern *et al*. (28) extracted I-RNA separately from the peripheral blood lymphocytes of 5 "cured" melanoma patients, 4 patients with colon cancer, 3 patients with breast carcinoma, 1 patient with hypernephroma, and 5 normal volunteers. These I-RNA preparations were extracted from lymphocytes harvested with the continuous blood flow cell separator. Each I-RNA preparation was incubated separately with aliquots of the same batch of normal, allogeneic lymphocytes collected on the blood cell separator from another healthy volunteer and the lymphocytes were then assayed for cytotoxic activity against tumor target cells *in vitro*. The experiment demonstrated specific cytotoxicity of the melanoma target cells by all 5 I-RNA preparations extracted from the peripheral blood lymphocytes of melanoma patients. RNA's from lymphocytes of normal volunteers or from patients with other tumor types were inactive. Three of 4 I-RNA's extracted from the peripheral blood lymphocytes of colon cancer patients mediated cytotoxic immune responses against colon cancer cells and 2 of 3 I-RNA's from the lymphocytes of breast cancer patients mediated reactions against breast cancer cells. Only the specific I-RNA produced cytolysis of tumor target cells and RNA from normal volunteers or from patients from other tumor types was not effective. All of these patients were male and none had been transfused, and it therefore seems unlikely that they could have been sensitized to HLA antigens or other human transplantation antigens in vivo. Cytotoxic immune reactions were shown to be directed only against tumor target cells of the same histologic tumor type as the RNA donor. These experiments provide evidence that the RNA extracted from peripheral blood lymphocytes of cancer patients mediates cytotoxic immune reactions directed against common tumor-associated antigens specific for the tumor type of the I-RNA donor.

One potential hazard of subjecting cancer patients to leukophoresis in order to harvest I-RNA is the possibility of diminishing the cellular immunocompetence of the donor following removal of a large number of lymphocytes, from which I-RNA is prepared. However, Waldman (60) did not detect a change in the skin test reactivity of cancer patients to DNCB or common skin test antigens following a single leukophoresis. Lymphocyte mediated cytotoxicity to tumor cells as assayed in vitro, decreased transiently in a few patients but returned to normal within 24 hours after leukophoresis.

However, the extraction of allogeneic Immune RNA from lymphocytes of human donors has several disadvantages. First, donor selection and donor availability are limited. Second, it is uncertain that any human can provide lymphocytes which will produce an optimally immunoreactive I-RNA extract. Human tumors may be more immunogeneic when inoculated into animals than they are in their host of origin. Third, the concern that repeated extraction of lymphocytes from "cured" cancer patients may result in sufficient immunosuppression to cause exacerbation of the donors malignant disease requires cautious application of this methodology.

These laboratory studies provided a background for the extension of I-RNA immunotherapy to the clinical setting. Immunotherapy with I-RNA offers theoretical advantages over other methods of adoptive immunotherapy. Since allogeneic human leukocytes are not transfused, sensitization of the recipient to foreign histocompatibility antigens is avoided. (Immune RNA itself does not contain transplantation antigens.) The possibility of inducing a graft versus host reaction in immunodeficient or immunosuppressed patients is eliminated. Repeated injections of I-RNA would not be expected to sensitize the recipient since RNA is not itself immunogeneic. Purification and isolation of human tumor-specific transplantation antigens is not necessary for immunotherapy with Immune RNA. Finally, it is conceivable that Immune RNA might be effective despite certain types of host anergy (primarily afferent limb anergy).

Several methods of utilizing I-RNA for immunotherapy are suggested by the studies described above. I-RNA might be derived from the lymphocytes of cured cancer patients (allogeneic I-RNA) or from lymphoid tissues of specifically immunized animals (xenogeneic I-RNA). Routes of administration might be by direct injection of I-RNA, or by the incubation of autologous lymphocytes with I-RNA in vitro followed by reinfusion.

The development of the continuous blood flow cell separator has provided a method for harvesting circulating lymphocytes for incubation in vitro with Immune RNA and subsequent reinfusion. Waldman et al. (60) did not detect any clinically significant alteration in hematologic or immunologic parameters after a single leukophoresis in normal volunteers and cancer patients. The peripheral blood leukocyte count fell transiently but returned to normal within 1 to 2 days. This approach has the obvious advantage of direct exposure of the lymphocytes to I-RNA with little danger of degradation of the RNA by ribonucleases. Toxicity is potentially greater since some RNA will be injected intravenously.

Clinical Trials

RATIONALE. The mediation of cellular immune responses to human tumor-associated antigens in vitro by I-RNA extracted from the lymphoid organs of immunized animals (xenogeneic) provided a logical basis for the immunotherapy of cancer with xenogeneic I-RNA. Xenogeneic I-RNA offers several distinct theoretical advantages over other methods of immunotherapy. First, large quantities of Immune RNA can be produced in quantity from relatively inexpensive and plentiful animals without dependence upon human donors. Second, since histologically similar human tumors appear to share common, group specific tumor-associated antigens, many patients with the same tumor type can be treated with I-RNA from an animal immunized with a single patient's tumor.

Because the accumulated laboratory studies strongly suggested that I-RNA could induce antitumor immune responses, and because of the many potential advantages of this form of immunotherapy, preliminary clinical trials were undertaken to examine the feasibility of I-RNA im-

munotherapy of human malignancy. The primary aims of these preliminary studies were to assess toxicity and to establish dose-response relationships associated with I-RNA therapy rather than to document any
clinical effect. It also was intended to follow any changes in host immunity which might be due to Immune RNA therapy. It therefore appeared
appropriate to treat only patients with gross recurrent and/or metastatic
disease and especially patients for whom no effective therapy was available or in whom all standard therapy had failed. It is known that such
patients have little chance of responding to immunotherapy of any type
and therefore clinical responses, although sought, were not expected.
Similarly, controls were not included since therapeutic response was not
a major determinant of the study. Later some patients who were rendered
free of clinically detectable disease, but who had a significant probability
of developing tumor recurrence and/or metastases (minimum residual
disease) were included. In these patients tumor-free interval was determined as well as changes in immunologic parameters. These patients
were included only after a significant number of patients with metastatic
disease had been treated and were found to develop no toxicity.

METHODS. Xenogeneic Immune RNA was extracted from the
lymphoid tissues of sheep which were immunized with human tumor
tissue in the following manner. A thick suspension of viable tumor cells
prepared in 3 ml of medium was emulsified in an equal volume of complete Freund's adjuvant and injected intradermally into all 4 extremities
of a sheep at weekly intervals for 3 consecutive weeks. Ten days after the
last injection the animals were sacrificed and the spleens and mesenteric
lymph nodes excised and immediately frozen in dry ice. I-RNA was extracted from the frozen lymphoid tissues as previously described (50). The
I-RNA was reprecipitated twice from solutions made 2M with respect to
potassium acetate, treated with pronase (to remove contaminating protein), again reprecipitated from 2M potassium acetate, dialyzed against
sterile distilled water, sterilized by passage through a 0.22-micron milli-
pore filter and lyophylized. The lyophylized I-RNA was resuspended in
normal saline prior to injection.

All I-RNA preparations were assayed for RNA, DNA, and protein concentration. The pronase treatment and reprecipitation method reduced
the protein concentration to very low levels. However, traces of sheep
protein remained, possibly complexed to the RNA. Sterility of each preparation of RNA was determined by routine bacterial and fungal cultures. In
no instance was any preparation of I-RNA found to be contaminated. The
integrity of the RNA was determined by sucrose density gradient analysis
and by disc gel electrophoresis. Preparations which were found to be

degraded were discarded, although this was a rare occurrence. The I-RNA was usually stored to $-75°C$ although lyophylized preparations stored at room temperature for 30 days were found to have undergone no degradation.

ADMINISTRATION OF RNA.   Immediately before administration, the I-RNA was resuspended in sterile saline and injected intradermally in multiple wheels of 0.1 ml near lymph node bearing areas (groins or axillae). When possible, each patient received I-RNA prepared against autologous tumor tissue. If this was not feasible, I-RNA prepared against allogeneic tumor tissue of the same histologic type was used. Doses of I-RNA ranged from 2 mg/week to 60 mg/week in single or divided doses but were usually 4 or 8 mg/week. No patient received any other form of antitumor therapy (surgery, radiotherapy, chemotherapy or other form of immunotherapy) while receiving I-RNA.

As noted above, one purpose of the initial Phase I study was to determine dose/response relationships. As far as could be determined, there was no significant difference in response of patients to small or large doses. However since measurable objective responses were rare, as would be expected in patients with far advanced disease, assessment of proper dosage was difficult. Quantitative measurements by Pilch et al. of lymphocyte cytotoxicity in vitro mediated by I-RNA had suggested a relationship between the concentration of I-RNA and the magnitude of response (26, 29). Wang, et al. have also reported a dose/response curve based on in vitro cytotoxicity (B. S. Wang, P. J. Deckers, and J. A. Mannick, unpublished data). Further clinical experience is necessary before optimal in vivo dose schedules can be determined.

IMMUNOLOGIC MONITORING.   Immune responses of treated patients were monitored by testing cutaneous reactions to DNCB and common recall antigens and by measuring changes in lymphocyte mediated cytotoxicity to tumor target cells. Patients were sensitized and subsequently challenged with DNCB according to the method of Eilber and Morton (13). They were retested at 8–12 week intervals with DNCB and common antigens throughout their treatment. Lymphocyte cytotoxicity to tumor target cells was determined by a microcytotoxicity test which has been previously reported (43). Peripheral blood samples were obtained serially prior to and during the course of therapy. Lymphocytes were isolated on Ficoll-isopaque gradients and were frozen in the vapor phase of liquid nitrogen at 1°C per minute. Viability of the frozen lymphocytes were varied from 60% to 80%. The target cells for the microcytotoxicity assay were allogeneic tumor cells of the same histologic type as the tumor of the patient under study, the nature and propogation of which have been described (48).

Immunotherapy of Advanced Disease

MALIGNANT MELANOMA. Patients in the advanced disease category had either unresectable local or regional recurrence, visceral metastases, or both. Over half the patients had failed one or more chemotherapeutic regimens. I-RNA immunotherapy consisted of weekly intradermal injections of 4–8 mg of Immune RNA. In several cases where a patient's autologous tumor tissue was available, the I-RNA was extracted from lymph nodes and spleens of sheep immunized with the patient's own tumor. In other instances, the I-RNA administered was from sheep immunized with melanoma tissue obtained from another patient. Patients were treated for a minimum of 2 months, and therapy was continued thereafter until progression occurred.

A total of 15 patients with advanced melanoma received Immune RNA. Progression occurred within 2 months in 6 of the patients. One patient has shown no progression of his disease over a 7 month treatment interval and is alive. One patient had temporary stabilization of multiple pulmonary metastases for a 3-month period as indicated by serial chest X ray. His disease then slowly progressed and he died 10 months after the initiation of I-RNA therapy. One patient had slow progression of pulmonary metastases. He died with brain metastases 12 months after initiation of therapy. One patient had stabilization of his metastases for a period of 5 months, and died of brain metastases at 6 months. Of all 15 patients, 10 are dead at the time of this writing, 4 are alive with obviously progressive disease despite I-RNA therapy and 1 patient is alive with no progression of his disease after 7 months of therapy. There were no one-year survivors.

It is of interest that despite the advanced stage of disease in these patients when first seen, all reacted to DNCB skin tests prior to therapy. Two of the patients actually showed increasing reactivity to DNCB despite progression of their disease. Seven patients showed no change in cutaneous reactivity to DNCB when serially tested. The patient who had the most advanced disease with lung, brain, and intra-abdominal metastases was the only patient to become anergic to DNCB and showed no cutaneous reactivity when tested shortly before death.

All patients' lymphocytes were sampled prior to treatment and serially during therapy, and tested for cytotoxic activity against melanoma target cells. In all but one of these patients, the target cell was derived from the same allogeneic human melanoma cell line. A significant increase in lymphocyte cytotoxicity as compared to pretreatment levels was noted in 5 of the patients while they were receiving Immune RNA therapy, despite progressive tumor growth.

COLON CARCINOMA. Two patients with far advanced adenocarcinoma of the colon were treated. The I-RNA was obtained from lymphoid organs of sheep which had been immunized with human colon cancer tissue. One patient had pulmonary metastases and the other patient had intra-abdominal recurrence. The first patient was treated for two months. During this time, he had obvious clinical progression of disease. He was initially anergic to DNCB, but had a slight reaction when retested 8 weeks after the onset of I-RNA therapy. He is alive and receiving chemotherapy at this time.

A second patient, who underwent resection of an intra-abdominal recurrence of colon carcinoma was clinically stable for 6 months while receiving I-RNA. However, she then required surgery for another intra-abdominal recurrence that clearly had been progressing while she was receiving treatment. She reacted strongly to DNCB both prior to and while receiving I-RNA therapy. She is currently alive and receiving chemotherapy.

HYPERNEPHROMA. Twenty patients with metastatic hypernephroma (renal cell carcinoma) have been treated with Immune RNA. This I-RNA was obtained from sheep which had been immunized with allogeneic human hypernephroma tissue. Weekly intradermal doses of 4–8 mg of Immune RNA were given. Twelve patients had pulmonary metastases only while five had extrapulmonary metastases as well (to bone, brain, or liver). One patient had a large mass of metastatic hypernephroma in superior mediastinal lymph nodes proven by biopsy prior to the initiation of I-RNA therapy. Eight of the 20 patients presented with metastases at the time of original diagnosis and underwent palliative nephrectomy prior to receiving I-RNA treatment. The survival of these patients plotted by the "life table" method is depicted in Figure 5. Thirteen of the patients are still alive and receiving immunotherapy. Their mean survival has been 15 months from the time of diagnosis of metastases to the present. In this group, 3 patients have been under treatment for less than 4 months. The longest followup has been in the patient with biopsy-proven mediastinal lymph node involvement who is alive and well after 34 months. Seven patients have died, and their mean survival was 12.5 months from the diagnosis of metastases. Of the 8 patients who underwent palliative nephrectomy prior to receiving I-RNA therapy, 4 are alive with a mean survival of 13.5 months and 4 have died with a mean survival of 14.5 months. One patient who had a chest wall resection for metastatic disease was then begun on immunotherapy with Immune

RNA. He is not clinically free of the disease 25 months after initiation of I-RNA treatment. Survival appeared to correlate not only with extent of disease, but also with location of metastases. Those patients with metastases confined to the lungs had a better prognosis than those with metastatic involvement elsewhere. Four of 5 patients with extra-pulmonary involvement died with a mean survival of 8.5 months.

Ten patients with metastatic hypernephroma had serial mea-

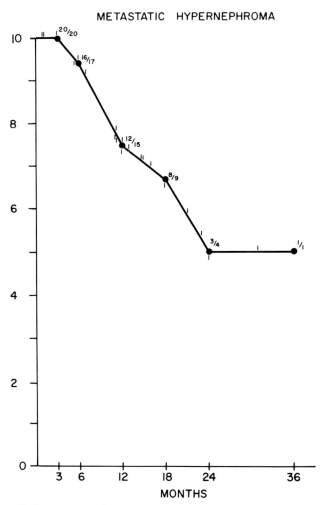

Fig. 5. Survival of patients with metastatic hypernephroma treated with Immune RNA.

surements of lymphocyte-mediated cytotoxicity against allogeneic hypernephroma target cells. In 6 of these patients, cytotoxicity did not increase at any time during therapy, which ranged from 5 to 19 months. Three of these patients are alive, 2 at 15 and 1 at 17 months, and 3 died, at 5, 11, and 12 months, respectively. Four other patients evidenced significant increases in lymphocyte cytotoxicity following initiation of I-RNA therapy. One of these patient's cytotoxicity index later decreased as progression of disease became rapid, and this patient died at 18 months. A similar pattern of decreased cytotoxicity which correlated with progressing metastatic disease was seen in another patient who is still alive at 11 months. Two patients have relatively stable metastatic disease and are alive at 7 and 31 months. In both of these patients the cytotoxicity index has remained high.

All patients were skin tested with DNCB. It is of interest that 10 of the patients with advanced metastatic disease did not respond to initial testing with DNCB. There appeared to be little correlation between this cutaneous anergy and tumor burden since patients with very small amounts of tumor as well as patients with extensive metastatic disease were included in this group. However, regardless of initial response, an increase in sensitivity to DNCB was correlated with stabilization of growth or unusual slow progression of metastases which was observed in 6 of 20 patients. The converse was not true since some patients who appeared to have temporary stabilization of growth of metastases did not have an increase in DNCB skin test reactivity.

MISCELLANEOUS TUMORS. Seven other patients have received Immune RNA for advanced malignancies. They include one patient with gastric carcinoma, 3 with sarcomas, 1 with metastatic lung cancer, and 1 patient with breast carcinoma. These patients were treated during the very early phase of our pilot study and it is not possible to draw any conclusions from review of their clinical courses.

Two of these patients, however, merit comment. A 9-year-old girl presented with an unresectable alveolar soft part sarcoma of the pelvic soft tissues and pulmonary metastases. She received I-RNA from a sheep immunized with her own tumor. Her pulmonary metastases did not progress at all while on therapy and a few decreased slightly in size. After 8 months and after this favorable clinical response, the patient was placed on chemotherapy and has had further regression. She is currently alive, 15 months after diagnosis. Her lymphocytes exhibited a moderate increase in cytotoxicity against allogeneic sarcoma target cells. Her DNCB reactivity also increased significantly during treatment.

One patient with lung cancer proven unresectable because of widespread disease at thoracotomy was treated with Immune RNA. His clinical course and chest X-rays remained excellent for 24 months, when he developed a brain metastasis. He currently is receiving chemotherapy and radiation therapy. This patient exhibited the greatest single increase in DNCB reactivity seen in this series, the reactivity increasing from an initial response of 0 to our highest recorded response noted at the time of his last testing, which was approximately 6 weeks before he clinically developed metastasis.

Adjuvant Immunotherapy

Patients in this category were at high risk for recurrence following potentially curative surgical resection of all clinical detectable tumor. Immunotherapy was initiated within 10 weeks of operation. All patients received 4 mg of I-RNA weekly. Whenever possible, each patient received Immune RNA from a sheep which had been immunized with his own, autologous tumor cells. Alternatively, each patient received Immune RNA from a sheep immunized with allogeneic tumor cells of the same histologic type. If progression of disease was noted, Immune RNA therapy was discontinued and alternative therapy instituted. If no recurrence developed, treatment continued for 2 years and was then stopped.

MALIGNANT MELANOMA. Ten patients with malignant melanoma, at high risk for recurrence, were included in this pilot study. Another patient had had multiple recurrences of tumor in the left axilla and chest wall. These had been locally excised 6 times within 4 years, the longest interval between recurrences being 8 months. An eighth patient was treated following excision of a mass of recurrent melanoma from the right groin less than one year after a groin dissection for lymph node metastases. Four patients were treated who did not have lymph node involvement. Two of these patients had not undergone node dissection and 2 had been subjected to node dissection and had no evidence of nodal involvement by microscopic exam. Of these 4 patients, one had a lower extremity melanoma with invasion to Clark's Level III and 3 had melanomas of the trunk with invasion to Clark's Level IV or V.

The survival free of disease (recurrence rate) of these 10 patients, plotted by the life table method, is presented in Figure 6. The median follow-up is 17 months and the mean follow-up is 18 months. Two patients have been treated for 24 months and their therapy has been discontinued. Only one patient has developed a recurrence. The patient from whose groin a mass of recurrent melanoma had been excised prior to entry into the study developed another recurrence in the same groin after 7 months of I-RNA immunotherapy. She was treated with radiation therapy

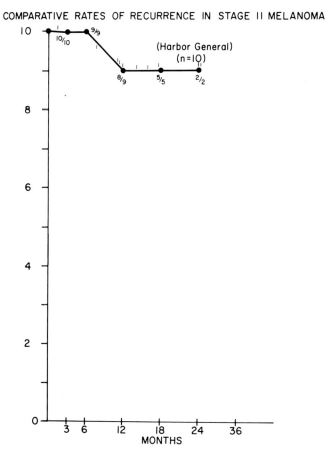

Fig. 6. Survival free of disease of patients with malignant melanoma receiving adjuvant immunotherapy with Immune RNA.

and chemotherapy and had a complete response. She remains alive and in complete remission over 1 year later.

In one of the melanoma patients receiving I-RNA immunotherapy, a 28-year-old white male with innumerable deeply pigmented nevi, a marked vitiliganous change developed in most of the nevi after one year of I-RNA treatment. Photographs of some of these nevi are presented in Figure 7. This is of interest, as vitiliganous change in pigmented nevi has occasionally been observed by other investigators in melanoma patients undergoing other forms of immunotherapy, and generally has been regarded as a favorable prognostic indicator.

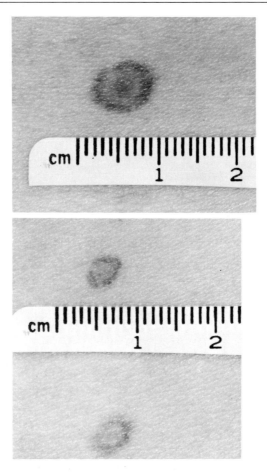

Fig. 7. Cutaneous nevi on the trunk of a melanoma patient showing vitiliganous change after 1 year of immunotherapy with Immune RNA.

All patients tested exhibited cutaneous responses to initial challenge doses of DNCB prior to beginning therapy, and in all patients the level of reactivity to subsequent DNCB challenges increased during therapy. Four of the 7 patients tested had significant increase in lymphocyte cytotoxicity during treatment, and 3 patients had no increase whatsoever.

HYPERNEPHROMA. All patients in this category underwent nephrectomy for hypernephroma and had associated findings at the time of surgery which indicated a high probability of recurrence, e.g., tumor resected from the diaphragm, invasion of the renal vein, metastases to regional lymph nodes, or involvement of the renal capsule. Patients who had undergone resection of local recurrence or metastatic deposits were also included in this group. Eight patients in this category, followed for 5, 6, 10, 11, 12, 14, 18, and 30 months, respectively, are alive without evidence of recurrence with a mean follow-up of 14.3 months.

In these patients, clinical course and the cytotoxicity index of peripheral blood lymphocytes for hypernephroma cells in vitro have shown little correlation. DNCB skin test responses were similarly of little prognostic value. One patient who died of metastatic disease, at 11 months had no increase in cytotoxicity index while on I-RNA therapy but had the greatest possible increase in response to sequential skin testing with DNCB. In the other patient who died of metastases, modest increases in responsiveness to DNCB were noted as was a slight increase in cytotoxicity index. Two of the patients who are clinically free of recurrence have never mounted a cutaneous response to DNCB while the remaining surviving patients have shown progressive increases in responses to sequential DNCB testing while on I-RNA therapy.

COLO-RECTAL CANCER. A prospectively randomized trial of adjuvant immunotherapy with Immune RNA in patients with colo-rectal cancer following potentially curative surgery was begun in September of 1975. Patients are eligible for admission to the study if, as determined following pathologic evaluation of the resected specimen, their tumor involves all layers of the bowel with or without positive nodes or their tumor does not penetrate through all layers of the bowel but one or more positive nodes are found in the resected specimen. Patients with metastatic disease or in whom residual tumor is known to remain following surgery are excluded.

Patients are randomized postoperatively into either "treatment" or "no treatment" groups. Treated patients receive 4 mg of I-RNA weekly. Treatment is initiated within 8 weeks of surgery and is continued for 2 years unless recurrence or metastases develop at which time immunotherapy is discontinued and appropriate alternative therapy instituted. Patients in the "no treatment" group are followed in an identical manner but receive no adjunctive therapy. To this date, 10 patients have been entered into this study—6 in the "treatment" group and 4 in the control group. The 6 patients receiving I-RNA have been followed for 2, 4, 7, 10, 12 and 16 months respectively without evidence of recurrence. Three of these patients are receiving I-RNA from sheep immunized with autologous tumor tissue, while the others are receiving I-RNA from sheep immunized with allogeneic colon cancer tissue. CEA levels in all of these patients have remained below 2.0. Of the 4 patients in the control group, one patient developed liver metastases 5 months after entering the study and the others remain free of disease at from 2 to 10 months. Obviously, the results of this study are inconclusive at this early date.

All patients had positive cutaneous reactions to DNCB at the time of entry to the study. All of the "treated" patients have evidenced moderate to marked increases in DNCB sensitivity.

Discussion

The numerous reports of the effective mediation of immune responses with I-RNA which have appeared in the literature during the past decade, the apparent absence of toxicity following administration of I-RNA in animal models, and the encouraging results observed in human systems in vitro seemed to us to be a logical foundation on which to base preliminary trials of Immune RNA immunotherapy in human cancer patients. We have reported here every patient to whom we have ever administered Immune RNA. In some of these patients, especially those treated early in our experience, patient selection was not ideal, treatment was tentative, and far advanced disease simply continued to advance. In some of the patients treated later, especially those with small or microscopic tumor burdens, there is a suggestion of therapeutic benefit that must await confirmation by further observation and randomized prospective trials.

Clearly, toxicity of Immune RNA has been absent or minimal. Over 700 doses of I-RNA have been administered. Total dosages of up to 600 mg (over 35 months) in one patient and single doses as high as 60 mg, including several intravenous doses of 60 mg, have not resulted in significant side effects. Three patients have reported mild, transient malaise and anorexia after I-RNA treatment, and one patient developed a transient low-grade fever. Transient flushing within 30 minutes after administration of I-RNA has been noted on 3 occasions. No patient has experienced any local skin reactions, no allergic or anaphalactoid reactions have occurred and in no instance has the dosage of I-RNA been modified or discontinued because of adverse reactions.

In previous animal experiments, it appeared desirable to administer Immune RNA in a medium containing the strong ribonuclease inhibitor, sodium dextran sulphate. There was some toxicity associated with this agent in our initial animal studies. However, appropriate dose reductions eliminated toxicity in animals. Approval to use this substance in man, however, has not yet been obtained from the Food and Drug Administration. The evaluation of other substances (such as Pyran Copolymer) which might inhibit circulating ribonucleases is presently being investigated in animal models. Thus we have not incorporated a ribonuclease inhibitor into our I-RNA preparations. Perhaps by so doing, we might significantly increase the efficacy of Immune RNA therapy in the future.

The incubation of normal lymphocytes *in vitro* with Immune RNA has been shown to induce such lymphocytes to effect antitumor immune responses *in vitro* and *in vivo*. Four weeks prior to this writing, 2 patients had been treated in this manner. Their autologous lymphocytes, collected on the continuous flow blood cell separator, were incubated for 30 minutes at 37° with 40 mg of I-RNA in 50 ml of saline, and the entire mixture was then reinfused intravenously. One patient developed a febrile response which lasted approximately 24 hours, but there has been no other apparent toxicity. Lymphocyte mediated cytotoxicity in one patient increased greatly after one week. It is obviously too early to have made any other observations on the effects of this treatment. However, this method of utilizing Immune RNA therapeutically may offer considerable future promise.

The influence of I-RNA therapy in patients with extensive disease is difficult to assess. Complete regression did not occur in any patient treated. Several patients, however, had temporary stabilization of growth of metastases which had been documented to be progressively growing prior to the initiation of Immune RNA therapy. Stabilization of growth of pulmonary metastases was noted in one patient with alveolar soft part sarcoma and in several patients with metastatic hypernephroma. However, the peculiar natural history of hypernephroma makes interpretation of such temporary changes in growth patterns difficult. Erratic growth of pulmonary nodules with periods of growth arrest is known to occur in patients receiving no therapy and occasional spontaneous regressions have also been reported (14).

The survival of patients with metastatic hypernephroma has not been shown to be influenced by any currently available methods of therapy. Johnson et al. (23) reported approximately 25% one-year survival in 93 patients with metastatic hypernephroma. The two-year survival was 13%. Rafla (47) reported a higher two-year survival—28%. However, Mostofi (40), in a review of 1700 cases of patients with metastatic renal carcinoma, reported only 2 survivors after 2 years in patients who had metastases at the time of diagnosis, regardless of therapy. When compared with these published statistics, the patients with metastatic hypernephroma treated with Immune RNA seem to have had an increase in survival from the time of onset of metastases. The comparison of these patients with matched retrospective controls in the same institutions from which the treated patients were derived is under way. It appears that patients whose metastatic hypernephroma is confined to the lungs and who are treated with Immune RNA may well have a greater survival than matched untreated patients. However, only by prospectively randomized studies can any true alteration of survival or growth of metastases be attributed directly to Immune RNA therapy.

The failure of Immune RNA therapy to influence extensive disease, with the possible exception of hypernephroma, is not surprising since immunotherapy of any form may be effective only in the presence of minimal tumor burden. As in any trial of a new and unproven therapeutic agent, it is necessary, initially, to treat patients with advanced disease who have failed all established forms of therapy. This was done in the early phases of this series. However, patients with minimum residual disease and patients with a high probability of recurrence following potentially curative surgery are more suitable candidates for immunotherapy. Twenty-four patients in this category (10 melanoma, 6 colon carcinoma, 8 hypernephroma) have received adjuvant immunotherapy with Immune RNA and have been observed from 2 to 25 months. Only 2 of these patients have developed evidence of recurrence during this period. Our preliminary results in the adjuvant immunotherapy of malignant melanoma with I-RNA suggest a decreased recurrence rate. While our initial results are encouraging, the number of patients is small and longer follow-up is necessary. Furthermore, factors such as patient selection, histology and thoroughness of surgical excision influence the probability of recurrence. Again the definitive determination of the efficacy of Immune RNA immunotherapy in this category of patients awaits the results of randomized clinical trials, such as the one in progress in patients with Dukes' B_2 and Dukes' C colo-rectal cancer.

Evidence for stimulation of host immunity by Immune RNA was assessed through skin test responses to DNCB and assessment of lymphocyte mediated cytotoxicity to tumor target cells in vitro. In most patients, a decreased DNCB response correlated with progression of disease. Initial skin test responses in hypernephroma patients, however, often did not correlate with tumor burden. Furthermore, the subsequent clinical course, in many cases, was not reflected by changes in DNCB response. In all patient groups, increases in skin test responses were frequently noted after the institution of I-RNA therapy.

Changes in lymphocyte mediated cytotoxicity values are difficult to interpret. Increases in cytotoxicity indices in some patients were clearly attributable to I-RNA therapy; but in others, no significant changes were noted. In addition, there was no good correlation between changes in lymphocyte mediated cytotoxicity and clinical course.

The mechanism of action of Immune RNA remains unclear. Identification of the active fraction and the mechanism by which it transfers immunologic information may be necessary before rapid advances in the field are possible. Furthermore, the specific aspect of host immunity which is influenced by Immune RNA must be elucidated. If this could be determined, appropriate *in vitro* assays could be used to identify which patients would be the best candidates for Immune RNA therapy and to monitor the effects of therapy which are relevant to *in vivo* responses.

Finally, it is apparent that Immune RNA, when prepared as described above and administered intradermally in the doses and schedules described, is virtually free of significant local or systemic toxicity and is very well tolerated. There is a suggestion that it might be of clinical benefit in metastatic hypernephroma, and that it might be useful in preventing recurrences in patients with melanoma, colon cancer and hypernephroma who have high likelihood of recurrence following potentially curative surgery. Definitive answers to these questions will require continued follow-up of the patients already treated and must await the results of prospectively randomized clinical trials.

ACKNOWLEDGMENTS

This work was supported in part by the Medical Research Service of the Veterans Administration and by the following grants and contracts from the National Institutes of Health: NIH-CA-21664, NIH-CA-12582-06, USPHS-5-P01-CA-16042-02, and NIH-4-444992-32691.

REFERENCES

1. Alexander, P., Delorme, E. J., Hamilton, L. D. G., *et al.* 1967. Effect of nucleic acids from immune lymphocytes on rat sarcomata. *Nature* 213: 569–572.

2. Askonas, B. A., and Rhodes, J. M. 1965. In J. Starzl (ed.), *Molecular and Cellular Basis of Antibody Formation*, p. 502. Acacemic Press, New York.

3. Bondevik, H., and Mannick, J. A. 1968. RNA-mediated transfer of lymphocyte vs. target cell activity. *Proc. Soc. Exp. Biol. N.Y.* 129: 264–268.

4. Brower, P. A., deKernion, J. B., and Ramming, K. P. 1976. Immune cytolysis of human renal carcinoma mediated by immune RNA. *J. Urol.* 115: 243–245.

5. Brown, R. E., and Katz, M. 1967. Passive transfer of delayed hypersensitivity reaction to Tuberculin in children with protein and calorie malnutrition. *J. Pediatr.* 70: 126–238.

6. Cheema, A. R., and Hersh, E. M. 1972. Local tumor immunotherapy with *in vitro* activated authchthonous lymphocytes. *Cancer* 29: 982–986.

7. deCarvalho, S. 1963. Preliminary experimentation with specific immunotherapy of neoplastic disease in man. *Cancer* 16: 306–330.

8. Deckers, P. J., and Pilch, Y. H. 1971. Transfer of immunity to tumor isographs by the systemic administration of xenogeneic "immune" RNA. *Nature New Biol.* 231: 181–183.

9. Deckers, P. J., and Pilch, Y. H. 1972. Mediation of immunity to tumor-specific transplantation antigens by RNA: Inhibition of isograft growth in rats. *Cancer Res.* 32: 839–846.

10. Deckers, P. J., Pilch, Y. H., and Ramming, K. P. 1973. The transfer of tumor immunity with syngeneic RNA. *Ann. N.Y. Acad. Sci.* 207: 442–453.

11. Deckers, P. J., Wang, B. S., and Mannick, J. A. 1976. Immunotherapy of murine tumors with immune RNA, in D. M. Southam and H. Friedman, (eds.), *International Conference on Immunotherapy of Cancer,* pp. 575–591. New York Academy of Sciences, New York.

12. deKernion, J. B., Kern, D. H., Lovrekovich, H., *et al.* 1974. Intracellular localization of antitumor immune RNA. *Surg. Forum* 25: 123–125.

13. Eilber, F. R., Nizze, J. A., and Morton, D. L. 1975. Sequential evaluation of general immunocompetence in cancer patients: Correlation with clinical course. *Cancer* 35: 748–755.

14. Everson, T. C., and Cole, W. H. 1976. *In* M. A. Fink (ed.), *Spontaneous Regression of Cancer,* pp. 11–87. Saunders Co., Philadelphia.

15. Fishman, J. 1961. Antibody formation *in vitro. J. Exp. Med.* 114: 837–856.

16. Fishman, M., and Adler, F. L. 1963. Antibody formation initiated *in vitro.* II. Antibody synthesis in X-irradiated recipients of diffusion chambers containing nucleic acid derived from macrophages incubated with antigen. *J. Exp. Med.* 117: 595–602.

17. Fudenberg, H. H. 1976. Dialyzable transfer factor in the treatment of human osteosarcoma: An analytic review, in D. M. Southam and H. Friedman (eds.), *International Conference on Immunotherapy of Cancer,* pp. 545–557. New York Academy of Sciences, New York.

18. Fukushima, M., Machida, S., Hokama, A., *et al.* 1974. Passive transfer of the resistance to tumor with RNA. *Tohoku J. Exp. Med.* 112: 115–163.

19. Friedman, H. 1976. Protective immunity in leukemic mice treated with specific immunogenic RNA, in D. M. Southam and H. Friedman (eds.), *International Conference on Immunotherapy of Cancer,* pp. 708–715. New York Academy of Sciences, New York.

20. Hellström, I., Sjögren, H. O., Werner, G., *et al.* 1971. Blocking of cell mediated tumor immunity by sera from patients with growing neoplasms. *Int. J. Cancer* 7: 226–237.

21. Jensen, K., Patnode, R. A., Townsley, H. C., *et al.* 1962. Multiple passive transfer of delayed type hypersensitivity in humans. *Am. Rev. Resp. Dis.* 85: 373–377.

22. Jewell, W. R., Thomas, J. H., Morse, P., and Humphrey, L. J. 1976. Comparison of allogenic tumor vaccine with leukocyte transfer and transfer factor treatment of human cancer, in C. M. Southam and H. Friedman (eds.), *International Conference on Immunotherapy of Cancer,* pp. 516–552. New York Academy of Sciences, New York.

23. Johnson, D. E., Kaesler, K. E., and Samuels, M. L. 1975. Is nephrectomy justified in patients with metastatic renal carcinoma? *J. Urol.* 114: 27–29.

24. Kennedy, C. T., Cater, D. B., and Hartveit, F. 1969. Protection of C3H mice against BP-8 tumor by RNA extracted from lymph nodes and spleens of specifically sensitized mice. *Acta. Pathol. Microbiol. Scand.* 77: 796–799.

25. Kern, D. H., Chow, N., and Pilch, Y. H. 1976. Kinetics of synthesis and immunologically active fraction of anti-tumor Immune RNA. *Cell Immunol.* 24: 58–68.

26. Kern, D. H., Drogemuller, C. R., and Pilch, Y. H. 1974. Immune cytolysis of rat tumor cells mediated by syngeneic "Immune" RNA. *J. Natl. Cancer Inst.* 52: 299–302.

27. Kern, D. H., Fritze, D., Drogemuller, C. R., and Pilch, Y. H. 1976. Mediation of cytotoxic immune responses against human tumor-associated antigens by xenogeneic Immune RNA. *J. Natl. Cancer Inst.* 57: 97–103.

28. Kern, D. H., Fritze, D., Schick, P. M., Chow, N., and Pilch, Y. H. 1976. Mediation of cytotoxic immune responses against human tumor-associated antigens by allogeneic Immune RNA. *J. Natl. Cancer Inst.* 57: 105–109.

29. Kern, D. H., and Pilch, Y. H. 1974. Immune cytolysis of murine tumor cells mediated by xenogeneic "Immune" RNA. *Int. J. Cancer* 13: 679–688.

30. Lawrence, H. S. 1955. The transfer in humans of delayed skin sensitivity to Streptococcal M substance and to Tuberculin with disrupted leukocytes. *J. Clin. Invest.* 34: 219–230.

31. Lawrence, H. S. 1970. Transfer factor and cellular immune deficiency diseases. *N. Engl. J. Med.* 283: 410–411.

32. Lawrence, H. S., and Pappenheimer, A. M., Jr. 1956. Transfer of delayed hypersensitivity to Diptheria toxin in man. *J. Exp. Med.* 104: 321–326.

33. Lawrence, H. S., and Valentine, F. T. 1970. Transfer factor and other mediators of cellular immunity. *Amer. J. Pathol.* 60: 437–551.

34. McKahnn, C. F. 1972. Immunobiology of cancer, *in* J. S. Majarian and R. L. Simmons (eds.), *Transplantation,* p. 297. Lea and Febiger, Philadelphia.

35. Mannick, J. A., and Deckers, P. J. 1973. Mechanism of RNA-mediated transfer of cellular immunity. *Ann. N.Y. Acad. Sci.* 207: 398–405.

36. Mannick, J. A., and Egdahl, R. H. 1962. Transformation of nonimmune lymph node cells to a state of transplantation immunity by RNA. *Ann. Surg.* 156: 356–366.

37. Moore, G. E. 1972. Cultured human lymphocytes. *J. Surg. Oncol.* 4: 320–353.

38. Moore, G. E., and Gerner, R. E. 1970. Cancer Immunity—Hypothesis and clinical trial of lymphocytotherapy for malignant diseases. *Ann. Surg.* 172: 733–739.

39. Morton, D. L., Eilber, F. R., Joseph, W. L., *et al.* 1970. *Ann. Surg.* 172: 740–749.

40. Mostofi, F. K. 1967. Pathology and spread of renal cell carcinoma, *in* J. S. King (ed.), *Renal Neoplasia,* p. 41. Little, Brown, Boston.

41. Nadler, S. H., and Moore, G. E. 1966. Clinical immunologic study of malignant disease: Response to tumor transplants and transfer of lymphocytes. *Ann. Surg.* 164: 482–490.

42. Ohno, R., Esaki, K., Kodera, Y., *et al.* 1973. Experimental models in the role of RNA in immunotherapy of leukemia. *Ann. N.Y. Acad. Sci.* 207: 430–441.

43. Pilch, Y. H., Fritze, D., Ramming, K. P., deKernion, J. B., and Kern, D. H. 1976. The mediation of immune responses by I-RNA to animal and human tumor antigen, *in* M. A. Fink (ed.), *Immune RNA in Neoplasia,* pp. 149–175. Academic

Press, New York.

44. Pilch, Y. H., and Kern, D. H. 1976. Immune RNA and tumor immunity, in E. P. Cohen (ed.), *Immune RNA*, pp. 71–107. C.R.C. Press, Cleveland.

45. Pilch, Y. H., Myers, G. H., Sparks, F. C., and Golub, S. H. 1975. *Prospects for the Immunotherapy of Cancer. Part II: Current Status of Immunotherapy*, p. 9. Year Book Medical Publishers, Chicago.

46. Pilch, Y. H., Ramming, K. P., and Deckers, P. J. 1973. Studies in mediation of tumor immunity with "immune" RNA, in H. Busch (ed.), *Methods in Cancer Research*, pp. 195–254. Academic Press, New York.

47. Rafla, S. 1970. Renal cell carcinoma. Natural history and results of treatment. *Cancer* 25: 26–40.

48. Ramming, K. P., and deKernion, J. B. 1976. Immune RNA therapy for renal cell carcinoma: Survival and immunologic monitoring. *Ann. Surgery* (in press).

49. Ramming, K. P., and Pilch, Y. H. 1970. Mediation of immunity to tumor isographs in mice by heterologous ribonucleic acid. *Science* 168: 492–493.

50. Ramming, K. P., and Pilch, Y. H. 1970. Transfer of tumor specific immunity with RNA; demonstration by immune cytolysis of tumor cells *in vitro*. *J. Natl. Cancer Inst.* 45: 543–553.

51. Ramming, K. P., and Pilch, Y. H. 1971. Transfer of tumor specific immunity with RNA: Inhibition of growth of murine tumor isografts. *J. Natl. Cancer Inst.* 46: 735–750.

52. Rigby, P. G. 1968. Propagation of survival of tumor bearing animals by transfer of immune RNA with DEAE dextran. *Nature* 221: 968–972.

53. Sabbadini, E., and Sehon, A. H. 1967. Acceleration of allograft rejection induced by RNA from sensitized donors. *Int. Arch. Allergy Appl. Immunol.* 32: 55–63.

54. Schlager, S. I., and Dray, S. 1975. Antitumor activity of RNA extracts *in vivo*. *Proc. Am. Assoc. Cancer Res.* 16: 22.

55. Seigler, H. F., Buckley, C. E., Sheppard, L. B., Horne, B. J., and Shingleton, W. W. 1976. Adoptive transfer and specific active immunization of patients with malignant melanoma, in C. M. Southam and H. Friedman (eds.), *International Conference on Immunotherapy of Cancer*, pp. 522–532. New York Academy of Sciences, New York.

56. Spitler, L. E., Fudenberg, H. H. 1975. Transfer factor I. Methods of therapy. *Birth Defects* 11(1): 445–448.

57. Spitler, L. E., Levin, A. S., Blois, M. S., *et al.* 1972. Lymphocyte responses to tumor-specific antigens in patients with malignant melanoma and results of transfer factor therapy. *J. Clin. Invest.* 51: 92a.

58. Sumner, W. C., and Foraker, A. G. 1960. Spontaneous regression of human melanoma, clinical and experimental study. *Cancer* 13: 79–81.

59. Veltman, L. L., Kern, D. H., and Pilch, Y. H. 1974. Immune cytolysis of human tumor cells mediated by xenogeneic "Immune" RNA. *Cell. Immunol.* 13: 367–377.

60. Waldman, S. R., Roth, J. A., Kern, D. H., and Pilch, Y. H. 1975. Effects on cancer patients of leukophoresis using the continuous flow blood cell separator. II. Immunologic parameters, *in vitro*. *J. Lab. Clin. Med.* 86: 950–961.

CHAPTER 11

IMMUNOLOGY AND IMMUNOTHERAPY OF MELANOMA

Gary M. Stuhlmiller
H. F. Seigler

Department of Microbiology
and Immunology
Department of Surgery
Duke University Medical Center
Durham, North Carolina 27710
and Durham Veterans
Administration Hospital
Durham, North Carolina 27704

The immunogenicity of human melanoma is now well established. Through the use of sera from melanoma patients, melanoma-tumor-associated antigens (TAA) have been detected in the nucleolus and cytoplasm and on the cell membrane of melanoma cells. Heteroantisera against human melanoma have identified certain of these TAA as fetal antigens. A correlation exists between the extent of the disease and the presence of a demonstrable host antitumor immune response, suggesting a crucial role played by the immune response in the host-tumor interaction. Because of its natural immunogenicity, melanoma appears to be amenable to specific and nonspecific immunotherapy.

I. INTRODUCTION

Few human tumors can be as highly invasive of normal tissues or lead as rapidly to the death of the host as melanoma. Despite its highly malignant nature, melanoma appears to be immunogenic in the host, and thus, potentially susceptible to elimination by the host immune response. According to the theory of immune surveillance, the immune response might have evolved as a mechanism for destroying cells which have undergone malignant transformation. Any immunogenic tumor cells would thus be readily destroyed and only in the event of failure or circumvention of the immune response would a tumor become detectable. The fact that melanoma accounts for only 1 to 3% of all clinically detected human tumors may be a reflection of the usual efficiency of the host's immune response to destroy such immunogenic tumor cells.

Since its description in the nineteenth century, melanoma has been of great interest to the medical world, in part because of its sometimes bizarre and unpredictable behavior, suggestive of some form of host control mechanism. Eberman reported a series of cases in which the primary tumor had undergone regression while regional lymph node metastases persisted (29). A number of similar cases have since been reported (24, 82, 112, 120, 123). Another unusual feature of the disease is the finding that some primary and metastatic lesions undergo regression coincident with the development of new metastases at other sites. The most compelling evidence for the presence of a host antitumor immune response comes from reports describing the regression of established and widespread metastatic tumor (47, 113). These latter reports are clearly of great clinical significance and strongly suggest that the host immune response is capable of eliminating even large amounts of tumor, although this capability is only infrequently fully realized in the melanoma patient.

Also suggestive of a host control mechanism over melanoma is the appearance of metastatic tumor long after the primary tumor has been "completely" removed. Such behavior is most typical of primary ocular melanoma in which the development of metastases has been delayed as long as thirty years after removal of the primary tumor with no clinically detectable disease in the intervening years. It is probable that some tumor remained undetected but without growth during this "disease-free" period.

The immune destruction of a tumor is dependent upon an interaction between elements of the immune response and tumor associated antigens

(TAA) on the tumor cell membrane. The regression of a tumor is thus suggestive evidence for cell membrane TAA. In the case of human melanoma, cytoplasmic and nucleolar TAA have also been described. In this chapter, we will describe the melanoma TAA and how they have been defined. We will also attempt to indicate the possible role(s) of these TAA in the host-tumor interaction and their potential for use in immunodiagnostic assays or immunotherapeutic regimens.

II. MELANOMA ANTIGEN SITES

A. Melanoma Cell Membrane TAA Defined by Melanoma Patient Sera

Lewis provided the first serological evidence for a host anti-melanoma immune response (65). He found that melanoma patient sera, when added to autologous melanoma cells growing in tissue culture, had a cytotoxic effect upon the cells. No such effect was observed against allogeneic melanoma cells. Subsequently, Lewis (66) and Lewis and Phillips (67) evaluated melanoma patient sera for anti-cell membrane TAA antibody by immunofluorescence and the complement-dependent antibody cytotoxicity assay. They detected antibody reactive with cell membrane TAA found only on autologous melanoma cells. Results from these studies thus suggested that each melanoma possessed individually unique (non-cross-reactive) cell membrane TAA, a situation analogous to that which had been described for carcinogen-induced rodent tumors (99).

Morton, however, also evaluated the sera of melanoma patients for their content of anti-melanoma cell membrane TAA antibodies using immunofluorescence (85). He demonstrated significant reactivity of the sera in 4/5 (80%) autologous serum: cell combinations and in 36/63 allogeneic serum: cell combinations. In addition, 7/53 (13%) normal sera gave positive reactions. Qualitatively similar results were obtained by Romsdahl and Cox (130) and by Fossati (34) using immunofluorescence and by Gray (41) using complement-dependent antibody cytotoxicity. These results are clearly suggestive of cross-reactivity among the cell membrane TAA of different melanomas and thus, in direct conflict with the results obtained by Lewis and his colleagues. Such a situation is more reminiscent of that encountered with the RNA tumor virus-induced tumors in which all tumors induced by a given virus possess TAA characteristic of that virus.

Whether or not all human melanomas share certain cross-reactive cell membrane TAA is of crucial importance for the potential success of a specific immunotherapeutic and immunoprophylactic regimens. Clearly, both active immunotherapy and immunoprophylaxis using, for instance, a melanoma cell membrane TAA isolated from a single melanoma, would be feasible only if all melanomas shared the same or highly cross-reactive cell membrane TAA. Likewise, the potential success of passive serotherapy using an anti-melanoma antiserum would depend upon the presence of the same TAA on the immunizing and target melanoma cells. Rather than helping to answer this question, the early studies using melanoma patient sera to detect the melanoma cell membrane TAA raised the question as to why different groups, working with essentially the same techniques and comparable reagents, had reported such conflicting results.

The most reasonable explanation for this controversy relates to the necessarily subjective manner in which the data from these studies, and in particular, those employing immunofluorescent techniques, must be interpreted. Each investigator must decide what intensity of the fluorescence will be considered a positive result. Although attempts have been made to quantitate these results through the use of a fluorescence index, considerable subjectivity is inherent in the interpretation of the results. Although the interpretation of results from cytotoxicity assays is more objective, the investigator must still choose a level of base cytotoxicity above which a reaction will be called positive. Variations in what different investigators consider a positive reaction may thus cause considerable variation in the reported results, especially when weak cross-reactivities are involved.

In those studies mentioned above, it appears as though Lewis and his colleagues selected much more stringent criteria for classifying a reaction as positive than did other investigators. In doing so, however, they may have overlooked certain positive reactions. On the other hand, the criteria used by Morton and others may have been sufficiently non-selective such that certain reactions due to the presence, in the sera, of antibodies other than those directed against the melanoma TAA were considered positive. In view of the fact that Bloom (6) has demonstrated the presence of blood group antigens on human melanoma cells, the possibility that natural anti-blood group antibodies were being detected in certain instances must be considered. The fact that 13% of the normal sera examined by Morton were positive against melanoma target cells, whereas none of the normal sera tested by Lewis and colleagues were positive, adds support to this possible explanation for the discrepant results.

The weight of evidence now supports the contention that the cell membrane TAA of different melanomas, as detected by the sera of melanoma patients, possess some degree of cross-reactivity, although there is still some question as to whether or not each melanoma may possess individually unique TAA in addition to those cross-reactive with the TAA of other melanomas. Nairn, for example, has reported cross-reactivity among the cell membrane TAA of different melanomas but also found an element of individual specificity (91). Bodurtha reports a strong individual specificity with weaker cross-reactivity of the sera with allogeneic melanomas (9). Gupta and Morton eluted antibody from a melanoma and found it to react with solubilized melanoma TAA from five different melanomas in complement-fixation assays (43). DeVries (27) also detected cross-reactivity using immuno adherence techniques, as did Macher (70).

An outstanding feature of these studies has been the lack of any data to suggest a complete cross-reactivity of the cell membrane TAA from different melanomas. No single melanoma patients serum has yet been shown to react with all target melanomas. Thus, in this system, the extent of cross-reactivity of the cell membrane TAA cannot be fully evaluated. In a subsequent section, evidence will be presented to indicate that certain cell membrane TAA can be detected on all melanomas using antimelanoma heteroantisera. Two other techniques have been utilized to detect a humoral immune response of melanoma patients against their tumors. Kodera and Bean employed the antibody dependent cell-mediated cytotoxicity assay and found the sera of 4/16 melanoma patients to have significant reactivity with autologous tumor cells (61). No allogeneic serum cell combinations were examined in this study. Irie detected antibody and complement bound on fresh suspended melanoma cells through the use of mixed hemadsorption techniques (58).

B. Melanoma Cytoplasmic TAA Defined by Melanoma Patient Sera

That sera from some melanoma patients also reached with an antigen located in the cytoplasm of melanoma cells was initially reported in 1968 by Morton (85) and by Oettgen (92) and subsequently by several other investigators (66, 88, 91, 103). Demonstration of this TAA by immunofluorescence required fixation of the target cells prior to their exposure to fluorescein-labeled antibody. Through the use of absorption analysis, Lewis and Phillips were able to separate antibody reactive with cytoplasmic TAA from that reactive with cell membrane TAA and thus to demonstrate that these TAA were distinct (68). Whereas a controversy existed regarding the cross-reactivity of the cell membrane TAA of different melanomas, the results from studies of the cytoplasmic TAA showed considerable agreement and strongly suggested some degree to cross-reactivity between the cytoplasmic TAA of different melanomas. Thus, the serum of a melanoma patient which was reactive with the cytoplasmic TAA of homologous melanoma cells was usually reactive against cytoplasmic TAA of allogeneic melanomas as well. The extent of this reported cross-reactivity was somewhat variable depending upon the investigator.

There is some question as to the specificity of the cytoplasmic antigen for melanoma. For example, Morton found that the sera of 13% of the normal donors tested also reacted with an antigen located in the melanoma cell cytoplasm (85). Oettgen reported that 10% of the sera from patients with other forms of cancer and from 11% of patients with various nonmalignant disorders contained antibody reactive with such an antigen (92). Wood and Barth compared three groups of sera for their content of anti-melanoma cytoplasmic antigen activity; sera from melanoma patients, sera from patients with other tumors, and sera from normal donors (127). They found no significant differences between the groups with regard to the percentage of positive sera. Rather, they found that the titer of the antibody was much greater in the sera of melanoma patients. In contrast, Elliott was unable to detect any antibody against melanoma cytoplasmic antigen in the sera of 150 donors with various pigmented and non-pigmented skin lesions (30). Copman, however, did detect such antibody in the sera of donors who had halo nevi (20).

As of the present, a very important aspect of this problem appears to have been largely neglected. Emphasis thus far has been placed upon determining the distribution, among various groups of donors, of antibody reactive with antigen present in the cytoplasm of melanoma cells. In view of the fact that a relatively large number of sera from donors other than melanoma patients react with some cytoplasmic melanoma antigen, studies to determine the tissue distribution of the melanoma cytoplasmic TAA, as detected by melanoma patient sera in autologous tumor cells, should be performed. Nairn performed a very limited study in this regard and found that sera from melanoma patients did react with the cytoplasm of 1/4 squamous cell carcionomas (91). Muna and his collaborators were unable to demonstrate any reactivity of melanoma patient sera against benign nevus cells, HeLa cells or human kidney cells (88). However, this group also failed to detect any anti-melanoma activity in the sera of 22 normal donors and even the reactivity of melanoma patient sera with melanoma cells was extremely weak (titer 1:2). The system used thus seems to have been relatively insensitive and the possibility that some positive reactions were not detected cannot be eliminated. Lewis and Sheikh approached this problem indirectly by demonstrating that the antibody reactive with the cytoplasmic melanoma TAA could be removed from melanoma patient sera by absorption with homogenates of melanoma but not of normal pigmented and non-pigmented tissues (69). This result would suggest some degree of melanoma specificity for this antigen.

Clearly, much more extensive investigation into the tissue distribution of this TAA in the population as a whole is required. One point which is of particular importance is to determine whether or not the sera of melanoma patients and that of other donors react with the same antigen(s) in the melanoma cell cytoplasm. A situation analogous to the ABO blood group antigen-antibody system might exist. Thus, natural antibody reactive with some cytoplasmic alloantigen, totally distinct from the melanoma TAA defined by autologous serum, might be present in the sera of many normal donors and could thus account for the observed reactivity of such sera against melanoma cells. While purely a hypothetical situation, the analogy does illustrate the necessity of determining which antigen is being detected by the sera of melanoma patients, and which by the sera of other donors.

C. Melanoma Nuclear TAA Defined by Melanoma Patient Sera

Morton (85) and Oettgen (92) briefly mentioned that sera from melanoma patients also reacted with an antigen found in the nucleus of melanoma cells. Oettgen dismissed this finding as being non-specific but failed to elaborate on this point. Morton found the sera of 61% of the melanoma patients and 20% of normal donors to react with this antigen. McBride further localized this antigen to the nucleolus and demonstrated that it was widely cross-reactive among the melanomas (78). Of the melanoma patient sera examined, 15% contained antibody reactive with autologous tumor cells but 45% of the tested melanomas could be shown to contain this antigen. Bowen extended this study and found that the presence of the nucleolar antigen did not correlate with the presence of cytoplasmic antigen (10). Reactive sera from two melanoma patients were examined for reactivity with the nucleus of a variety of fresh tumors and with cells from normal and malignant tissue culture cell lines. These sera reacted with a nuclear antigen present in cells from Hodgkin's disease, carcinoma of the liver, osteosarcoma and adenocarcinoma of the colon. Thus, this antigen is not totally specific for melanoma.

III. MELANOMA TAA DEMONSTRATED BY MELANOMA PATIENT CELLULAR IMMUNE RESPONSES

Histological evidence suggestive of some form of host response against melanoma was provided as early as 1907 by Handley who reported that melanomas localized to the upper layers of the dermis often contained a dense lymphocytic infiltrate similar to that observed in inflammatory responses (47). The significance of this response, as it related to a specific antitumor immune reaction, was not to be appreciated until much later, however. Abundant documentation of such a specific cell-mediated immune response of melanoma patients against their tumors has since been provided. One of four basic techniques has usually been employed to demonstrate this cell-mediated immunity: (1) delayed cutaneous hypersensitivity; (2) lymphocyte stimulation in vitro; (3) measurement of some in vitro parameter of lymphocyte recognition of melanoma TAA other than stimulation, i.e., migration inhibition, and (4) cell-mediated cytotoxicity of target tumor cells in vitro.

Before the development of suitable in vitro methods for measuring cell-mediated immunity, the only available technique for evaluating patient cell-mediated immunity was the delayed cutaneous hypersensitivity reaction. Consequently, the earliest investigations of melanoma patient CMI to melanoma TAA were performed using this technique. Hughes provided the first meaningful results to demonstrate this immunity (56). Numerous other investigators have confirmed and extended his findings (7, 14, 15, 19, 33, 54, 55, 94, 104, 116). In most such studies, a solubilized melanoma TAA preparation has been shown to elicit much stronger delayed cutaneous hypersensitivity reactions in melanoma patients than in patients with other histological forms of tumor. Control antigen material prepared from normal skin, muscle, etc., does not elicit such a response. Such findings are then interpreted as meaning that melanoma patients have been pre-sensitized to the melanoma TAA. Because patients with other forms of tumor do not respond as vigorously to the TAA preparation as do melanoma patients, the results also suggest that the reaction is specific for melanoma TAA in the skin test preparations. Hughes (56), Stewart (116), Fass (33), Cooper (19) and Oren and Heberman (94) demonstrated hypersensitivity of melanoma patients to KCL extracts or homogenates of autologous tumor. That factors other than sensitization to melanoma TAA could effect the response of melanoma patients to antigen was demonstrated by Bluming who reported that certain melanoma patients also reacted against a control antigen prepared from normal skin (7). Hollingshead reported that solubilized melanoma TAA were able to elicit a hypersensitivity reaction in some breast cancer patients in addition to melanoma patients (55). Furthermore, these authors also found that antigen prepared from normal black skin caused a hypersensitivity response in some melanoma patients.

In vitro lymphocyte stimulation has proven to be a useful assay for cell-mediated immunity. Jehn demonstrated that soluble extracts of melanoma cells were stimulatory to peripheral blood lymphocytes (PBL) of melanoma patients (16). Tumor cyst fluid and urine from melanoma patients were also shown to stimulate melanoma patient PBL in vitro.

This latter finding is of potentially great significance as it suggests that melanoma TAA may be found in soluble form in the body fluids. As a result, it should be possible to develop immunodiagnostic assays for the melanoma TAA. Nagel (90), Seigler (107), Mavligit (76) and Hersh (54) have also successfully utilized this technique for measuring anti-melanoma cell mediated immunity.

A variety of in vitro assays have been developed which measure lymphocyte responses secondary to the primary event of antigen recognition. Of these, the most widely used has been the leukocyte migration inhibition assay (8, 15, 16, 17, 53, 71, 79, 105). Theoretically, lymphocytes exposed to an antigen to which they have been pre-sensitized in vivo are unable to migrate away from that particular antigen, whereas a control antigen to which the individual has not been sensitized has no such effect. A very similar assay, the monocyte spreading inhibition assay, has also been employed (77). The leukocyte adherence inhibition assay has also been utilized to measure anti-melanoma cell mediated immunity (46).

Before proceeding further, it is important that one serious limitation of the aforementioned cell-mediated immunity assays be mentioned. As already discussed, at least three distinct melanoma TAA have been described serologically through the use of melanoma patient sera. Through the natural process of cell death, the "internal" melanoma TAA could be released. As a result, the host immune system would be exposed, and presumably, presensitized to these TAA, as well as to the cell membrane TAA. In all of the studies mentioned, the test antigen preparation is likely to have contained not only cell membrane TAA, but also the "internal" TAA. Thus, the responses measured by delayed hypersensitivity reactions, lymphocyte stimulation, leukocyte adherence inhibition, etc., may be due, in part, or in toto, to a reaction with the "internal" TAA. Immune destruction of a tumor cell is dependent upon an interaction between elements of the immune response and cell membrane TAA on the tumor cell. Thus, although the host may respond against "internal" TAA, this response would have no known effect on the viable tumor cell. Because these various assays are unable to distinguish between responses against cell membrane TAA and those against internal TAA, the clinical significance of this demonstrated immunity is very difficult to evaluate. In contrast, specific cell-mediated cytotoxicity of target tumor cells is dependent upon the interaction between cell membrane TAA and PBL sensitized to these cells. For this reason, this type of assay has the advantage of measuring a cell-mediated immune reaction which is of potentially great significance in the host-tumor interaction. Using this assay, the Hellströms and their colleagues have been able to demonstrate that PBL of a large proportion of melanoma patients were cytotoxic to melanoma target cells in *vitro.* Allogeneic as well as autologous melanoma cells were killed, thus providing evidence for the cross-reactivity of the cell membrane TAA of different melanomas (48, 50). PBL from normal black donors were also cytotoxic for melanoma cells (49). DeVries has demonstrated that this cytotoxic activity resides in the T cell subpopulation and that short term cultures of melanoma cells are more susceptible to cytolysis than cells from melanoma cell lines (26, 27, 28). Nairn (91), Heppner (51), Currie (21), Embleton and Price (31) and Berkelhammer (4) have also successfully demonstrated cell-mediated immunity of melanoma patients against melanoma using this assay.

In spite of the fact that this assay has been widely employed to measure anti-TAA cell mediated immunity, questions have arisen regarding its specificity and reproducibility. Takasugi found that in certain instances, PBL from normal donors were as reactive or more reactive against melanoma target cells than were the PBL of some melanoma patients (121). Similar findings have been reported by Peter (97) and by Pavie Fischer (96). Furthermore, Takasugi has also demonstrated that PBL from melanoma patients show no histological specificity as previously claimed by the Hellströms (122). Rather, PBL reactive against melanoma targets were also reactive against cells from a number of histologically different tumors. Heppner found that markedly different results were obtained when the same target-effector cell combinations were repeatedly tested (52). In addition, in direct contrast to the findings of DeVries (26), Heppner demonstrated that melanoma cells from established lines were more susceptible in this assay than were cells from short-term cultures.

It is evident that the situation encountered in evaluating anti-melanoma cell-mediated immunity by cell-mediated cytotoxicity is complex. Several factors which have contributed, in part, to the conflicting results presented include the varying of the assay conditions, source of target cells, and possible allogeneic effects. Several modifications of the techniques have been employed and factors such as incubation times, effector-cell:target-cell ratio, and preparation of effector cells have varied widely. As in the case of serological studies of melanoma TAA, different interpretation of the data could also cause considerable variation and conflict in the results reported by various investigators.

IV. MELANOMA TAA DEFINED BY HETEROANTISERA

Interest in the use of heteroantisera for the study of melanoma TAA has arisen because of two problems encountered in the use of melanoma patient sera for this purpose. When the cell membrane melanoma TAA have been studied, it has been found that no single serum from any melanoma patient will react with all target melanomas. Secondly, the titer of such sera is usually low (42, 88, 107). Consequently, these sera are of limited usefulness for definition and isolation of the TAA, for immunodiagnosis or for passive serotherapy. Heteroantisera have the advantages of being, in most cases, higher titered and of broader reactivity than patient sera. The major problem associated with the use of heteroantisera for the study of human TAA is, obviously, specificity. In addition to responding against TAA, immunized animals also respond against many human species, tissue, allo- and isoantigens, and it is only after antibodies reactive with these "normal" human antigens are removed that the anti-melanoma TAA activity of such antisera may be realistically evaluated. Even in the most carefully controlled study, the possibility that what is considered to be specific anti-TAA antibody might, in reality, react with an antigen present on only a small subpopulation of normal cells and on tumor cells cannot be totally eliminated. As a consequence, results obtained using heteroantisera against human TAA must be interpreted with this limitation in mind. In spite of this shortcoming, the use of heteroantisera for the study of melanoma TAA has provided valuable insight into the nature of these TAA, and, for this reason, our discussion here will go into considerable detail.

Viza and Phillips (124) immunized rabbits with a papain solubilized melanoma TAA preparation. The antisera so produced were absorbed with lyophilized normal human serum, papain solubilized "HLA" antigens and with inactivated papain until the antisera did not react with these antigens by immunodiffusion analysis. One such antiserum retained reactivity against soluble extract from the immunizing tumor and against one of two extracts prepared from "pooled" melanomas. An antigenically identical determinant was detected in extracts of human embryo and human leukemia. Further absorption of the antiserum with the embryo extract removed all detectable reactivity against embryo, melanoma and leukemia extracts from the antiserum. Although several aspects of this study may be subject to criticism, we have included it in this discussion as it is, to our knowledge, the first study in which an association of fetal antigens with melanoma has been demonstrated. In subsequent studies these authors utilized this reagent to demonstrate the presence of soluble melanoma TAA in the serum of melanoma patients (125, 126).

Goodwin and his colleagues immunized rabbits with melanoma tissue from a single human donor (40). Following absorption with either whole skin, cell-free extract of skin, cell-free extract of lymph node, or kidney powder, this antiserum reacted with antigen present in 23/26 target melanomas. Subcellular localization of this antigen(s) could not be determined. The antiserum did not react with benign pigmented moles, mesenchymal sarcoma or with carcinomas of the thyroid or colon.

The presence of soluble melanoma TAA in the urine of melanoma patients was demonstrated by Carrell and Theilkaes (13). These authors immunized rabbits with TAA extracted from solid tumor or with urine from melanoma patients. Both antisera were shown to react with an antigen present in the urine of 29/32 melanoma patients. Of 72 urine samples from normal donors or patients with various malignant and non-malignant disorders, only three were found to contain this antigen. Two of these samples were from patients with neuroblastoma and the third from a patient with ganglioneuroma. This finding is significant because these tumors, as well as melanoma, are of neuro-ectodermal origin and suggests that the antigen detected may be fetal antigen.

Further evidence to support the association of fetal antigens with melanoma is provided by Avis and Lewis, who immunized rabbits with perchloric extracts of human fetus (1). Following absorption of the antiserum with normal human tissue, the antiserum did not react with normal adult lymphocytes, skin, gut, or buccal squame cells. However, it did react with cell membrane antigens of a number of human tumors, including melanoma, teratoma, carcinomas of the colon, breast, and kidney, neuroblastoma, and Wilm's tumor, in addition to fetal cells. A very significant aspect of this study was the demonstration that the rabbit antihuman fetus antiserum did not block the cell membrane TAA detected by melanoma patient serum. Such a finding strongly suggests the presence of at least two distinct TAA on the melanoma cell membrane, one of these being of fetal origin and shared with other human tumors.

Guinea pigs have also been utilized to raise antisera against human melanoma TAA (37, 38). These antisera reacted with cells from melanoma cell lines and with human fetal skin in a complement dependent microcytotoxicity assay, but not with cells from carcinomas of the ovary, colon or stomach. Absorption of the antisera with fetal skin cells removed all detectable anti-melanoma and anti-fetal activity from the antiserum. Ghose immunized goats with human melanoma. Discussion of this report will be presented in a subsequent section (39).

In order to avoid the stimulation of potent immune response against normal human antigens, we have utilized non-human primates for the production of anti-melanoma antisera. Because of their phylogenic proximity to man, non-human primates share many antigens which are cross-reactive with their human counterparts. As a result, the primate immune response against these normal human antigens is much weaker than that of other more commonly employed species thus permitting a stronger, more specific anti-TAA response. Metzgar first demonstrated that monkeys immunized with cells from melanoma cell lines maintained in tissue culture responded with the production of antisera which, following absorption with human RBC and PBL, were specifically reactive with melanoma cell membrane TAA (80). Normal PBL and skin fibroblasts were not lysed by these absorbed antisera. Further absorption of the antisera with cells from a single melanoma removed all reactivity against all target melanomas tested. These results strongly suggested that all melanomas possessed certain shared or highly cross-reactive melanoma cell membrane TAA.

In a more extensive study, we immunized a chimpanzee with fresh tumor from a single donor. Following absorption with RBC and PBL of the tumor donor, this antiserum reacted against cell membrane TAA found on all melanomas tested (14/14) but not with tumor cells from eight different types of tumor. In addition, this antiserum reacted with cell membrane antigens of human fetal fibroblasts. Absorption of the antiserum with cells from any one of eight different melanomas removed all detectable reactivity against melanoma cells and fetal cells. Comparable absorption with fetal cells removed all anti-fetal reactivity and some, but not all, of the anti-melanoma activity from the antiserum. This does not appear to reflect quantitative differences in antigen expression on melanoma and fetal cells as additional absorptions of the antiserum with fetal cells failed to further reduce the anti-melanoma titer of the antiserum (118). We have interpreted these results as indicating that at least two distinct TAA are expressed on the melanoma cell membrane. One of these is shared with fetal fibroblasts and the other apparently unique to melanoma cells. In this regard our results confirm the previous findings of Avis and Lewis (1). We have also utilized melanoma cells obtained from a melanoma cell line for immunization of a chimpanzee with essentially comparable results. Dent (25) and Levy (64) have also shown non-human primates to be useful for the production of antihuman primates to be useful for the production of anti-melanoma antiserum.

Using the chimpanzee antihuman melanoma antiserum, we have been able to demonstrate that the melanoma cell membrane TAA are released from the cell membrane in an antigenically active form spontaneously as a result of membrane turnover (119). We have also found that these TAA are susceptible to proteolytic digestion with pronase and trypsin, as a treatment of melanoma cells with these enzymes renders the cells refractory to cytolysis by the antiserum. Preliminary results suggest that these TAA are released from the cell in an antigenically active form (unpublished results).

The results obtained from the study of melanoma TAA using heteroantisera are thus significant for two reasons. (1) In studies in which the cell membrane TAA are investigated, heteroantisera appear to detect a common or highly cross-reactive TAA on all melanomas. (2) Included among the melanoma TAA are fetal antigens which may or may not be shared by other histological types of tumor. In the case of the cell membrane TAA, fetal antigens are distinct from the TAA unique to melanoma. This latter finding suggests that specific immunodiagnostic procedures for melanoma using heteroantisera might be developed. Further studies using heteroantisera will be included where appropriate in subsequent sections.

V. CORRELATION BETWEEN EXTENT OF DISEASE AND PRESENCE OF DEMONSTRABLE HOST ANTITUMOR RESPONSE

Results from several investigations suggest that a correlation exists between the presence of a detectable host anti-tumor immune reaction and the extent of the disease. This was first observed by Lewis, who noted that only those sera from patients with localized tumor contained antibody cytotoxic for target melanoma cells (65). In a subsequent study, Lewis confirmed this early observation and extended it by demonstrating that antibody reactive with cytoplasmic melanoma TAA could be detected in the sera of only those patients with localized tumor (66). Gray (41) and Dent (25) have reported that cytotoxic antibody reactive against melanoma cells is found in the sera of patients with localized tumor more frequently than in sera from patients with disseminated disease. The inverse relationship has been observed with regard to antibody reactive with the nucleolar TAA in that this antibody appears in the latter stages of the disease. However, this may be explained by the observation that this TAA does not appear until the latter stages of disease (10).

The question of crucial importance is whether the loss of detectable anti-melanoma TAA antibody, and in particular, the reactivity against melanoma cell membrane TAA, precedes tumor dissemination. If loss of detectable antibody preceeded tumor dissemination, this would suggest some failure of the immune response not necessarily related to tumor growth. If, however, the antibody disappeared as a result of tumor growth and dissemination, it would suggest that the tumor in some way, specifically or non-specifically actively turned off the immune response.

Cell-mediated immune reactions against melanoma TAA have also been found to correlate with the extent of the disease. Fass found that melanoma patients with localized tumor were able to mount a delayed hypersensitivity response against aqueous extract of autologous tumor (33). Patients with widespread disease failed to mount this response. Hollingshead reported similar results as 17/22 patients with early stage disease but only 7/19 patients with later stage disease responded against a soluble melanoma TAA skin test reagent (54).

Significant insight into a possible explanation for this in vivo correlation has been provided by the work of the Hellströms and their colleagues. When the PBL of melanoma patients having localized or disseminated tumor were examined for their ability to effect cytolysis of melanoma target cells in vitro, no significant differences between the two groups were detected (48). However, if serum from patients with growing tumors was included in the assay in place of normal human serum, the cytotoxic activity of the PBL was abrogated. Furthermore, this "blocking" was specific in that only sera from melanoma patients had this effect. Sera from patients with other forms of tumor had no inhibitory effect in the melanoma system. Likewise, the sera of melanoma patients had no inhibitory effect on the cytolysis of other types of tumor cells by appropriately presensitized PBL. Others who have observed this blocking phenomenon are DeVries (28), Currie (21), Heppner (51) and Halliday (46).

Because of the specificity of the inhibition, blocking factor was originally thought to be host-derived antibody which, in effect, masked the cell membrane TAA of the target cells preventing their interaction with effector cells. Sjögren presented evidence to suggest that blocking factor was actually an antibody-TAA complex (110). Sera with blocking activity were fractionated into two weight classes by molecular filtration at low pH. Neither the high molecular weight fraction (greater than 100,000 daltons) nor the low molecular weight material (less than 100,000 daltons), when tested alone, had blocking activity. When these fractions were recombined at physiological pH, blocking activity was again detected. Free TAA have also been postulated to have blocking activity. Embleton and Price have shown that papain solubilized melanoma TAA are able to block cytotoxicity of PBL for target melanoma cells (31). Although it is impossible to state conclusively that blocking, as detected in vitro, is responsible for the in vivo growth of tumor. Studies in an analogous system suggest that such a mechanism might function in vivo. Myburgh and Smit have presented evidence that baboon histocompatibility antigens, in either the form of free antigen or of immune complexes, were able to markedly prolong the survival of kidney allografts (84).

For such a blocking mechanism to function in vivo, large amounts of antigen would have to be released from the tumor cell membrane into the body fluids. Fine has shown that such in vivo shedding of cell membrane histocompatibility antigens does occur. Long surviving kidney allografts were found to bind specific anti-allotype antibody and then to quickly release it in the form of immune complexes (35). We have demonstrated that melanoma cell lines maintained in tissue culture spontaneously release detectable levels of TAA into the culture medium (117). Grimm has found that melanoma TAA released into serum-free medium are effective skin test reagents (42). The presence of soluble melanoma TAA in the serum (125, 126) and urine (13, 60) supports the belief that this shedding mechanism also functions in vivo. Further data to suggest the existence of this correlation comes from studies of macrophage function. Although its precise role in the destruction of tumor has yet to be determined, the macrophage appears to be an important element of the host antitumor immune response. Snyderman has demonstrated abnormal macrophage chemotaxis in a significantly large number of melanoma patients (114). In many cases, this response returned to within normal limits following surgical removal of tumor or immunotherapy with BCG. Of the patient who had normal chemotactic responses during this study, 18/20 were clinically free of tumor.

VI. NATURE OF MELANOMA TAA

Before we proceed to a discussion of the immunotherapy of melanoma, we will speculate somewhat as to the possible origin of the melanoma TAA. The association between melanoma TAA and fetal antigens as detected by heteroantisera produced against either of these antigen types has already been described. In addition, rabbit antisera prepared against a soluble extract of carcinoma of the colon reacts with an antigen common to a number of types of tumor, including melanoma cells and with fetal cells. Because of its beta electrophoretic mobility, this antigen has been termed "beta oncofetal antigen" (36). It is distinct from the more commonly described fetal antigens, alpha-feto-protein (AFP) and carcino-embryonic antigen (CEA). From the studies of Martin (74) and Mihalev (81) it appears as though CEA and AFP are not associated with melanoma, as elevated serum levels of these fetal antigens were detected in only 1/11 and 2/10 melanoma patients respectively.

A possible viral origin of the melanoma TAA is suggested by results from studies of human, murine and hamster melanomas. Dalton and Felix studied the S-91 melanoma of CBA mice by electronmicroscopy and found virus-sized particles associated with internal membranes of these cells (23). More recently, particles with features characteristic of RNA tumor viruses have been induced from B16 murine melanoma cells growing in tissue culture by incubation of these cells in medium containing 5-BUDR (108). Ito and Mishima (59) have demonstrated the presence of virus particles in cells from melanoma of the golden hamster, and Epstein (32) was able to transmit this melanoma to 9/11 hamsters using a cell free filtrate from these cells.

Reid reported that human occular melanoma cells contained a reverse transcriptase similar to that found in RNA tumor viruses (102). Subsequently, Parsons reported finding particles characteristic of RNA tumor viruses in human melanoma cell lines (95). Most recently, Birkmayer has detected both virus particles and reverse transcriptase in the cytoplasm of fresh melanoma cells (15). When sub-cellular fractions were assayed for their content of reverse transcriptase activity, the greatest activity was detected in the fractions containing the virus particles. Rabbit antiserum prepared against the enzyme-containing fraction reacted with the cytoplasm of melanoma cells to a much greater extent than with the cytoplasm of normal cells. There is thus some marginally suggestive evidence that RNA tumor viruses may be involved in the etiology of melanoma. If this is true, it would not be unreasonable to presume that certain of the melanoma TAA are structural components of the virus of virus-coded enzymes as has been demonstrated in a number of other virus-induced animal tumor systems. However, these latter studies have been severely criticized and, at present, most tumor virologists contend that these results were due to contamination of the materials used in the study.

VII. IMMUNOTHERAPY OF MELANOMA

We have devoted the first portion of this chapter to the definition of the melanoma TAA and their subcellular localization. In addition, we have discussed the various methods employed to detect these TAA and the immune responses of melanoma patients and heteroimmunized animals to these TAA. From this discussion, it is evident that the host anti-melanoma immune response, and in particular the response against the cell membrane TAA, may play a crucial role in the host-tumor interaction. In the tumor bearing host, the antitumor immune response is ineffective at destroying what is known to be a tumor of relatively potent immunogenicity. Often tumor growth occurs in spite of a demonstrable systemic host anti-tumor immune reaction. It is believed that local failure of inhibition of the immune response might permit the tumor to grow unchecked. Immunotherapy is based upon the premise that immunity towards a TAA may be augmented by adjuvant activity of a non-specific agent or by specific immunization. The major goal of immunotherapy is thus to potentiate the host response against his tumor, thus enabling the host to destroy the tumor.

We will not attempt to review all of the literature which has been forthcoming from immunotherapy studies in patients with melanoma. Several reviews of this subject have been written and the reader is referred to these for more in-depth discussion (3, 75, 84). Instead, we will provide an overview of the subject, discussing the theory behind the various protocols which have been employed and, when possible, reasons for success or failure of a particular immunotherapeutic regimen. At the outset, it should be noted that because immunotherapy is a very new therapeutic modality for melanoma, results obtained to date are largely inconclusive. Furthermore, the wide variation of protocols and status of the patients entered into these protocols makes comparison between results from different laboratories extremely difficult. Most of the immunotherapy regimens developed utilize one or more of three basic approaches: (1) nonspecific immunopotentiation using stimulants such as BCG, Corynebacterium parvum or vaccinia; (2) specific immunization with melanoma cells or extracts of melanoma cells; and (3) specific adoptive immunotherapy using sensitized lymphocytes, transfer factor, or immune RNA.

The original observation that bacterial toxins injected intratumor produced an antitumor inflammatory reaction was made at the turn of the century (18). Subsequently, BCG, an attenuated bovine tubercule bacillus, was found to have a similar effect in various animal tumor models (93, 128). BCG therapy for melanoma was first employed by Morton who found that subcutaneous lesions injected with BCG often underwent regression (87). Occasionally, distant noninjected lesions also regressed, suggesting that BCG was stimulating a systemic antitumor immune response. The use of BCG for immunotherapy of melanoma has become increasingly more popular following these early reports. The clinical experience with BCG thus far has paralleled that in experimental rodent tumors in that BCG has proven effective, in a large number of cases, in causing regression of limited amounts of tumor such as subcutaneous tumor nodules injected with BCG (44, 86, 106). Such findings suggest that contact between the BCG and melanoma TAA may be required for this anti-tumor effect to be manifested. In most instances, immunotherapy with BCG has not been of any significant benefit to patients with widely disseminated tumor or large tumor volumes. Although BCG and other such immunostimulants are generally thought to provide an adjuvant effect, thereby potentiating the immunogenicity of the TAA, recent work by Minden suggests that certain of the melanoma TAA are cross-reactive with antigens of the BCG (83). Such an antigenic relationship would certainly help to explain the finding that uninjected nodules will occasionally regress when distant nodules receive BCG. Whether or not this cross-reactivity alone causes all of the anti-tumor effects of BCG remains to be determined.

The use of BCG is not without complications. Patients receiving BCG often become febrile and/or nauseous and develop painful ulcers at the site of BCG administration. In addition, patients occasionally develop mycobacterial pneumonia or granulomatous hepatitis following BCG administration. Minden's findings of cross-reactive antigens between BCG and melanoma are significant as they indicate that it may be possible to isolate this antigen from the BCG and to use it for immunotherapy. As such, the patient would derive maximum benefit from the treatment while, hopefully, avoiding the complications associated with the use of whole BCG. Obviously, much more investigation in this area is required.

Ikonopisov (57) and Currie (22) demonstrated that melanoma patients immunized with autologous tumor cells showed a transient rise in the titer of serum-borne anti-melanoma antibody and in the ability of PBL from these patients to effect in vitro cytolysis of autologous melanoma target cells, respectively. From these results, it appeared as though melanoma patients could be immunized against their own tumors. Why this immunization was able to stimulate the host immune response while the growing tumor did not is not known, although local immunosuppressive effect of the tumor may have contributed to this failure. In view of these findings, several immunotherapy regimens have utilized immunization with autologous or allogeneic melanoma TAA either as whole cells or as cell extracts. The success of immunization with allogeneic melanoma obviously depends upon the existence of cell membrane TAA which are cross-reactive among the melanomas. BCG has often been mixed with these TAA inoculums in an effort to further increase their immunogenicity. Numerous studies in rodent tumor systems have revealed that tumor cells treated with neuraminidase are more immunogenic than untreated cells (2, 109). For this reason, melanoma cells have been pretreated with neuraminidase prior to their administration in some immunotherapy protocols (106, 107).

The ability of lymphocytes to respond in vitro against antigenically dissimilar cells in reactions such as the mixed lymphocyte culture is the basis for immunotherapy regimens which utilize adoptive transfer of sensitized lymphocytes. Briefly, peripheral blood lymphocytes are collected from a patient, exposed in vitro to autologous or allogeneic melanoma cells and then administered back to the patient. The theory is that these lymphocytes, once stimulated against melanoma TAA in vitro, will be more efficient antitumor effector cells in vivo. Because patient sera have often been found to contain blocking activity, the lymphocytes are usually incubated in vitro in medium containing normal human AB serum. Results from such studies have been variable. However, some benefit appears to be derived from this procedure when the patient PBL are sensitized against autologous tumor cells and his tumor volume is small (73, 107).

Because of recent results, interest in the use of "immune RNA" for immunotherapy has increased considerably. Mannick and Egdahl demonstrated that normal PBL could become sensitized to specific alloantigens by incubation in vitro with RNA extracted from lymphoid organs of animals immunized against those alloantigens (72). Ramming and Pilch subsequently observed a similar phenomenon when normal PBL were incubated with RNA extracted from lymphoid tissues of animals immune to certain tumors (100, 101). These in vitro sensitized PBL were specifically cytotoxic to tumor cells bearing the TAA to which they had been sensitized. Pilch and his co-workers extended this observation to human melanoma by demonstrating that normal human PBL became "killer cells" specifically reactive against human melanoma target cells following their in vitro incubation with "immune RNA" from sheep or guinea pigs immunized with human melanoma cells (98). RNA extracted from PBL of "cured" melanoma patients also converted normal human PBL into "killer cells" reactive against melanoma target cells. In a recent report, Brower described a case history of a patient with renal carcinoma who had been treated with sheep "immune RNA." Following therapy, PBL from this patient demonstrated an increased in vitro cytotoxic activity against target renal carcinoma cells (12). In view of these results, it is possible that immunotherapy of melanoma using immune RNA may prove an effective therapeutic modality.

Transfer factor was originally described by Lawrence as a dialysable factor, present in extracts of antigen-sensitized PBL, which had the ability to transfer antigen-specific systemic cell-mediated immunity to normal individuals (63). Its application for immunotherapy of melanoma has been limited, but results from preliminary studies have demonstrated a beneficial host response to this therapy in several cases (11, 62, 111, 115). Several features distinguish transfer factor from immune RNA, among them the facts that transfer factor is dialysable and species-specific, whereas immune RNA is non-dialysable and effective across species barriers. The initial results obtained using these substances in immunotherapy regimens clearly warrant further more extensive study.

From the above discussion, it is evident that, under certain conditions, immunotherapy may be of some benefit for the melanoma patient. The extent of dissemination of tumor and the tumor volume appear to be crucial factors which determine how successful immunotherapy will be. Best results have been obtained when patients have been free of visceral metastases and have had small tumor loads. As such, immunotherapy may prove to be of great benefit as a follow-up to surgery for localized tumor. Some current protocols have combined immunotherapy and chemotherapy to achieve the maximum anti-tumor effect (54). In view of the fact that certain of the anti-tumor agents are also immunosuppressive, the beneficial and potentially detrimental effects of such combined therapy must be carefully weighed.

Because of the specificity displayed in antigen antibody interactions, there has long been interest in using tumor-specific antibody to concentrate antitumor agents on tumor cells. In doing so, much lower concentrations of the drug would be effective and adverse side effects might be avoided. Such studies have usually proven unsuccessful, in most cases because the antibody lacked suitable specificity for TAA. One study was very successful, however, and deserves further comment. The globulin fraction of a goat-antihuman melanoma antiserum was conjugated with the alkylating agent, chlorambucil, and administered to a melanoma patient with disseminated tumor (39). Shortly after treatment, the tumor systemically regressed. Thus, although only limited success has been achieved using this approach, it might become a useful mode of therapy if antisera with greater specificity for melanoma cell membrane TAA can be produced.

VIII. FUTURE CONSIDERATIONS

The central problem which has emerged from our discussion of the immunology of melanoma is that we know relatively little about melanoma TAA, their biochemical nature and the host response against them. In stating that certain of the melanoma TAA appear to be fetal antigens, we have only said that they are transiently expressed normally during the gestational period. We have said nothing about the possible role or function of these antigens in the cell. One possibility which cannot be ignored is that TAA are merely normal host components which have been somehow modified such that the host's immune response recognizes them as foreign. The possible association between histocompatibility antigens and TAA is currently of great interest. One approach to solving this problem is to isolate the melanoma TAA for study apart from other molecular species. Studies in this area are currently underway in several laboratories.

Aside from their use in biochemical analyses, melanoma TAA may prove effective in immunotherapeutic and, perhaps, immunoprophylactic regimens. However, the major usefulness for isolated TAA appears to be for immunodiagnosis. Because soluble melanoma TAA are found in the serum and urine of melanoma patients, it should be possible to monitor the presence of these TAA by radioimmunoassay and thus to detect new or recurrent disease prior to its clinical manifestation. In addition, such an assay would be useful for evaluating the effectiveness of immunotherapy and chemotherapy. Finally, it should be possible to produce more highly specific anti-melanoma heteroantisera using isolated melanoma TAA.

One final area for future study is solid tumor diagnosis. Although diagnosis of melanoma is usually straightforward, occasional cases arise in which no primary lesion is located and regional nodal metastases are highly undifferentiated. In such cases, the pathologist, having little upon which to base his diagnosis, is forced to say only "undifferentiated carcinoma." Because current results in therapy of tumors suggest differential responsiveness of various histological types of tumor to different therapeutic agents, the need for an absolute diagnosis is crucial. In such cases, highly specific hetero-antisera might be useful for diagnosis. We have reported two such cases in which the tumor cells were lysed by our chimpanzee anti-melanoma antisera (117). The serological results correlated with histochemical analysis to provide a definitive diagnosis of melanoma.

REFERENCES

1. Avis, P., and Lewis, M. G. 1972. Tumor-associated fetal antigens in human tumors. *J. Natl. Cancer Inst.* 51: 1063–1066.

2. Bagshawe, K. D., and Currie, G. A. 1968. Immunogenicity of L1210 murine leukemia cells after treatment with neuraminidase. *Nature (London)* 218: 1245–1255.

3. Bast, R. C., Zbar, B., Borsos, T., and Rapp, H. 1974. BCG and cancer. *N. Engl. J. Med.* 290: 1413–1458.

4. Berkelhammer, J., Mastrangelo, M. J., Laucius, J. F., Bodurtha, A. J., and Prehn, R. T. 1975. Sequential *in vitro* reactivity of lymphocytes from melanoma patients receiving immunotherapy compared with the reactivity of lymphocytes from healthy donors. *Int. J. Cancer* 16: 571–578.

5. Birkmayer, G. D., Hammer, C., Eberhard, H. D., and Brendel, W. 1975. A tumor-specific antigen associated with reverse transcriptase. *Behr. Inst. Mitt.* 56: 107–115.

6. Bloom, E. T., Foley, J. L., Peterson, I. A., Geering, G., Bernhard, M., and Trempe, G. 1973. Anti-tumor activity in human serum: Antibodies detecting blood-group-A-like antigen on the surface of tumor cells. *Int. J. Cancer* 12: 21–31.

7. Bluming, A. Z., Vogel, C. L., Ziegler, J. L., and Kiryabwire, J. W. M. 1972. Delayed cutaneous sensitivity reactions to extracts of autologous malignant melanoma: A second look. *J. Natl. Cancer Inst.* 48: 17–24.

8. Boddie, A. W., Urist, M. M., Chee, D. O., Holmes, E. L., and Morton, D. L. 1976. Detection of human tumor associated antigens by the leukocyte migration in agarose assay. *Int. J. Cancer* 18: 161–167.

9. Bodurtha, A. J., Chee, D. O., Laucius, J. F., Mastrangelo, M. J., and Prehn, R. T. 1975. Clinical and immunological significance of human melanoma cytotoxic antibody. *Cancer Res.* 35: 189–193.

10. Bowen, J. M., McBride, C. M., Hersh, E. M., Miller, M. F., and Dmochowski, L. 1975. Nucleolar antigens in tumor cells of patients with malignant melanoma, in *Immunological Aspects of Neoplasia*, pp. 223–239. Williams and Wilkins, Baltimore.

11. Brandes, L. J., Galton, D. A. G., and Wiltshaw, E. A. 1971. A new approach to immunotherapy of melanoma. *Lancet* 2: 293–295.

12. Brower, P. A., DeKernion, J. B., and Ramming, K. P. 1976. Immune

cytolysis of human renal carcinoma mediated by xenogeneic immune ribonucleic acid. *J. Urol.* 115: 243–245.

13. Carrel, S., and Theilkaes, L. 1973. Evidence for a tumor-associated antigen in human malignant melanoma. *Nature* 242: 609–610.

14. Char, D., Hollinshead, A., Cogan, D. G., Ballintine, E. J., Hogan, M. J., and Herberman, R. B. 1974. Cutaneous delayed hypersensitivity reactions to soluble melanoma antigen in patients with ocular melanoma. *N. Engl. J. Med.* 291: 274–277.

15. Chee, D. O., Boddie, A. W., Roth, J. A., Holmes, E. C., and Morton, D. L. 1976. Production of melanoma-associated antigens by a defined malignant melanoma cell strain grown in chemically defined medium. *Cancer Res.* 36: 1503–1509.

16. Cochran, A. J., Jehn, U. W., and Gothoskar, B. 1972. Cell mediated immunity in malignant melanoma. *Lancet* 1: 1340–1341.

17. Cochran, A. J., Mackie, R. M., Thomas, C. E., Grant, R. M., Cameron-Mowat, D. E., and Spilg, W. G. S. 1973. Cellular immunity to breast carcionoma and malignant melanoma. *Brit. J. Cancer* 28. Suppl 1: 77–81.

18. Coley, W. B. 1925. Some clinical evidence in favor of the extrinsic origin of cancer. *Surg. Gynecol. Obst.* 59: 353.

19. Cooper, H. L. 1970. Lymphocyte stimulation in malignant melanoma. *N. Engl. J. Med.* 283: 369–370.

20. Copeman, P. W. M., Lewis, M. G., Phillips, T. M., and Elliott, P. G. 1973. Immunological associations of the halo nevus with cutaneous malignant melanoma. *Brit. J. Derm.* 88: 127.

21. Currie, G. A. 1973. Effect of active immunization with irradiated tumor cells on specific serum inhibitors of cell-mediated immunity in patients with disseminated cancer. *Brit. J. Cancer* 28: 25–35.

22. Currie, G. A., Lejeune, F., and Hamilton-Fairley, G. 1971. Immunization with irradiated tumour cells and specific lymphocyte cytotoxicity in malignant melanoma. *Brit. Med. J.* 2: 305–310.

23. Dalton, A. J., and Felix, M. D. 1956. The electron microscopy of normal and malignant cells. *Ann. N.Y. Acad. Sci.* 63: 1117–1140.

24. DasGupta, T., Dowden, L., and Berg, T. W. 1963. Malignant melanoma of unknown primary origin. *Surg. Gynec. Obst.* 117: 341.

25. Dent, P. B., Liau, K. K., McCulloch, P. G., and MacNamara, J. 1976. Melanoma antigens on cultured melanoma cell lines detected by xeno- and allo-antibody. *Proc. Amer. Assoc. Cancer Res.* 17: 311.

26. deVries, J. E., Cornain, S., and Rumke, P. H. 1974. Cytotoxicity of non-T versus a T-lymphocyte from melanoma patients and healthy donors on short and long-term cultured melanoma cells. *Int. J. Cancer* 14: 427–434.

27. deVries, J. E., Cornain, S., and Rumke, P. H. 1975. Humoral and cellular immunity in melanoma patients. *Behr. Inst. Mitt.* 56: 148–156.

28. deVries, J. E., Rumke, P. H., and Bernheim, J. L. 1972. Cytotoxic lymphocytes in melanoma patients. *Int. J. Cancer* 9: 567–576.

29. Eberman, A. A. 1896. Beitrag zur Casiustik der melanotischen Geschwulste. *Dtsch. Z. Chir.* 11: 498.

30. Elliott, P. G., Thurlow, B., Needham, P. R. G., and Lewis, M. G. 1973. The specificity of the cytoplasmic antigen in human malignant melanoma. *Eur. J. Cancer* 9: 607–610.

31. Embleton, M. J., and Price, M. R. 1975. Inhibition of *in vitro* lymphocytotoxic reactions against tumor cells by melanoma membrane extracts. *Behr. Inst. Mitt.* 56: 157–160.

32. Epstein, W. L., Fukuyama, K., Benn, M., Keston, A. S., and Brandt, R. B. 1971. Transmission of a pigmented melanoma in golden hamsters by cell-free ultrafiltrate. *Nature* 219: 979–980.

33. Fass, L., Ziegler, J. L., Herberman, R. B., and Kiryabwire, J. W. M. 1970. Cutaneous hypersensitivity reactions to autologous extracts of malignant melanoma cells. *Lancet* 1: 116–118.

34. Fine, R. N., Batchelor, J. R., French, M. E., and Shumak, K. H. 1973. The uptake of ^{125}I-labeled rat alloantibody and its loss after combination with antigen. *Transplantation* 16: 641–648.

35. Fossati, G., Colnaghi, M. I., Della Porta, G., Cascinelli, N., and Veronesi, U. 1971. Cellular and humoral immunity against human malignant melanoma. *Int. J. Cancer* 8: 344–350.

36. Fritsche, R., and Mach, J. P. 1975. Identification of a new oncofetal antigen associated with several types of human carcinomas. *Nature* 258: 734–737.

37. Fritze, D., Kern, D. H., Drogemuller, C. R., and Pilch, Y. H. 1976. Production of antisera with specificity for malignant melanoma and human fetal skin. *Cancer Res.* 36: 458–466.

38. Fritze, D., Kern, D. H., and Pilch, Y. H. 1975. Serologic evidence for cross-reacting tumor associated antigens in two chemically induced murine sarcomas and in human malignant melanoma. *Behr. Inst. Mitt.* 56: 90–97.

39. Ghose, T., Norvell, S. T., Guclu, A., Cameron, D., Bodurtha, A., and MacDonald, A. S. 1972. Immunotherapy of cancer with chlorambucil-carring antibody. *Brit. Med. J.* 3: 495–499.

40. Goodwin, D. P., Hornung, M. O., Leong, S. P. L., and Krementz, E. T. 1972. Immune responses induced by human malignant melanoma in the rabbit. *Surgery* 72: 737–743.

41. Gray, B. K., Mehigan, J. T., and Morton, D. L. 1971. Demonstration of antibody in melanoma patients cytotoxic to human melanoma cells. *Proc. Amer. Assoc. Cancer Res.* 12: 79.

42. Grimm, E. A., Silver, H. K. B., Roth, J. H., Chee, D. O., Gupta, R. K., and Morton, D. L. 1976. Detection of tumor-associated antigen in human melanoma cell line supernatants. *Int. J. Cancer* 17: 559–564.

43. Gupta, R., and Morton, D. L. 1975. Suggestive evidence for *in vivo* binding of specific antitumor antibodies of human melanoma. *Cancer Res.* 35: 58–62.

44. Gutterman, J. V., Mavligit, G. M., Reed, R. C., Burgess, M. A., McBride, C. M., and Hersh, E. M. 1975. Adjuvant immunotherapy with BCG for recurrent malignant melanoma. *Behr. Inst. Mitt.* 56: 199–206.

45. Gutterman, J. V., Mavligit, G. M., Gottlieb, J., Burgess, M. A., McBride, C. M., Einhorn, L., Freireich, E. J., and Hersh, E. M. 1975. Chemoimmunotherapy of disseminated melanoma with dimethyl triazo imadizole carboximide (DTIC) and bacillus Calmette-Guérin (BCG). *Behr. Inst. Mitt.* 56: 235–250.

46. Halliday, W. J., Maluish, A. E., Little, J. H., and Davis, N. C. 1975. Leukocyte adherence inhibition and specific immunoreactivity on malignant melanoma. *Int. J. Cancer* 16: 645–658.

47. Handley, W. S. 1907. The pathology of melanocytic growths *Lancet* 1: 927.

48. Hellström, I., Hellström, K. E., Sjögren, H. O., and Warner, G. A. 1971. Demonstration of cell-mediated immunity of human neoplasms of various histological types. *Int. J. Cancer* 7: 1–16.

49. Hellström, I., Hellström, K. E., Sjögren, H. O., and Warner, G. A. 1973. Destruction of cultivated melanoma cells by lymphocytes from healthy black (North American Negro) donors. *Int. J. Cancer* 11: 116–122.

50. Hellström, I., Warner, G. A., Hellström, K. E., and Sjögren, H. O. 1973. Sequential studies on cell-mediated tumor immunity and blocking serum activity in ten patients with malignant melanoma. *Int. J. Cancer* 11: 280–292.

51. Heppner, G. H., Stolbach, H., Byrne, M., Cummings, F. J., McDonough, E., and Calabresi, P. 1973. Cell-mediated and serum blocking reactivity to tumor antigens in patients with malignant melanoma. *Int. J. Cancer* 11: 245–260.

52. Heppner, G., Stolbach, H. L., Cummings, F., McDonough, E., and Calabresi, P. 1975. Problems in the clinical use of the microcytotoxicity assay for measuring cell-mediated immunity to tumor cells. *Cancer Res.* 35: 1931–1937.

53. Herberman, R. B., Hollingshead, A., Char, D. J., Oldham, R., McCoy, J., and Cohen, J. 1975. In vivo and in vitro studies of cell-mediated immune response to antigens associated with malignant melanoma. *Behr. Inst. Mitt.* 56: 131–138.

54. Hersh, E. M., Gutterman, J. V., Mavligit, G. M., Granatek, C. H., Reed, R. C., Ambus, V., and McBride, C. 1975. Approaches to the study of tumor antigens and tumor immunity in malignant melanoma. *Behr. Inst. Mitt.* 56: 139–147.

55. Hollinshead, A. C., Herberman, R. B., Jaffurs, W. J., Alpers, L. K., Minton, J. P., and Harris, J. E. 1974. Soluble membrane antigens of human malignant melanoma. *Cancer* 34: 1235–1243.

56. Hughes, L. E., and Lytton, B. 1964. Antigenic properties of human tumors: Delayed cutaneous hypersensitivity reactions. *Brit. Med. J.* 1: 209–212.

57. Ikonopisov, R. L., Lewis, M. G., Hunter-Craig, I. O., Bodenham, D. C., Phillips, T. M., Cooling, C. I., Proctor, J., Fairley, H. G., and Alexander, P. 1970. Autoimmunization with irradiated tumor cells in human malignant melanoma. *Brit. J. Med.* 2: 752–754.

58. Irie, K., Irie, R. F., and Morton, D. L. 1975. Detection of antibody and complement-complexed *in vivo* on membranes of human cancer cells by mixed hemadsorption techniques. *Cancer Res.* 35: 1244–1248.

59. Ito, R., and Mishima, Y. 1967. Particles in the cisternae of the endoplasmic reticulum of Fortner's amelanotic and melanotic melanomas. *J. Invest. Derm.* 48: 268–272.

60. Jehn, U. W., Nathanson, L., Schwartz, R. S., and Skinner, M. 1970. In vitro lymphocyte stimulation by a soluble antigen from malignant melanoma. *N. Engl. J. Med.* 283: 329–333.

61. Kodera, Y., and Bean, M. A. 1975. Antibody-dependent cell-mediated cytotoxicity for human monolayer target cells bearing blood group and transplantation antigens and for melanoma cells. *Int. J. Cancer* 16: 579–592.

62. Krementz, E. T., Mansell, P. W. A., Hornum, M. O., Samuel, M. S., Sutherland, C. A., and Benes, E. N. 1974. Immunotherapy of malignant disease: The use of viable transfer factor prepared from sensitized lymphocytes. *Cancer* 33: 394–401.

63. Lawrence, H. S. 1954. The transfer of delayed skin sensitivity to streptococcal or substance and to tuberculin with disrupted leukocytes. *J. Clin. Invest.* 34: 219–230.

64. Levy, N. L. 1976. Functional subfractionation of human melanoma antigens. *Proc. Am. Assoc. Cancer Res.* 17: 86.

65. Lewis, M. G. 1967. Possible immunological factors in human malignant melanoma in Uganda. *Lancet* 2: 921–922.

66. Lewis, M. G., Ikonopisov, R. L., Nairn, R. C., Phillips, T. M., Hamilton-Fairley, G., Bodenham, D. C., and Alexander, P. 1969. Tumour-specific antibodies in human malignant melanoma and their relationship to the extent of the disease. *Brit. Med. J.* 3: 547–552.

67. Lewis, M. G., and Phillips, T. M. 1972a. The specificity of surface membrane immunofluorescence in human malignant melanoma. *Int. J. Cancer* 10: 105–111.

68. Lewis, M. G., and Phillips, T. M. 1972b. Separation of two distinct tumor-associated antibodies in the serum of melanoma patients. *J. Natl. Cancer Inst.* 49: 915–917.

69. Lewis, M. G., and Sheikh, M. A. 1975. Evidence for tumor specific antigen in human malignant melanoma. *Behr. Inst. Mitt.* 56: 78–82.

70. Macher, E., Muller, C. H. R., Sorg, G., Gossen, A., and Sorg, C. 1975. Evidence for cross-reacting membrane associated specific melanoma antigens as detected by immunofluorescence and immune adherence. *Behr. Inst. Mitt.* 56: 86–90.

71. Mackie, R. M., Spilg, W. G. S., Thomas, C. E., and Cochran, A. J. 1972. Immunity in patients with malignant melanoma. *Brit. J. Derm.* 87: 523–528.

72. Mannick, J. A., and Egdahl, R. H. 1964. Transfer of heightened immunity to skin homografts by lymphoid RNA. *J. Clin. Invest.* 43: 2166.

73. Mansell, P. W. A., Kremwentz, E. T., and Deluzio, N. R. 1975. Clinical experiences with immunotherapy of melanoma. *Behr. Inst. Mitt.* 56: 256–262.

74. Martin, E. W., Kibbey, W. E., DeVecchia, L., Anderson, G., Catalano, P., and Minton, J. P. 1976. Carcinoembryonic antigen: Clinical and historical aspects. *Cancer* 37: 62–81.

75. Mastrangelo, M. J., Bellet, R. E., Laucius, J. F., and Berkelhammer, J. 1976. Immunotherapy of malignant melanoma: A review, in P. F. Engstrom and A. I. Sutnick (eds.), *Recent Developments in Medical Oncology.* University Park Press, Baltimore.

76. Mavligit, G. M., Hersh, E. M., and McBride, C. M. 1974. Lymphocyte blastogenesis induced by autochthonous human solid tumor cells: Relationship to stage of disease and serum factors. *Cancer* 34: 1712–1721.

77. Mazuran, R., Mujagic, H., Malenica, B., and Silobrcic, V. 1976. In vitro detection of cellular immunity to melanoma antigens in man by the monocyte spreading inhibition test. *Int. J. Cancer* 17: 14–20.

78. McBride, C. M., Bowen, J. M., and Dmochowski, L. 1972. Anti-nucleolar

antibodies in sera from patients with malignant melanoma. *Surg. Forum* 23: 92–93.

79. McCoy, J. L., Jerome, L. F., Dean, J. H., Perlin, E., Oldham, R. K., Char, D. H., Cohen, M. H., Felix, E. L., and Herbermann, R. B. 1975. Inhibition of leukocyte migration by tumor associated antigens in soluble extracts of human melanoma. *J. Natl. Cancer Inst.* 55: 19–23.

80. Metzgar, R. S., Bergoc, P. M., Moreno, M. A., and Seigler, H. F. 1973. Melanoma specific antibodies produced in monkeys by immunization with human melanoma cell lines. *J. Natl. Cancer Inst.* 50: 1065–1068.

82. Mihalev, A., Tzingilev, D., and Sirakov, L. M. 1976. Radioimmunoassay of alpha-fetoprotein in the serum of patients with leukemia and malignant melanoma. *Neoplasma* 23: 103–107.

83. Minden, P., Sharpton, T. R., and McClatchy, J. K. 1976. Shared antigens between human malignant melanoma cells and mycobacterium bovis (BCG). *J. Immunol.* 116: 1407–1414.

84. Morton, D. L. 1974. Cancer immunotherapy: An overview. *Seminars Oncology* 1: 297–310.

85. Morton, D. L., Malmgren, R. A., Holmes, E. C., and Ketcham, A. S. 1968. Demonstration of antibodies against human malignant melanoma by immunofluorescence. *Surgery* 68: 158–240.

86. Morton, D. L., Eilber, R. F., Holmes, E. C., Hunt, S. S., Ketcham, A. S., Silverstein, M. J., and Sparks, F. C. 1974. BCG immunotherapy of malignant melanoma: Summary of a seven year experience. *Ann. Surgery* 180: 635–643.

87. Morton, D. L., Eilber, F. R., Malmgren, R. A., and Wood, W. C. 1970. Immunological factors which influence response to immunotherapy in malignant melanoma. *Surgery* 68: 158–164.

88. Muna, N., Marcus, S., and Smart, C. 1969. Detection by immunofluorescence of antibodies specific for human malignant melanoma cells. *Cancer* 34: 1712–1721.

89. Myburgh, J. A., and Smit, J. A. 1975. Prolongation of liver allograft survival by donor-specific soluble transplantation antigens and antigen-antibody complexes. *Transplantation* 19: 64–71.

90. Nagel, G. A., Piessens, W. F., Stilmont, M. M., and Lejeune, F. 1971. Evidence for tumor-specific immunity in human malignant melanoma. *Eur. J. Cancer* 7: 41–47.

91. Nairn, R. C., Nind, A. P. P., Guli, be. p. g., davies, D. J., Little, J. H., Davis, N. C., and Whitehead, R. H. 1972. Anti-tumor immunoreactivity in patients with malignant melanoma. *Med. J. Australia,* 1: 397–403.

92. Oettgen, H. F., Aoki, T., Old, L. J., Boyse, E. A., DeHarven, E., and Mills, G. M. 1968. Suspension culture of a pigment-producing cell line derives from a human malignant melanoma. *J. Natl. Cancer Inst.* 41: 827–831.

93. Old, L. J., Bennaceraf, B., Clarke, D. A., and Carswell, E. A. 1961. The role of the reticuloendothelial system in the host response to neoplasia. *Cancer Res.* 21: 1281–1300.

94. Oren, M. E., and Herberman, R. B. 1971. Delayed cutaneous hypersensitivity reactions to membrane extracts of human tumor cells. *Chem. Exp. Immunol.* 9: 45–56.

95. Parsons, P. G., Goss, P., and Pope, J. H. 1974. Detection in human melanoma cell lines of particles with some properties in common with RNA tumor viruses. *Int. J. Cancer* 13: 606–618.

96. Pavie-Fischer, J., Kourilsky, F. M., Banzet, P., Puissant, A., and Levy, J. P. 1975. Investigation of cell-mediated immune reactions in malignant melanoma using the chromium release test. *Behr. Inst. Mitt.* 56: 160–167.

97. Peter, H. H., Diehl, V., Kalden, J. R., Seeland, P., and Eckert, G. 1975. Humoral and cellular cytotoxicity *in vitro* against allogeneic and autologous human melanoma cells. *Behr. Inst. Mitt.* 56: 167–177.

98. Pilch, Y. H., Fritze, D., and Kern, D. H. 1975. Immune cytolysis of human melanoma cells mediated by immune RNA. *Behr. Inst. Mitt.* 56: 184–196.

99. Prehn, R. T., and Main, J. M. 1957. Immunity to methyl-cholanthrene-induced sarcomas. *J. Natl. Cancer Inst.* 18: 769–778.

100. Ramming, K. P., and Pilch, Y. H. 1970. Mediation of immunity to tumor isographs in mice by heterologous ribonucleic acid. *Science* 168: 492–492.

101. Ramming, K. P., and Pilch, Y. H. 1976. Transfer of tumor specific immunity with RNA. Demonstration of immune cytolysis of tumor cells *in vitro*. *J. Natl. Cancer Inst.* 45: 543–553.

102. Reid, T., and Albert, D. M. 1972. RNA-dependent DNA polymerase activity in human tumors. *Biochem. Biophys. Res. Comm.* 46: 383–390.

103. Romsdahl, S. A., and Cox, I. S. 1970. Human malignant melanoma antibodies demonstrated by immunofluorescence. *Arch. Surgery* 100: 491.

104. Roth, J. A., Holmes, E. C., Reisfeld, R. A., Slocum, H. K., and Morton, D. L. 1976. Isolation of a soluble tumor associated antigen from human melanoma. *Cancer* 37: 104–110.

105. Segall, A., Weiler, O., Genin, J., Lacour, J., and Lacour, F. 1972. *In vitro* study of cellular immunity against autochthonous human cancer. *Int. J. Cancer* 9: 417–425.

106. Seigler, H. F., Shingleton, W. W., Metzgar, R. S., Buckley, C. E., and Bergoc, P. M. 1973. Immunotherapy in patients with melanoma. *Ann. Surgery* 178: 352–359.

107. Seigler, H. F., Shingleton, W. W., Metzgar, R. S., Bergoc, P. M., Miller, D. S., Fetter, B. F., and Phaup, M. B. 1972. Non-specific and specific immunotherapy in patients with malignant melanoma *Surgery* 72: 162–174.

108. Silagi, S., Beju, D., Wrathall, J., and Deharven, E. 1972. Tumorgenicity immunogenicity and virus production in mouse melanoma cells treated with 5-bromodeoxyuridine. *Proc. Natl. Acad. Sci.* 69: 3443–3447.

109. Simmons, R. I., and Rios, A. 1971. Combined use of BCG and neuraminidase in experimental tumor immunotherapy. *Surg. Forum* 22: 99.

110. Sjögren, H. O., Hellström, I., Bansal, S. C., and Hellström, K. E. 1971. Suggestive evidence that the "blocking antibodies" of tumor bearing individuals may be antigen-antibody complexes. *Proc. Natl. Acad. Sci.* 68: 1372–1375.

111. Smith, G. V., Mores, P. A., Deraps, G. D., Raju, S., and Hardy, J. D. 1973. *Immunotherapy of patients with cancer. Surgery* 74: 59–68.

112. Smith, J. L., and Stehlin, J. S. 1965. Spontaneous regression of primary malignant melanoma with regional metastases. *Cancer* 18: 1399–1415.

113. Smithers, D. W. 1967. Spontaneous regression of cancer. *Ann. Royal College Surg. England* 41: 160–162.

114. Snyderman, R., Seigler, H. F., and Meadows, L. 1976. Abnormalities of monocyte chemotaxis in patients with melanoma: Effects of immunotherapy and tumor removal. *J.N.C.I.* (in press).

115. Spittler, L. E. 1973. Cellular immunity to melanoma antigens in malignant melanoma. *Clinical Res.* 21: 654.

116. Stewart, T. H. M. 1969. The presence of delayed hypersensitivity reactions in patients toward cellular extracts of their malignant tumors. I. The role of tissue antigen, non-specific reactions of nuclear material and bacterial antigen as a cause for this phenomenon. *Cancer* 23: 1368–1379.

117. Stuhlmiller, G. M., Boylston, J. A., Seigler, H. F., and Fetter, B. F. 1976. Immunodiagnosis of melanoma using chimpanzee anti-human melanoma antiserum. *Amer. J. Clin. Path.* (in press).

118. Stuhlmiller, G. M., and Seigler, H. F. 1975. Characterization of a chimpanzee anti-human melanoma antiserum. *Cancer Res.* 35: 2132–2137.

119. Stuhlmiller, G. M., and Seigler, H. F. 1976. Enzymatic susceptibility and spontaneous release of human melanoma associated antigens. *J. Natl. Cancer Inst.* (in press).

120. Summer, W. C., and Foraker, A. G. 1960. Spontaneous regression of human melanoma—clinical and experimental studies. *Cancer* 13: 79–81.

121. Takasugi, M., Mickey, M., and Teraski, P. I. 1973. Reactivity of lymphocytes from normal persons on cultured tumor cells. *Cancer Res.* 33: 2898–2901.

122. Takasugi, M., Mickey, M., and Terasaki, P. I. 1974. Studies on Specificity of Cell-Mediated Immunity to Human Tumors. *J.N.C.I.* 53: 1527–1538.

123. Todd, D. W., Spencer-Payne, W., Farrow, G. M., and Winklemann, R. K. 1966. Spontaneous regression of primary malignant melanoma with regional metastases: Report of a case and photographic documentation. *Proc. Mayo Clin.* 41: 10–17.

124. Viza, D., and Phillips, J. 1971. Extraction and solubilization of cell surface antigens from malignant melanomas. *Rev. Instit. Pasteur Lyon* 4: 339–342.

125. Viza, D., and Phillips, J. 1975. Identification of an antigen associated with malignant melanoma. *Int. J. Cancer* 16: 312–317.

126. Viza, D., Phillips, J., and Bourgoin, J. J. 1973. Detection of specific antigens in the serum of melanoma patients. *Rev. Instit. Pasteur Lyon* 6: 321–324.

127. Wood, G. W., and Barth, R. F. 1974. Immunofluorescent studies of the serologic reactivity of patients with malignant melanoma against tumor-associated cytoplasmic antigens. *J.N.C.I.* 53: 309–316.

128. Zbar, B., and Tanaka, T. 1971. Immunotherapy of cancer—regression of tumors after intralesional injection of living microbacterium bovus. *Science* 172: 271–273.

CHAPTER 12

IMMUNOBIOLOGY OF INTRACRANIAL TUMORS

William H. Brooks
Thomas L. Roszman

Neurosurgical Service
Veterans Administration Hospital
Division of Experimental Pathology
Department of Pathology
and College of Medicine
University of Kentucky
Lexington, Kentucky 40506

Three basic conclusions can be drawn from this review. First, although primary neoplastic processes occurring within the central nervous system may not be freely accessible to the host's immunologic effectors, i.e., a "privileged" site, studies indicate that cellular and humoral cytotoxic responses are detectable in the peripheral blood of patients with brain tumors. The specificity of these responses, however, is not clear. Secondly, the general immunologic response of these patients is not normal. Cutaneous delayed-type hypersensitivity, antibody titers, and in vitro correlates of cell-mediated immunity are broadly depressed. The interactions of the central nervous system with the immune response accounting for these observations also remains to be elucidated. Thirdly, clinical trials have clearly shown that immunotherapy, as currently utilized, is not advantageous in the treatment of brain tumors.

Introduction

The immunologic features of most neoplasms have been extensively studied with perhaps the exception of primary tumors arising within the brain. Unique features of the central nervous system (CNS) and autochthonous malignant tumors have been the major obstacles to sustained and productive investigations of the immunobiology of brain tumors. First, the brain has been considered to be an "immunologically privileged site" (15, 16, 23) with a blood-brain barrier and absence of lymphatic channels. Second, neoplasia of the brain represents a small percentage (3–5%) of all solid tumors occurring in human beings. Finally, the mean survival time of patients with malignant tumors is very short, therefore precluding long-term follow-up studies. Nevertheless, observations have been made which suggest the presence of humoral and cell-mediated immunologic responses against malignant brain tumors. This chapter is a review of these findings and of current concepts regarding the relationship between the immune response and malignant primary intracranial tumors.

The Brain as an Immunologically Privileged Site

Medawar (23) demonstrated that the brain does not reject allogenic skin implanted in the cerebrum and thus may be considered a "privileged site" hidden from the immune response. This implies that the afferent arc of the immune response is blocked and would indicate that neoplasias arising in the brain are protected from any type of immune surveillance mechanism. This concept of "immunologic privilege" has been recently reexamined by Scheinberg and co-workers (28–31). In a series of experiments they demonstrated that (a) a methylcholanthrene-induced ependymoblastoma obtained from a C57BL/6J mouse could be successfully transplanted intracerebrally 100% of the time into other C57BL/J6 mice, but only 10–35% of the time into allogenic mice; (b) transplantation of the ependymoblastoma into the brains of syngeneic mice which were then cured by irradiation resulted in rejection of subsequent tumor implants into either the brain or skin; similarly, subcutaneous transplantation of the tumor into syngeneic mice followed by irradiation cure rendered a significant number of animals refractory to subsequent intracerebral or subcutaneous tumor implants; and (c) prior immunization of the mice with ependymoblastoma cells incorporated in complete Freund's adjuvant resulted in inhibition of growth in 85% of subsequent tumor implants. Others have confirmed these results (9, 19, 27).

Thus, the original concept of "immunologic privilege" has been altered to "partial privilege," explaining the retarded and incomplete rejection of tumors and allografts by the CNS. The fact that malignant tumors spontaneously arising within human brain can revoke an immune response, further indicates that the CNS is not immunologically privileged. However, it is quite possible that the normally intact and impermable blood-brain-barrier is broken by tumor implantation or neoplastic changes. Loss of this barrier may result in loss of "privilege" by allowing exit of tumor antigens and/or entrance of immunologic effectors.

Organ- and Tumor-Specific Antigens

There have been numerous studies attempting to characterize the antigenic properties of brain tumors and normal brain. One of the first studies concerned with immunologic specificity of brain tumors was performed by Siris (33). He demonstrated that glioblastoma multiforme and normal brain share antigens which were not found in other tissues. More recent studies (42, 44) also indicate that there is an antigenic relationship between human fetal and adult brain, rabbit brain and human malignant gliomas. In these studies rabbits were immunized with an homogenate of normal human brain and the sera collected at the time when the rabbits were experiencing symptoms of experimental autoimmune encephalitis (EAE). This antibrain sera, after absorption with homogenates from non-CNS tissue, reacted only with the glial specific membrane antigens (malignant and normal brain tissue) as evidenced by direct immunofluorescent experiments. These studies indicate that malignant brain tumors do not possess tumor specific antigens.

To the contrary, other investigators have reported that tumor associated antigens can be demonstrated on human astrocytomas (7, 8). In these experiments antiserum to a human astrocytoma cell line was cytotoxic only for these brain tumors and not non-CNS tumors. Moreover, when this antiserum was absorbed with either human adult or fetal brain it did not lose its cytotoxicity, suggesting that this antibody was directed against specific tumor associated astrocytoma antigens and not against brain organ specific or oncofetal brain antigens. It should be pointed out that these antibodies were produced by intravenous injection of whole tumor cells while in most other studies of this type the antigen is injected along with complete Freund's adjuvant. Similar results have been reported for a rat astrocytoma (21). Antibodies to this tumor reacted only to soluble, membrane derived astrocytoma antigens and not to antigens from rat liver or brain.

It is evident that the question of whether tumor specific antigens are present on malignant brain tumors is as controversial as it is with most other malignant tumors. Unique to investigation of CNS tumors is the fact that an autoimmune response can be elicited to the organ-specific brain antigens. Further progress in this area is in part dependent on establishing a reliable animal model which is an accurate reflection of the human situation.

Humoral Immune Response to Brain Tumors

Brain tumor patients have antibodies which can react with either their autologous tumors or allogenic tumors. Various immunologic procedures such as cytotoxicity, immunodiffusion and immunofluorescence have been employed to detect these antibodies using either whole cells or cellular fractions. Kornblith and co-workers (17, 26) used a microcytotoxicity assay to examine the serum from 26 patients with astrocytomas and found that sera from 17 of these patients produced significant cytotoxicity against an established human astrocytoma cell line. In addition, the astrocytoma patients sera was cytotoxic for other allogeneic astrocytoma cell lines indicating the reactivity of the antibodies was not directed against HLA antigens. Employing a microimmunodiffusion assay, Winter and Rich (45) used soluble antigens from human meningiomas to screen brain tumor patients sera for antibodies. The antigen preparation not only reacted with sera from 63% of meningioma patients but 53% of glioma patients and 17% of patients with various other types of brain tumors. More importantly, only 6% of the sera from normal patients reacted with these antigens. It is of interest that in the study of Kornblith et al. (17), none of the 4 sera from meningioma patients reacted in the microcytotoxicity assay with the astrocytoma cells. This may in part be due to the small number of patient sera tested, the difference in assay techniques or the nature of the antigens. Winters and Rich (45) were able, based on immunodiffusion patterns, to determine that at least 3 different antigens were present in the homogenates. Antigen A reacted with sera from meningioma patients, antigen B reacted with glioma sera, and antigen C with sera from patients with nonneural tumors. These findings are similar to those obtained by others employing an immunofluorescence assay to detect antibodies in meningioma and glioma patients' sera (6, 10).

In contrast to these in vitro observations, it has been demonstrated by immunoperoxidase techniques that in vivo antibody is present on the surface of membranes of human glioblastomas (35). Studies that utilize antisera to detect "cytotoxic" or "blocking" antibodies on tumor cells must be critically reviewed because human IgG can bind nonspecifically via the Fc fragment to myelin, glia cells, and neurons (1). This difficulty can be overcome by the use of (Fab ')₂ reagents.

The reports that antibodies react with histologically similar brain tumors from different individuals suggest that these tumors may be virally induced. It must be rigorously proven, however, that these antibodies have specificity for tumor specific and not organ specific antigens. Moreover, further characterization of these antibodies is required with regards to the immunoglobulin class and quantity present in the blood.

Cell-Mediated Immune Response to Brain Tumors

Various investigations (3, 4, 14) have demonstrated that brain tumor patients have cell-mediated immunity to autochthonous—and, in many instances, to allogenic—brain tumors—as well. Thus, in vitro studies have shown that patients with primary intracranial tumors have peripheral blood lymphocytes which have specific cytotoxicity against autologous and allogenic tumor cells (20). Similar findings were reported by Kumar et al. (18). However, it is important to emphasize that peripheral blood lymphocytes from patients with malignant gliomas have been found to be cytotoxic to cultured autologous tumor cells as well as to adult and fetal glial cells (43). Moreover, it has been demonstrated that 2 soluble antigens isolated from normal human brain extracts could stimulate lymphocytes from 9 out of 14 malignant glioma patients to undergo blastogenesis (41). Interestingly, both of these antigens could induce EAE when they were incorporated in complete Freund's adjuvant and injected into guinea pigs. These results indicate that antigens from malignant brain tumors may gain entrance into the general circulatory vasculature resulting in the sensitization of lymphocytes to organ specific glial antigens. Glioma cells have in fact been reported in the peripheral blood of brain tumor patients (24). The rarity of malignant brain tumor metastases may be a consequence of an efficient immune response directed against organ specific antigens.

Impaired General Cell-Mediated Immunity

Impairment of cell-mediated immunity is a general consequence of malignancy particularly in those patients with wide-spread metastases (11). Patients with malignant brain tumors have been shown to have impaired cutaneous reactivity to ubiquitous antigens such as tuberculin, candida, trichophyon, mumps, and streptokinase (3, 4, 22). In addition, they exhibit a reduced ability to become sensitized to dinitrochloroben-zene (3, 4) and keyhole limpet hemocyanin (unpublished data). Using in vitro correlates of cell-mediated immunity such as lymphocyte reactivity to mitogens and mixed lymphocyte cultures it has been found that brain tumor patient lymphocytes are much less responsive than normal lym-phocytes (3, 4, 38, 46). In part, this anergy may be a result of serum blocking factor(s) present in the sera of patients with malignant gliomas. However, Wahlstrom (41) did not find any difference in the in vitro re-sponse of lymphocytes from patients with astrocytomas and epen-dymonas to purified protein derivative when cultured in either autolog-ous serum or normal control sera.

While the role of serum blocking factors remains to be clarified, other explanations for the impaired cell-mediated immunity detected in pa-tients with malignant brain tumors must be sought. Mahaley et al. (22) have demonstrated that patients with malignant brain tumors have de-pression of their peripheral blood lymphocyte counts which continues throughout the course of the disease. We have compared the percentage of thymus-dependent cells (T cells) in the peripheral blood of patients with malignant brain tumors to those values obtained from normal individuals and patients with nonmalignant CNS disease (5). Brain tumor patients had significantly fewer T cells than did the control groups. Furthermore, those patients who were unresponsive to DNCB had fewer T cells than did those patients which did react to DNCB indicating a correlation between depressed cell-mediated and reduced numbers of T cells. We are currently determining the percentages of T cells, bone marrow-derived lympho-cytes (B cells), complement receptor lymphocytes (CRL), and Fc-receptor lymphocytes (FcR) in the peripheral blood of patients with malignant brain tumors. The results confirm the finding that brain tumor patients have diminished numbers of T cells but in addition indicate that they have elevated numbers of CRL (unpublished data). The B cell and FcR populations remain unaltered.

Investigations into other aspects of the immune response of patients with malignant brain tumors are needed. The observed depression in cell-mediated immunity in these patients may be the result of increased numbers of more efficient suppressor cells (12). New techniques are be-coming available to study the suppressor cells in the peripheral blood of human subjects which can be applied to cancer patients (32). The role of the macrophage in patients with malignant brain tumors needs to be established. It is clear that in certain malignancies the function of the macrophage is depressed (34).

Impaired Humoral Immunity

There is not much information on the status of the humoral response in patients with malignant brain tumors. This is also true for other types of malignancies and probably results from the concept that cell-mediated immunity is far more important. Mahaley et al. (22) studied the serum tetanus and influenza antibody titers of patients with glioblastomas. Although the antibody titers rose after initial postoperative booster injection, subsequent sequential injections failed to boost antibody levels. A progressive decline in responsiveness was detected in most patients despite repeated bi-monthly boosting and tended to parallel clinical deterioration. The quantitative immunoglobulin levels were within normal ranges for all patients with the exception of higher mean preoperative levels of bigM in patients with glioblastoma. The IgM levels remained elevated for 2 months but declined progressively thereafter. Tokumaru and Catalano (39) have recently reported elevated IgM serum levels (up to 1700 mg%, mean of 420) in 15 patients with meningiomas as compared with a range of 40–250 mg % (mean, 145) for controls. More studies of general humoral immunocompetence in brain tumor patients are clearly warranted.

Immunotherapy

An immunotherapeutic approach to gliomas is highly speculative and, considering the evidence of shared antigens between tumor cells, normal brain, and lymphoid tissue (13), may be detrimental to the patient. Nevertheless, this treatment modality has been tried with varying results.

Takakura et al. (37) have transfused normal adult bone marrow into children with a variety of malignant intracranial tumors. Approximately 50 ml of bone marrow aspirate was transfused into ABO and Rh compatible patients following surgery, radiation, and chemotherapeutic trials. The average survival of this group of patients was 32 months. A control group was not reported. This same team (36) also has reported the infusion of purified white blood cells into the tumor space following operation. The intratumoral instillation of 10^{10} cells resulted in average survivals of 25.7 months. These reports are difficult to interpret because immunotherapy was used in conjunction with more conventional modes of adjunctive therapy, the studies were not well controlled nor randomized, and no effort was made to limit the investigations to one specific type of tumor. Nevertheless, the reports of Takakura stating that the addition of immunotherapy to surgery, radiation, and chemotherapy has increased the survival of his patients with "malignant brain tumors" from 49 days to one year are encouraging.

Trouillas (40) has reported the efficacy of adjunctive therapy to surgery in a randomized study comparing immunotherapy, cobalt therapy, and combination therapy. Postoperatively, those patients receiving immunotherapy were injected with a mixture of saline extract from their own tumor and Freund's adjuvant. Four to ten injections were made dependent upon the amount of tumor tissue available. Adjunctive immunotherapy increased the survival from 3.4 months, obtained with surgery alone, to 7.4 months. There was no significant difference in survival between patients receiving radiation (7.1 months) and immunotherapy (7.4 months). However, the combination of surgery, radiation, and immunotherapy increased the survival of the group to 10.1 months. Although promising, the inherent danger of this form of immunotherapy is illustrated by a single occurrence of allergic encephalitis in the immunotherapy group. This is probably related to antibody cross-reactive between glioma tissue and normal brain.

Bloom and his co-workers (2) reported the results of a trial designed to assess the value of immunotherapy in patients receiving irradiation and chemotherapy. One milliliter of the patient's own irradiated tumor cells were injected into the thigh as soon as possible following craniotomy. During the course of radiation therapy, additional injections were made. Contrary to the trial of Trouillas, (40) the results of this study clearly demonstrate that this form of active specific immunotherapy does not improve the survival of patients treated by surgery and radiotherapy. Fourteen percent of the patients receiving only surgery and irradiation survived 36 months, whereas patients receiving immunotherapy were all dead by 30 months. Furthermore, one patient may have developed allergic encephalitis.

Although nonspecific immunotherapy using BCG has been used in a variety of solid tumors, little has been done in patients with brain tumors. Ommaya (25) has recently completed a small prospective study combining chemotherapy and/or immunotherapy with maximal resection and irradiation. Although immunotherapy with BCG and autochthonous tumor cells stimulated an in vivo immune response as emidenced by lymphocytic infiltration of neoplastic tissue, all patients had tumor recurrence within 12 months.

Future Considerations

Thorough study of the immunobiological responses of malignant brain tumors will require elucidation of the unique inter-relation between the host's immune system and his brain. Does "immunological privilege" exist to any degree? In human beings, what is the significance of the antigenic relationship between the brain and T cells. Does the antigenicity of neoplastic brain cells differ from normal brain cells? Do patients with cell-mediated tumor immunity have immunological evidence of EAE? These important questions must be clearly answered before the observed phenomenon of impaired cellular and humoral immunity in patients with intracranial malignancies can be appropriately evaluated and the feasibility of immunotherapy considered.

ACKNOWLEDGMENTS

This work was supported in part by grants from U.S.P.H.S. (CA18234) and the American Cancer Society (IM-92).

REFERENCES

1. Aarli, J. A., Aparicio, S. R., Lumsden, C. E., and Tonden, O. 1975. Binding of normal human IgG to myelin sheaths, glia and neurons. *Immunology* 28: 171–185.

2. Bloom, H. H. G., Peckham, M. J., Richardson, A. E., Alexander, P. A., and Payne, P. M. 1973. Glioblastoma multiforme: A controlled trial to assess the value of specific active immunotherapy in patients treated by radical surgery and radiotherapy. *Brit. J. Cancer* 27: 253-2-7.

3. Brooks, W. H., Netsky, M. G., Normansell, D. E., and Horwitz, D. A. 1972. Depressed cell-mediated immunity in patients with primary intracranial tumors. *J. Exp. Med.* 136: 1631–1647.

4. Brooks, W. H., Caldwell, H. D., and Mortara, R. H. 1974. Immune responses in patients with gliomas. *Surg. Neurol.* 2: 419–423.

5. Brooks, W. H., Roszman, T. L., and Rogers, A. S. 1976. Impairment of rosette-forming T lymphocytes in patients with primary intracranial tumors. *Cancer* 37: 1869–1873.

6. Catalano, L. W., Jr., Harter, D. H., and Hsu, K. C. 1972. Common antigen in meningioma-derived cell cultures. *Science* 175: 180–182.

7. Coakham, H. 1974. Surface antigen(s) common to human astrocytoma cells. *Nature* 250: 328–330.

8. Coakham, H. B., and Lakshmi, M. S. 1975. Tumour-associated surface antigen(s) in human astrocytomas. *Oncology* 31: 233–243.

9. Dixit, S. P., and Coppola, E. D. 1969. The fate of intracerebral grafts in the dog. *Arch. Surg.* 99: 352–355.

10. Eggers, A. E. 1972. Autoradiographic and fluorescence antibody studies of the human host immune response to gliomas. *Neurology* 22: 246–250.

11. Eilber, F. R., and Morton, D. L. 1970. Impaired immunologic reactivity and recurrence following cancer surgery. *Cancer* 25: 362–367.

12. Gershon, R. K. 1974. T cell control of antibody production. *Contemp. Topics Immunol.* 3: 1–35.

13. Golub, E. S. 1971. Brain-associated theta antigen. Reactivity of rabbit anti-mouse brain with mouse lymphoid cells. *Cell. Immunol.* 2: 353–361.

14. Grace, J. T., Jr., Perese, D. M., Metzgar, R. S., Sasabe, T., and Holdridge, B. 1961. Tumor autograph responses in patients with glioblastoma multiforme. *J. Neurosurg.* 18: 159–167.

15. Greene, H. S. N. 1951. Transplantation of tumors to brains of heterologous species. *Cancer Res.* 11: 529–534.

16. Greene, H. S. N. 1953. Transplantation of human brain tumors to brains of laboratory animals. *Cancer Res.* 13: 422–426.

17. Kornblith, P. L., Dohan, Jr., F. C., Wood, W. C., and Whitman, B. O. 1974. Human astrocytoma: Serum-mediated immunologic response. *Cancer* 33: 1512–1519.

18. Kumar, S., Taylor, G., Steward, J. K., Waghe, M. A., and Morris-Jones, P. 1973. Cell-mediated immunity and blocking factors in patients with tumours of the central nervous system. *Int. J. Cancer* 12: 194–205.

19. Lance, E. M. 1967. A functional and morphological study of intracranial parathyroid allografts in the dog. *Transplantation* 5: 1471–1483.

20. Levy, N. L., Mahaley, Jr., M. S., and Daz, E. D. 1972. In *vitro* demonstration of cell-mediated immunity to human brain tumors. *Cancer Res.* 32: 477–482.

21. Lim, R., and Kluskins, L. 1972. Immunological specificity of astrocytoma antigens. *Cancer Res.* 32: 1667–1670.

22. Mahaley, M. S., Jr., Brooks, W. H., Roszman, T. L., Bigner, D. D., Dudka, L., and Richardson, S. 1977. Immunobiology of primary intracranial tumors I. Studies of the cellular and humoral general immune competence of brain tumor patients. *J. Neurosurg.* 46: 467–476.

23. Medawar, P. B. 1948. Immunity to homologous grafted skin. III. Fate of skin homografts transplanted to brain, to subcutaneous tissue, and to anterior chamber of eye. *Brit. J. Exp. Path.* 29: 58–69.

24. Morley, T. P. 1961. Discussion: Tumor autograft responses in patients with glioblastoma multiforme by J. J. Grace, D. M. Perese, R. S. Metzgar, T. Sasabe, and B. Holdridge. *J. Neurosurg.* 18: 159–167.

25. Ommaya, A. K. 1976. Immunotherapy of gliomas: A review. *Adv. Neurol.* 15: 337–359.

26. Quindlen, E. A., Dohan, F. C., Jr., and Kornblith, P. L. 1974. Improved assay for cytotoxic anti-glioma antibody. *Surg. Forum.* 25: 464–466.

27. Ridley, A., and Cavanaugh, J. C. 1969. The cellular reactions to heterologous, homologous and autologous skin implanted into brain. *J. Path.* 99: 193–203.

28. Scheinberg, L. C., Suzuki, K., Edelman, F., and Davidoff, L. M. 1963. Studies in immunization against a transplantable cerebral mouse of glioma. *J. Neurosurg.* 20: 312–317.

29. Scheinberg, L. C., Edelman, F. L., and Levy, W. A. 1964. Is the brain an "immunologically privileged site?" 1. Studies Based on Intracerebral Tumor Homotransplantation and bisotransplantation to Sensitized Hosts. *Arch. Neurol.* 11: 248–264.

30. Scheinberg, L. C., Levy, A., and Edelman, F. 1965. Is the brain an "immunologically privileged site"? 2. Studies in Induced Host Resistance to Transplantable Mouse Glioma Following Irradiation of Prior Implants. *Arch. Neurol.* 13: 283–286.

31. Scheinberg, L. C., Kotsilimbas, D. G., Karpf, R., and Mayer, N. 1966. Is the brain an "immunologically privileged site"? III. Studies Based on Homologous Skin Grafts to the Brain and Subcutaneous Tissues. *Arch. Neurol.* 15: 62–67.

32. Shou, L., Schwartz, S. A., and Good, R. A. 1976. Suppressor cell activity after concanavalin A treatment of lymphocytes from normal donors. *J. Exp. Med.* 143: 1100–1110.

33. Siris, J. H. 1936. Concerning the immunological specificity of glioblastoma multiforme. *Bull. Neurol. Inst. N.Y.* 4: 597–601.

34. Synderman, R., and Stahl. 1975. Defective immune effector function in patients with neoplastic and immune deficiency diseases, in J. A. Bellanti and D. H. Dayton (eds.), *The Phagocytic Cell in Host Resistance,* pp. 267–281. Raven Press, New York.

35. Tabuchi, K., and Kuschi, W. M. 1976. Detection of IgG on glioblastoma cell surfaces. Presented at Amer. Assoc. Neurol. Surgeons, San Francisco, Calif.

36. Takakura, K. 1975. Immunotherapy can aid in brain tumor treatment. *Med. World News.* 16: 39.

37. Takakura, K., Miki, Y., and Kubo. 1975. Adjuvant immunotherapy for malignant brain tumors in infants and children. *Child's Brain* 1: 141–147.

38. Thomas, D. G. T., Lannigan, C. B., and Behan, P. O. 1975. Impaired cell-mediated immunity in human brain tumours. *Lancet* 1: 1389.

39. Tokumaru, T., and Catalano, L. W. 1975. Elevation of serum immunoglobulin M (IgM) level in patients with brain tumors. *Surg. Neurol.* 4: 17–21.

40. Trouillas, P. 1973. Immunology and immunotherapy of cerebral tumors. Current status. *Rev. Neurol.* 128: 23–38.

41. Wahlstrom, T. 1973. Sensitivity to normal brain antigens of blood lymphocytes from patients with gliomas. *Acta Path. Microbiol. Scand.* 81: 763–767.

42. Wahlstrom, T., Linder, E., and Saksela, E. 1973. Glia-specific antigens in cell cultures from rabbit brain, human foetal and adult brain, and gliomas. *Acta. Path. Microbiol. Scand.* 81: 768–774.

43. Wahlstrom, T., Saksela, E., and Troupp, H. 1973. Cell-bound antiglial immunity in patients with malignant tumors of the brain. *Cell. Immunol.* 6: 161–170.

44. Wahlstrom, T., Linder, E., Saksela, E., and Westermark, B. 1974. Tumor-specific membrane antigens in established cell lines from gliomas. *Cancer* 34: 274–278.

45. Winters, W. D., and Rich, J. R. 1975. Human meningioma antigens. *Int. J. Cancer* 15: 815–822.

46. Young, H. F., Sakales, R., and Kaplan, M. 1975. Inhibition of cell-mediated immunity in patients with brain tumors. *Surg. Neurol.* 5: 19–23.

CHAPTER 13

IMMUNOTHERAPY OF HUMAN GLIOMAS

Harold F. Young
Alan Kaplan

Division of Neurosurgery
Department of Surgery
and Department of Microbiology
MCV/VCU Cancer Center
Medical College of Virginia
Virginia Commonwealth University
Richmond, Virginia 23298

Cancer of the brain has thus far been relatively resistant to presently employed therapeutic combinations of surgery, X-ray therapy, and chemotherapy. All three of these treatment modalities must necessarily be restricted in their application to the treatment of brain cancer because of injurious effects on the central nervous system. A fourth treatment modality, immunotherapy, has been used in the treatment of brain cancer in only a limited number of trials without striking success. Here we look at previous attempts at brain tumor immunotherapy as well as recent data obtained by treating post-surgery glioma patients with intra-tumor autologous leukocyte infusions. The results suggest this form of therapy may be effective in those patients with a small tumor burden.

I. INTRODUCTION

The crude incidence rate of brain cancer is 4.5/100,000, with a male/female ratio of 57:43 (71). Tumors of the brain and central nervous system are the second most common cancer in children of both sexes under the age of 15 years, surpassed in incidence only by leukemia. The etiology of intracranial tumors is unknown; a few relatively rare forms, such as acoustic neuroma and neurofibroma appear to be hereditary. Different forms of brain cancer have different biologic, kinetic, and metabolic characteristics, making it difficult to discuss this field as a single entity. The most common brain cancer is the highly malignant glioblastoma multiforme with an adult age distribution between 40 and 60 years. This tumor is the most important of the gliomas or astrocytoma series which comprises about 50% of all intracranial tumors. Astrocytomas constitute 0.6% of all autopsied deaths and 4.5% of all primary tumors (53, 55). Glioblastomas have a high mitotic index and consequently a rapid growth rate (43).

Non-central nervous system malignant neoplasms display variable aggressiveness, and in rare cases, complete and permanent regressions have been documented. Over the past few decades there have been rare reports of complete and permanent regressions in many types of cancer, including neuroblastoma, choriocarcinoma, lymphosarcoma, melanoma and hypernephroma (15). By contrast, complete regressions of glioblastomas in humans have not been documented (79, 80). Glioblastomas almost never metastasize outside the central nervous system unless there has been previous surgery (1). This phenomenon is surprising since malignant cells have been recovered from venous blood draining cerebral gliomas (45) and autografting experiments of viable tumor tissue have revealed that typical glioma can in fact grow at peripheral implantation sites (4, 23).

Failure of glioblastomas to metastasize may be related to the relatively short survival of patients following diagnosis or to mechanical rather than immunological factors since rapidly growing deposits have occurred following ventriculopleural or ventriculo-peritoneal shunts (68, 75).

These observations would suggest several hypotheses: It appears that in certain systemic cancers, there are host defenses which may infrequently result in regressions of the cancer. These host defenses are apparently inoperative or unable to be activated in malignant gliomas (57). The fact that brain tumors are uncommon may be due to some form of host surveillance mechanism, although this phenomenon may also be explained by the low mitotic activity of the CNS.

Cellular immune responses are generally believed to be more important in the rejection of solid tumors than humoral antibodies, and a hallmark of the rejection response is invasion of foreign tissue by mononuclear cells. Lymphocytic infiltration around gliomas had been noted by Bertrand and Mannen in 1960 (3) but without consideration of its relevance. In a postmortem study, Ridley and Cavanaugh (52) studied 93 cases of gliomas and found that 30% of gliomas showed significant lymphocytic infiltration, 28% slight infiltration and 42% no lymphocytic reaction. They discussed this as evidence for a possible immune response by the host to the tumor. The low percentage of glioblastoma patients in whom mononuclear cell infiltration can be detected is of interest with respect to approaches to immunologic intervention.

There is evidence for tumor-specific antigens in rats with astrocytomas (39). Moreover, Mahaley and Day (41), using labeled ^{125}I-rabbit antihuman glioma antibody, could localize high concentrations of the labeled antibody over the glioma cells, suggesting the existence of a specific glioma antigen. In contrast, Wickremesinghe and Yates (74) have demonstrated a loss of normal cellular antigens in malignant glioma tissue and Delpech et al. (11) were unable to detect anti-tumor autoantibodies in the sera from patients with glioblastoma. However, Kornblith et al. (32) could detect antibody to glioblastoma cells in the sera of 17 of 26 glioblastoma patients.

II. CURRENT STATUS OF THERAPY FOR BRAIN TUMORS

Gliomas are usually not detected at an early stage, generally being more than 50 g in weight when diagnosed. Surgical resection is seldom adequate unless the tumor is located entirely within a resectable lobe of the brain. Among many neurosurgeons a therapeutic nihilism exists toward gliomas; if the tumor is located in the dominate hemisphere, often angiographic diagnosis without biopsy is followed by radiotherapy only (2). Commonly, a cortical incision to the tumor tissue and piecemeal removal by a combination of suction and tissue forceps technique is the type of therapy performed. Large amounts of tumor tissue remain. Yet it is recognized that wide resection of the tumor when possible affords the best prognosis (30), and it is recommended that en bloc resection of gliomas should be done whenever possible, especially when the tumor presents at the surface. This can usually be done safely without increasing neurological deficit when the tumor is located in either of the frontal or temporal lobes. Often, magnification surgery using the operating microscope or operating loops aids in defining a line of demarcation between the brain and tumor not seen by gross vision. Hopefully new noninvasive low risk techniques such as computerized tomography (CT) brain scanning will permit early diagnosis before the tumor has spread across midline structures such as the corpus callosum. This will permit greater reduction of tumor burden by surgery.

Although it is generally believed that radiation therapy increases the average post-operative lifespan of patients with malignant gliomas (21, 30, 63, 72), after 12 to 18 months there is little difference in the survival rate between the radiated and nonirradiated groups. The most favorable results have been reported after substantial tumor resections and high doses (5000 to 6000 rads) of radiation therapy with the one year survival rate approaching 50%. Recently, analysis of a prospective, controlled, randomized study of over 300 patients with glioblastomas has indicated that postoperative radiation of 6000 rads to the whole brain, significantly increases the median survival following operation (69).

Chemotherapy alone has thus far not been proven to be a significant additional form of therapy for brain tumors. Current reports concern the use of the nitrosoureas which are extremely lipid soluble and readily penetrate the brain and cerebro-spinal fluid; however, limited increased survival has been reported (51, 73). The combination of surgery and irradiation plus chemotherapy has resulted in a favorable response in a significant number of patients (6, 19).

Radiation therapy, chemotherapy and surgery have all been shown to cause general immunosuppression, and each alone or in combination have certain limitations when the treatment of malignant brain tumors is considered. X-ray therapy, though possessing the ability to destroy the tumor, may also greatly injure the brain (12, 48), and excessive use of any of these 3 modalities may result in increased neurological deficit or serious toxic side effects. Thus, an alternate non-toxic, non-invasive form of therapy may be necessary to control the last remaining tumor cells and thus produce a longer survival. Immunotherapy may offer such a form of therapy.

III. THE BLOOD BRAIN BARRIER AND THE BRAIN AS AN IMMUNOLOGICAL PRIVILEGED SITE

The terms blood-brain barrier and blood-CSF barrier have been used to describe the relative exclusion of various exogenous and endogenous compounds from the brain and CSF and their slow equilibration despite high concentration in blood and other tissue. The special permeability features of the brain and CSF depend on the characteristics of the multiple, complex membranes of the cerebral capillaries, glia, neurons, myelin, arachnoid, and choroid plexus, as well as on brain and choroidal metabolism, which serve to stabilize the chemical environment of the brain. The site of the barrier to the entry of large molecules like albumin is the capillary endothelim (20).

Brain scanning techniques, wherein radioisotopes "leak" or pass into a brain tumor, allowing their visualization, demonstrate the increased permeability of the blood-brain barrier or at least the blood-tumor barrier in patients with brain tumors; thus, cellular and humoral immune mechanisms may operate more readily. Moreover, Shuttleworth (60) has shown by electron microscopy that in gliomas the vascular endothelium is defective in parts, so that tumor cells are in direct contact with the blood. Even an intact blood-brain barrier may not prevent passage of sensitized lymphocytes which are known to be capable of migrating through normal vascular endothelium (22).

Medawar (44) introduced the idea that the brain was an "immunologically privileged site," meaning that antigens within the brain do not evoke an afferent response probably by virtue of their lack of lymphatic drainage. Yet cerebral tissue can be the site of effector mechanisms initiated by antigenic stimulation elsewhere. Shirai (59), Murphy and Sturm (46), and Green (24, 25) have demonstrated that transplanted tumors of mouse or man can grow actively in the brain of a wide variety of species while failing to grow subcutaneously or intramuscularly. This prolonged graft survival may relate to the lack of a demonstrable regional lymphatic drainage.

Scheinberg et al. (56) have shown that isologous mice previously sensitized peripherally to transplanted glioma via tumor-adjuvant immunization rejected syngeneic glioma grafts in the brain or in subcutaneous sites. The growth of gliomas in syngeneic mouse brain did not involve lymphocyte infiltration or an inflammatory response unless previous sensitization had occurred. Of particular interest was the observation that the spontaneous rejection that occurred after peripheral sensitization to transplanted glioma did not produce damage to normal adjacent brain tissue, although tumor rejection was mediated by a lymphocyte-mediated inflammatory reaction. This further suggested the presence of glioma-specific antigens in this system.

The concept of the brain functioning as an immunologically privileged site interacting with the general anti-tumor immune surveillance mechanism may be involved in the iatrogenically induced chronic immunosuppression employed in kidney transplant patients. These patients have an abnormally high incidence of central nervous system lymphomas (58). In this instance it appears that systemic suppression of immunocompetence during a period of chronic antigenic stimulation extends its effect in an exaggerated fashion to the brain and thus may tip the immunological balance in favor of neoplastic development.

The concept of immunological privilege is not yet carefully clarified, but the work of Kaplan and Streilein (31) may lead to a useful animal model to test immunotherapy on brain tumors in animals. In regard to immunologically privileged sites, they have demonstrated that allogeneic cells placed within the anterior chamber (AC) of the eye in Fisher rats were not isolated from the immunologic apparatus of the host but instead induced a primary immune response within the spleen, which altered the systemic immunologic response of the intact animal. Their data suggested that donor lymphocytes placed in the AC escape directly into the blood and thus reach the spleen. The spleen receives the majority of antigen presented to an animal intravenously, and the spleen has also been shown to be a major source of enhancing antibodies (18). Kaplan and Streilein, therefore, studied the effect of splenectomy on skin graft survival and demonstrated accelerated rejection after splenectomy, such as is found in specifically sensitized hosts b)31).

Their data suggest that in this system the spleen may function to modify cell-mediated responses. They proposed that the critical feature for an immunologically privileged site was to allow antigen direct access to the vasculature and blood without first meeting a lymph node. Therefore, the host's first exposure to antigen occurs mainly in the spleen, which directs what would be a cell-mediated cytotoxic response into an antibody-mediated response. This is often protective of the same target tissue possibly by stimulating T lymphocytes which cooperate with appropriate B cells rather than generating T cell effector function. The cell mediated cytotoxicity is then thwarted by preemption of helper T cells and competition between remaining T cells and antibodies. Though this splenic immunoregulation is of value for swift humoral response to infections, it may be detrimental for control of neoplasia for which cell-mediated responses are probably essential.

Thus, the spleen may be important in tipping the delicate immunological balance mechanism in "privileged" sites, in favor of neoplastic development and growth.

IV. PREVIOUS TRIALS OF IMMUNOTHERAPY OF BRAIN TUMORS

Previous trials of immunotherapy of human gliomas have been rare. However, four well documented trials have been reported in the literature and are worthy of review.

In 1972, Takakura et al. (62) reported allogeneic bone marrow cell transfusion or local intra-tumoral infusion of allogeneic or autologous peripheral white blood cells into 18 patients having malignant gliomas, after treatment by operation, radiation or chemotherapy. Bone marrow cell transfusion was conducted on 8 infants and children suffering from malignant brain tumors. Each patient received up to 10 transfusions of approximately 50 ml of bone marrow from healthy adults having the same ABO and Rh blood types. The donors of bone marrow blood were changed each time to avoid possible hypersensitivity reactions. Two cases of medulloblastoma were in fine condition 31 and 26 months after operation. Two patients with infantile optic astrocytoma and a patient with a third ventricle astrocytoma were doing well, more than 1 year after operation. A 10-year-old girl suffering from ectopic pinealoma in the chiasmal region was also doing fine, 15 months after operation. A case of pontine glioma (6-year-old girl) was not operated on and only radiation and 5-FU (I.V.) chemotherapy were given with a transfusion of 5×10^8 bone marrow cells. She died 10 months after the onset of symptoms. In these childhood brain tumors long term survivors have frequently been observed making it difficult to evaluate the role of supportive immunotherapy in these cases. Moreover, it is not clear in these studies whether the bone marrow was being used as supportive therapy to reduce the effects of chemotherapy or for its potential antitumor activity. In addition, evaluation of these results is further complicated by the presence of a potent antitumor immunomodulator, corynebacterium, in 70% of the bone marrow preparations.

Peripheral white blood cell infusion into the intracranial dead space of malignant brain tumors was conducted by Takakura et al. (62) on 10 patients with recurrent tumors. Patients were treated with from 2 to 12 infusions of phytohemagglutinin-treated leukocytes. A range of 150 ml in 2 infusions up to 4000 ml in 10 infusions was used in the 10 patients. Seven patients died 9 to 30 months following surgery. One patient with an oligodendroglioma was alive 37 months after initial operation, while two patients with glioblastomas were alive at 26 and 50 months post-surgery. Because of the small number of cases and the lack of controls it is difficult to interpret these results.

Trouillas (66) has used immunization of glioma patients with their own tumor to attempt to induce "rejection" of tumor cells remaining after surgery. Following operation, patients were given 4–10 injections of their own tumor cells emulsified with Freund's adjuvant. Sixty-five patients with glioblastoma were randomly divided into four groups. Ten patients received only postoperative immunotherapy, 18 received postoperative immunotherapy combined with cobalt therapy, 20 received postoperative cobalt therapy and 17 had no postoperative treatment. The patients were followed at least 24 months. Immunotherapy alone significantly increased the duration of remission and survival, median survival rose 35%, from 5.4 to 7.4 months. Cobalt therapy alone had a similar effect with survival increased to 7.5 months. Combined treatment increased survival time to 10.1 months.

Lymphocytic or plasmocytic infiltration of the tumor was demonstrated in 4 of 6 pathological studies in the post-operative immunotherapy group. The 2 negative samples were taken more than 7 months after immunotherapy, suggesting that the effect of treatment was not long term. Mononuclear cells were found both at the periphery and in the interior of the tumor.

All patients had a positive intradermal delayed hypersensitivity reaction to glioblastoma extract after immunization. Immunized patients reacted to extracts of other glioblastomas, suggesting the existence of a tumor-specific antigen(s) common to glioblastomas. Weaker reactions were observed with extracts of astrocytoma cell lines. The most striking aspect of immunotherapy was the appearance in serum of antibodies that caused lysis of glioma cells in culture in the presence of complement. These antibodies appeared to be tumor-specific as they did not react with normal glial cells in culture. The antibody levels rose during immunotherapy and fell after it was stopped. The same antigen was recovered in fetal brain, especially at 2–3 months. The new carcinoembryonic molecule was found to be a fetal lipoprotein.

Trouillas concluded that the efficacy of immunotherapy appeared to be a function of the number of tumor cells left to destroy, and should be used only after all other forms of therapy capable of reducing tumor mass have been carried out. The only side effect of immunotherapy was local induration and in one case a confusion syndrome and inflammatory response.

In 1973, Bloom et al. (5) reported the results of a randomized prospective clinical trial carried out to assess the value of specific active immunotherapy using irradiated autologous tumor cells in patients with glioblastoma multiforme treated by radical surgery and postoperative radiation. The results in 62 patients showed no statistically significant difference in survival between the group receiving adjuvant plus autologous tumor cells and those treated with surgery and radiotherapy alone. All 27 patients who received irradiated tumor cells were dead by 30 months, whereas 5 (14%) of the control group survived for more than 3 years, one patient still being alive at 72 months. The initial mortality was equally rapid in both groups. It is possible that normal brain tissue and thus normal brain-specific antigens may have been included in the injection along with the administration of irradiated autologous cells, but there was no evidence of allergic encephalomyelitis. Likewise, in the 10 patients in this series who had multiple injections of irradiated autologous tumor cells, none showed positive intradermal skin tests to indicate the development of a cell-mediated local reaction against the injected tumor. In most cases in this study, there was good clinical evidence of tumor recurrence which was proved histologically in 9 of 10 patients subject to autopsy, but since glioblastoma has such a high recurrence rate, the danger of enhancement of tumor growth by immunotherapy could not be resolved in this study. The results were sufficiently discouraging to abandon the trial on the grounds that there was sufficient evidence in this study that the administration of irradiated autologous cells was of no benefit to patients with glioblastoma.

Failure of immunotherapy and the lack of development of delayed hypersensitivity to the tumor tissue in this last study may be related to the fact that the tumor cells were heavily irradiated prior to innoculation and thus not a good source of antigen for immunotherapy or alternatively that an adjuvant was not used with the cells. Also, the potential effectiveness of immunotherapy may have been reduced by co-administration of radiotherapy. Alternatively, one must consider the possibility that this approach to brain-tumor immunotherapy simply does not work.

Recently Ommaya (49) reported pilot clinical studies conducted at the National Institutes of Health (NIH) according to an immunotherapy protocol designed as a prospective study to evaluate three modes of therapy for patients who had undergone maximal tumor resection and a full course (5000 to 6000 rads) of radiotherapy. All patients had a catheter implanted in the tumor cyst for drug administration. Patients were randomized to one of three groups: chemotherapy alone, immunotherapy alone, or immunochemotherapy. Two chemotherapeutic agents were used: CCNU and 8-Azaguanine. The 8-Azaguanine was given into the tumor cyst weekly for 6 weeks, then monthly, in a dose of 100 mg. CCNU was given orally, 130 mg per m^2 every 8 weeks.

Two patients received immunotherapy alone, which consisted of the administration of BCG, 10^7 organisms intradermally at monthly intervals, autochthonous tumor cells (10^6 cells treated with neuraminidase and mitomycin C) intradermally every other week and PPD, 0.1 ml of intermediate (5 TU) or second strength PPD (250 TU) injected into the tumor cyst implant at monthly intervals. BCG was given to enhance non-specific cellular immunity, which was depressed in these patients. Tumor cells were given to induce a specific lymphocytic sensitization to the patients' tumor antigens. PPD was given into the tumor cyst to recruit large numbers of sensitized immune cells into the tumor bed. Patients in the immunochemotherapy group received both immunotherapy and chemotherapy as described above.

Five patients received immunotherapy alone or in combination with chemotherapy and all developed recurrence of tumor within 12 months.

The first patient on immunochemotherapy had a tumor recurrence at 8 months. His initial NIH surgical specimen showed typical features of a malignant astrocytoma, while his post-therapy specimen showed necrosis and dense mononuclear cell infiltration. These cells were predominantly lymphocytes, but plasma cells were present in unusually large numbers.

To evaluate the degree of cellular immunity after therapy, radioactive ^{51}chromium release cytotoxic assays were performed on the three patients with recurrences. In each of these assays, the patient's lymphocytes were no more cytotoxic than were normal control lymphocytes. This was thought to possibly reflect a weak capacity for sensitization of the patients to their own tumor cells, either because of the weakness of the tumor antigens, low antigenicity of the cells treated with neuraminidase and mitomycin, or coating of fresh tumor cells by blocking factors.

As an adjunctive mode of therapy, immunotherapy in this study was no better than chemotherapy alone. Moreover, recurrence or remission did not correlate with skin DH responses to common skin antigens to dinitrochlorobenzene (DNCB) or lymphocyte responses to phytohemagglutinin (PHA). Immunotherapy complications were minimal. No instance of allergic encephalomyelitis was described and no severe local reaction to intracerebral PPD injections occurred.

V. IN VITRO CORRELATES OF IN VIVO GLIOBLASTOMA

A. Cell-Mediated Immune Reactivity to Gliomas

A number of investigators have demonstrated that central nervous system tissues could grow successfully in vitro (9, 26, 33, 54). Subsequently cell lines derived from gliomas were shown to be capable of indefinite proliferation in vitro (50). This capacity for successfully growing malignant glial cells in vitro has been a useful technique for demonstrating an efferent immune reaction wherein the in vitro cytotoxicity of lymphoid cells on autochthonous malignant glial cells could be demonstrated. In 1969, Ciembroniewicz and Kolar (10) reported clustering of lymphocytes around autologous and homologous glioblastoma cells in tissue culture.

In 1972 Levy et al. (38) demonstrated lymphocytoxicity directed against an antigen which was possibly shared by glioblastoma and melanoma cells. They reported that patients with glioblastoma and other intracranial neoplasms possessed peripheral blood lymphocytes specifically cytotoxic to cultured autologous tumor cells in vitro. They concluded that both anaplastic and well-differentiated tumors of the central nervous system can induce a tumor-specific, cell-mediated immune response in the host. However, previous attempts by this group to develop tumor specific antisera for treatment of glioblastoma were unsuccessful (40, 41, 42).

In 1973, Kumar *et al.* (36) reported the results on a study on 18 human brain tumors *in vitro* showing evidence of the presence of cellular and humoral immunity in the individuals having these tumors. This study showed the presence of both tumor-specific lymphocytotoxicity and an activity in the serum of some patients which was capable of abrogating this cytotoxicity. While the controls suggested that lymphocytotoxicity was tumor specific, it is impossible to evaluate the specificity of the blocking factors from the data presented. Increasing the proportion of lymphocytes from a patient with astrocytoma resulted in considerably increased killing of the tumor cells, whereas the increase was very much less when healthy donor's lymphocytes were used. The results of cross-over experiments confirmed that lymphocytes from patients with medulloblastomas were highly reactive against medulloblastoma as compared to astrocytoma. Similarly, lymphocytes from patients who had been treated for astrocytomas would inhibit autologous and allogeneic astrocytoma cells and had insignificant cytotoxicity against medulloblastomas. Serum samples of only 3 of 15 patients with central nervous system tumors had blocking activity. In a previous study Kumar and Taylor (37) had shown blocking factors in the sera of four out of five patients with clinically active CNS tumors while only one of fourteen patients clinically free of disease had similar activity. Again the specificity of blocking activity was not vigorously demonstrated.

In regard to humoral immunity, Kornblith *et al.* (32) found a serum-mediated response (humoral) in 17 of 26 patients with astrocytomas. They found that serum from these patients was cytotoxic to tumor cells grown in tissue culture.

Thus, the ability of lymphocytes to interact with glial tumor tissue *in vitro* has been demonstrated. The same phenomenon has thus far not been observed *in vivo*, as the general experience has been that adoptive immunotherapy with lymphoid cells is usually ineffective if instituted after a tumor is already clinically manifest (13, 14, 16, 17).

B. Serum Blocking Factors

Much of our current concept of serum blocking activity in human tumor systems is related directly to the findings of the Hellströms (29). Their pioneering work has indicated that many cancer patients have lymphocytes that are cytotoxic for tumor cells of the same histopathological type as the tumor of the patient. The presence of cytotoxic lymphocytes seem to be a relatively constant finding in most patients, except for those with extremely advanced disease and with this exception, appeared to be unrelated to the clinical status of the patient. They have found a strong correlation between the presence of blocking factors in the serum of patients and the clinical status of their disease. However, these findings have not been reproduced in other laboratories and the relationship between serum blocking factors, lymphocytotoxicity and prognosis certainly will require much additional work before an adequate interpretation can be made. Patients who had progressive disease had a higher incidence and higher levels of serum factors which would inhibit lymphocytotoxic activity than did patients who were apparently cured or tumor-free, whose sera manifested little or no blocking activity. At first, blocking was thought to be due to antibody, since blocking activity was found in the 7S fraction of serum. Later findings by Sjögren et al. (61) have suggested that blocking activity could be due to antigen-antibody complexes rather than antibody alone. Antigen-antibody complexes could provide a bifunctional type of blocking agent which could block efficient cytotoxic activity at the level of the tumor cell by masking the antigenic sites on the tumor cell surface or, at the level of the effector cell, by reacting with receptors for tumor antigen on the surface of the immune lymphocyte. Under either circumstance, the lymphocyte is prevented from interacting properly with the target tumor cell.

Brooks et al. (7) showed that patients with primary intracranial tumors have impaired cellular immunity. Patients with primary brain tumors demonstrated depressed cutaneous reactivity to common antigens, inability to become sensitized to dinitrochlorobenzene (DNCB) and impaired in vitro lymphocyte responsiveness to mitogens. They found that cell mediated immunity was broadly suppressed by the IgG fraction of serum obtained from patients with primary intracranial tumors, and also demonstrated that this humoral suppression was lost following surgical removal of the tumor only to appear with tumor recurrence (8). Furthermore Brooks demonstrated, in the mixed lymphocyte-tumor culture system (MLTC), specific sensitization of autologous lymphocytes to tumor associated antigens on the surface of the tumor cells. Autologous serum consistently inhibited lymphocyte activation by autochthonous cells in comparison with control cultures with normal human serum. This work suggested that there was a humoral factor in patients with primary brain tumors manifested as a defect in the immunocompetence of such patients, and this defect was related to tumor burden.

Patients with primary brain tumors have evidence of serum inhibitory factors as do other patients with other forms of cancer. Therefore, in 1973 we began a series of in vitro experiments to study the lymphocyte and plasma activity of patients with gliomas. The lymphocytes and plasma of patients with brain tumors were studied using the lymphocyte blast transformation technique to the mitogens phytohemagglutinin (PHA) and concanavallin A (Con A). We demonstrated that nearly 90% of patients with

glioblastoma demonstrated a strong plasma inhibitory effect on the blastogenesis of not only autologous lymphocytes but also of normal control
lymphocytes, and that this plasma effect could be correlated with the
clinical course of the patient (76). Lymphocytes from 50% of patients with
glioblastoma failed to undergo normal transformation when cultured in
normal plasma. Similar results have been published by Thomas et al. (64)
confirming these observations.

Those patients who had plasma inhibitory factor(s) could be divided
into two categories; those whose plasma inhibitory effect could be overcome by increasing mitogen concentration and those whose response to
mitogens was inhibited regardless of mitogen concentration. In the former
case we were presumably dealing with a trivial factor which competed for
mitogen with cell receptors or alternatively blocked mitogen cell receptors. The fact that preincubation of normal lymphocytes with inhibitory
plasma was unable to inhibit mitogen-induced blastogenesis (i.e., lymphocytes and inhibitory plasma had to be together during stimulation for
inhibition to occur) suggested that inhibitory plasma was not simply
blocking cell receptors. In the second category of patients, blastogenesis
was blocked regardless of the mitogen concentration and studies with
inhibitory plasma present at different time periods during the response to
PHA indicated that the events responsible for inhibition occurred early
after the initiation of cultures (unpublished observations).

When the presence of plasma inhibitory factor(s) was correlated with
lymphocyte function in a series of 15 patients with glioblastoma, a correlation coefficient of $r = 0.74$ was found, indicating that those patients
with plasma inhibitory factors were most likely to have inhibited lymphocyte function. In contrast, there was no relationship between either
lymphocyte function or the presence of plasma inhibitory factor(s) and
the number of peripheral T lymphocytes as measured by rosette formation
with sheep erythrocytes (78).

Whether the inhibitory factor in the plasma of glioblastoma patients is
of tumor cell origin or a host cell product is at present unknown. Moreover, whether this factor has any specificity with respect to its ability to
inhibit lymphocyte blastogenesis as opposed to DNA synthesis and/or
division in other cell populations is not known.

VI. IMMUNOTHERAPY WITH AUTOLOGOUS WHITE CELL INFUSION IN THE TREATMENT OF GLIOBLASTOMA MULTIFORME

Several facts suggested that infusion of autologous lymphocytes
into glioblastomas after surgery and radiation therapy might be beneficial.
Brooks et al. (7) have demonstrated the presence of lymphocytes specifi-

cally reactive to glioblastoma cells in the peripheral circulation but the reports of Ridley and Cavanaugh indicated that only 30% of patients with gliomas showed a significant lymphocyte infiltration of their tumor. We, therefore, reasoned that the direct delivery of peripheral lymphocytes into the tumor might either directly kill tumor cells or alternatively create a mild inflammatory response which would increase the number of potentially cytotoxic cells present in the tumor.

The transfusion of lymphocytes from allogeneic human donors to patients with cancer has been reported by Nadler and Moore (47). Two more studies were carried out by Krementz et al. (35, 36) and Israel et al. (28, 29) with improvement in patients with advanced cancer. Moreover, the study of Takakura et al. (62) suggested that leukocyte infusion may be of value in the post-surgical treatment of glioblastoma and the work of Trouillas (65) resulted in either no effect or the induction of perivascular lymphocyte-plasmocytic infiltrations at the tumor site.

Beginning in July 1974, we initiated a preliminary investigation of the effect of autologous leukocytes injected directly into the tumors of patients with proven glioblastoma multiforme. Over the next 27 months we treated a total of 18 patients with glioblastoma multiforme with 1 or more direct injections of autologous lymphocytes into the tumor bed via previously implanted Rickham reservoirs (Table 1). The autologous lymphocytes were isolated from peripheral blood and placed in direct contact with the tumor cells in an attempt to reproduce in vivo, the in vitro cytotoxicity previously described.

The continuous blood flow cell separator provided a method for the continuous collection of lymphocytes from the peripheral blood and the reinfusion of the remaining blood elements. In this series (77) no clinically significant changes in hematocrit and no evidence of systemic toxicity following the leukaphoresis of patients was noted. The peripheral blood leukocyte and lymphocyte counts fell transiently but returned to normal within 3 days. A potential danger of leukaphoresis in cancer patients is the possibility of decreased cellular immunocompetence following removal of the large number of peripheral lymphocytes. However, we have not detected any significant change in cell-mediated immunity as documented by serial lymphocyte transformation studies to the mitogens PHA and Con A, and therefore this aspect of the technique appears safe. However, final evaluation of changes in the immune function of these patients following leukaphoresis must be made by determining the tumor specific response before and after leukophoresis.

The initial patients in this study were selected because of recurrence of tumor and failure of all previous therapeutic modalities, including surgery, radiation therapy, and chemotherapy to control the tumor. Tumor recurrence was documented by clinical course and brain scan or computerized tomography (CT) scan. The initial objective was to assess the safety of intra-tumoral injections in regards to alterations of intracranial pressure and to the development of secondary reactions. Repeated biopsies and/or autopsy specimens were obtained and analyzed for development of acute allergic encephalomyelitis and hopefully any sign of lymphocytotoxicity to tumor cells. In this uncontrolled trial responses were judged to be positive if the patient's neurological status improved for over one month in association with regression or stabilization of tumor size by routine brain scan or CT scan. The initial patients had known large tumor burdens and, according to presently held immunological concepts, could not be expected to have dramatic responses to immunotherapy.

A total of 18 patients were treated (Table 1). The first five patients were critically ill with large tumor burdens. One of the first 5 patients (W.R.), who was comatose at the time of treatment and received 1 injection of autologous leukocytes (1×10^9 cells) into his tumor, improved within one week to a totally independent status, able to care for himself for 16 months while serial brain scans demonstrated regression in tumor size of approximately 50–70% without further treatment (77).

Another 10 of the 18 patients treated with autologous leukocytes had recurrent but smaller tumor burden than the first 5 patients. With the better clinical status in this group, there were 5 patients who following immunotherapy showed clinical improvement and regression of brain tumor size by scanning techniques for 1 to 5 months; however, 9 have expired and only one is alive and independent 1 month after treatment. Three other patients were given standard therapy of surgery and irradiation therapy followed by injection of autologous leukocytes directly into the tumor, before clinical deterioration, but when tumor was clearly visible on CT scan. These three patients are alive and well one year after surgical treatment, X-ray therapy, and two or more autologous leukocyte infusions (Table 1).

One of these last three patients, J.A., showed a stable clinical course 10 months following autologous lymphocyte infusion. A CT brain scan eight months after lymphocyte infusion did not reveal evidence of tumor (Fig. 1) compared to a CT scan taken before lymphocyte infusion (Fig. 1). Moreover, following lymphocyte infusion there has been a steady decline in the presence of plasma inhibitory factor(s) (Fig. 2).

It is important to appreciate the fact that 2 of 4 patients who improved or had long term stable courses after immunotherapy treatment certainly had small residual tumor burden at the time of treatment. These two patients may have done well without specific immunotherapy treatment as their tumors were located in the frontal lobes of the brain and were radically, but incompletely, resected at the time of surgery. The patient reported, J.A., had minimal resection because the tumor was located near

Table 1. Eighteen patients with supratentorial glioblastoma treated by immunotherapy. (All patients had initial surgical resection of the tumor.)

Patient	Age	Sex	Rx	Recurrence (months) from Rx	Clinical Status	Autologous Leukocytes (cell no.)	Results	Postlymph Survival (months)	Total Survival (months from diagnosis)
R.N.	52	M	6000R CCNU	11	Hemiparesis, confusion, memory loss	5×10^7	Unchanged	1wk.	11
W.D.	60	M	6000R	2	Comatose, dilated pupil	2×10^7	Unchanged	1wk.	2
J.S.	58	M	Steroids	—	Confused, aphasic	1.4×10^7	Unchanged	3	3
S.W.	57	M	Steroids	1	Hemiparesis	1.8×10^7	Unchanged	3	3
J.H., II	58	M	6000R	12	Hemiparesis	4.2×10^8 1.3×10^9	Unchanged	4	16
M.C.	48	F	—	—	Comatose	3×10^6	Unchanged	5	5
J.R.	63	M	6000R	8	Hemiparesis, aphasic	1.5×10^9 7×10^8 1.4×10^9	Unchanged	5	13
R.M.	67	F	Radiation	5	Ataxia, memory loss, incontinent	2×10^7	Hydrocephalus (shunt, mild improvement)	5	10
J.L.	64	M	6000R Steroids	2	Blind, confused, aphasic	2.6×10^7	Unchanged	12	14

	Age	Sex	Treatment		Clinical status	Cell dose	Response		
W.R.	49	M	6000R CCNU Steroids	6	Semicomatose, incontinent	5.0×10^7	Fully functional, 16 months	17	23
M.P.	20	M	6000R	4	Memory loss, headache	5.8×10^8 1.8×10^9	Improved, functionally independent, working,	13+	17+
A.T.F.	59	M	5040R BCNU	10	Aphasic, hemiparetic	1.2×10^9 1.8×10^9 1.2×10^9	Improved one month	8	18
J.A.	57	M	5000R	3	Aphasic, hemiparetic, confusion	4.5×10^8 7.8×10^8	Alert, speech improvement, (shunted), walks	12+ 8+ (pcst-shunt)	15+
R.S.	49	F	6000R	36	Seizure, confusion, mild hemiparetic	1.8×10^8 1.8×10^9 1.7×10^9	Functionally independent	13+	51+
J.H., I.	25	M	5000R CCNU Steroids	60	Aphasic, incontinent, drowsy, hemiparetic	3×10^7 3×10^7 4.2×10^8	Alert, functional, self-feeding, 11 mo.	12	72
R.S.	56	M	6000R	13	Drowsy, aphasic	2×10^9	More alert	6	19
A.M.	63	M	6000R	4	Aphasic, hemiparetic	1.9×10^8 1.8×10^9 1.7×10^9	Returned to work 1 mo.	4	8
I.B.	54	M	6000R Steroids BCNU	6	Headache, lethargy, hemiparesis	1×10^9 1×10^9	Alert, mild hemiparesis ambulatory	2	8

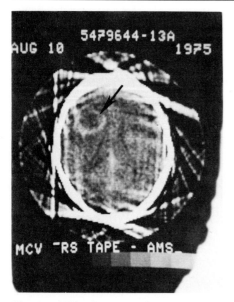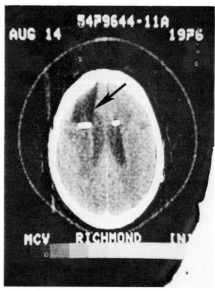

Fig. 1.   CT brain scans of patient J.A.'s tumor at time of diagnosis and after leukocyte infusion. *Left*—CT scan on patient J.A. at time of diagnosis on August 10,
1975, showing left frontal glioblastoma (*arrow*). *Right*—CT scan on patient J.A. 1
year later, showing cystic surgical decompression (*arrow*) with Rickham reservoir
on left (*white spot, L*) and shunt tube on right (*white spot, R*). No evidence of
enhanced tumor.

the speech area in the dominant hemisphere. It is precisely in this type of
patient who has had all gross tumor resected that immunotherapy may be
effective in preventing recurrence.

No clinical syndromes suggestive of acute allergic encephalomyelitis
have been demonstrated early or late following treatment. Repeated biopsies or autopsy specimens have been obtained in patients from one day to
6 months following injections. There has been no evidence of allergic
encephalomyelitis by detailed light and electron microscopic review of
specimens of brain, peripheral nerves or spinal cord. Mononuclear cell
infiltration was frequently seen in the periphery of the tumor near the
cystic cavity in specimens examined within 1 month of injection (Fig. 3).

Our preliminary results would suggest that white blood cell intratumoral infusion is relatively safe, and that it may benefit the patient
with a small tumor burden. The timing, amount, and frequency of treat-

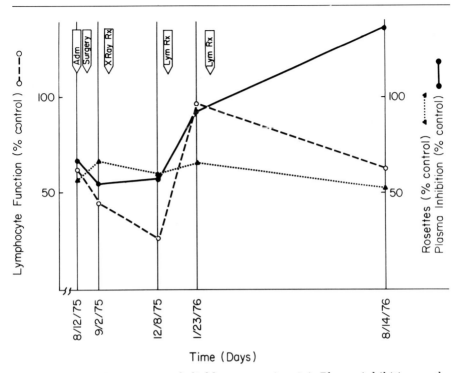

Fig. 2. Immunologic course of glioblastoma patient J.A. Plasma inhibition on the left ordinate represents stimulation by phytohemagglutinin (PHA) of normal lymphocytes in glioblastoma patient's plasma as a percent of PHA-stimulated normal lymphocytes in normal pooled plasma. Lymphocyte function on the right ordinate represents PHA stimulation of lymphocytes from patient J.A. in normal pooled plasma as a percent of the stimulation of control normal lymphocytes in normal pooled plasma. Rosettes are T cell sheep erythrocyte rosettes from peripheral blood of patient J.A. expressed as a percent of normal control values.

ments are yet to be defined, but many alterations of the technique are possible. Particularly it is important to correlate the *in vitro* cytotoxic capacity of lymphocytes with their *in vivo* function. Moreover, other cell types, particularly macrophages, may be of greater benefit than lymphocytes. The mechanism of action of tumor inhibition is unknown but may result either from the direct cytotoxic action of the infused lymphocytes or from the induction of an inflammatory response and the subsequent migration of cytotoxic cells into the tumor.

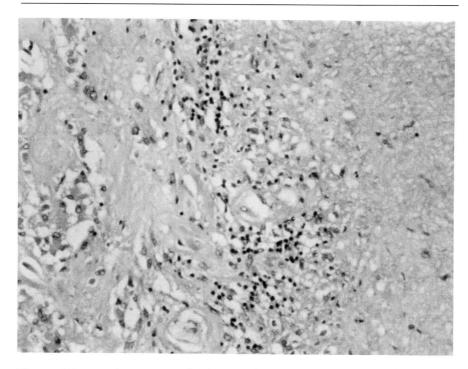

Fig. 3. Biopsy taken one week after autologous leukocyte infusion, showing brain on left and necrotic tumor on the right with small round mononuclear cells along brain-tumor interface.

VII. FUTURE OF HUMAN BRAIN TUMOR IMMUNOTHERAPY

Previous trials of immunotherapy of human brain tumors while generally not encouraging have in an anecdotal sense provided some suggestions of therapeutic effect. It is clear that if brain tumor immunotherapy is going to be adequately evaluated appropriate immunologic parameters as well as clinical parameters must be followed. Herein lies the major problem: there is at present no *in vitro* test which correlates in a prognostic sense with the *in vivo* course of the tumor-bearing patient. This is not only true of glioblastomas but for all tumors. Moreover, the relevance of animal data obtained with chemically and virally induced tumors to the human clinical situation is currently unclear. Certainly the spectrum of putative "tumor-associated antigens" thus far characterized in man differ in their distribution and specificity from mouse tumor antigens.

Despite these problems, in diseases such as glioblastoma where no definitive therapy is currently available immunotherapy trials will almost certainly continue. Therefore, it is of primary importance to develop protocols that can generate as much useful information as possible. This can best be achieved by limiting the number of treatments per patient, by rigidly controlling the protocols and by keeping the protocols as simple as possible. This may enable the acquisition of acceptable clinical data even in the absence of appropriate laboratory procedures. Perhaps, the single most agreed upon fact to emerge from animal tumor studies is the importance of minimal tumor burden for effective immunotherapy and this should certainly be considered in the development of clinical protocols.

With respect to the types of immunotherapy to use in brain tumors it may be important to keep in mind the lack of a significant inflammatory reaction and mononuclear infiltrate in the majority of glioblastomas. Moreover, at the same time one must consider the potential danger of changes in CSF pressure which frequently accompany inflammation in the CNS but which can be determined by use of an intracranial pressure monitor (67). As far as the infusion of lymphoid cells directly into the tumor cyst perhaps added benefit can be achieved by activation of lymphocytes in vitro with mitogens such as Concanavallin A or phytohemagglutin. Alternatively, activated macrophages which have been shown to be highly cytostatic and/or cytotoxic to tumor cells may be used. These methods may increase the effectiveness of direct infusion of effector cells and would tend to overcome the generally observed poor infiltration of mononuclear cells into gliomas. It is also possible that local use of agents like MIF or some of the other lymphokines might be useful in increasing the mononuclear cell infiltrate in the tumor. Moreover, it may be feasible to combine this latter method for directing mononuclear cells into the tumor bed with systemic macrophage activators, such as BCG or C. parvum. It should be apparent that these general approaches would be best evaluated in a glioblastoma animal model before being used clinically in man. Or these methods could be tested with human glioma material in the nude mouse model which has recently shown promise for evaluating several treatment modalities which function independently of thymus derived lymphocytes. In addition to focusing mononuclear cells in the tumor it is also possible that the nonspecific immunomodulators may be of value in overcoming the general immunodepression that has been demonstrated in glioma patients.

Unquestionably, much work in both animal studies and controlled clinical trials will be necessary to resolve these questions.

ACKNOWLEDGMENTS

This work was supported in part by U.S.P.H. Grant CA 16096 and an American Cancer Society Institutional Grant #IN-105.

REFERENCES

1. Anzil, A. P. 1970. Glioblastoma multiforme with extracranial metastases in the absence of previous craniotomy. Case Report. *J. Neur. Surg.* 33: 88–94.

2. Bartel, A. L., Heilbronn, Y. D., and Schiffer, J. 1973. Extensive resection of primary malignant tumor of the left cerebral hemisphere. *Surg. Neurol.* 1: 337–342.

3. Bertrand, I., and Mannen, H. 1960. Etude des réactions vasculaires dans les astrocytomas. *Revue Neurol.* 102: 3–19.

4. Bloom, W. H., Carstairs, K. C., Crompton, M. R., and McKissock, W. 1960. Autologous glioma transplantation. *Lancet* 2: 77.

5. Bloom, H. J., Peckham, M. J., Richardson, A. E., Alexander, P. A., and Payne, P. M. 1973. Glioblastoma multiforme: A controlled trial to assess the value of specific active immunotherapy in patients treated by radical surgery and radiotherapy. *Brit. J. Cancer* 27: 253–67.

6. Bloom, H. J. G. 1975. Combined modality therapy for intracranial tumors. *Cancer* 35: 111–120.

7. Brooks, W. H., Netsky, M. G., Normansell, D. E., and Horwitz, D. A. 1972. Depressed cell-mediated immunity in patients with primary intracranial tumors. *J. Exp. Med.* 136: 1631–1647.

8. Brooks, W. H., Caldwell, D. H., and Mortara, R. H. 1974. Immune responses in patients with gliomas. *Surg. Neurol.* 2: 419–423.

9. Buckley, R. C. 1929. Tissue culture studies of glioblastoma multiforme. *Amer. J. Path.* 5: 467–472.

10. Ciembroniewicz, J., Kolar, O. 1969. Tissue culture study of glioblastoma cells with addition of autologous lymphocytes. *Acta Cytol.* 13: 42–49.

11. Delpech, B., Delpech, A., Clement, J., and Lamonier, R. 1972. Immunochemical and immunological studies of human brain tumors. *Int. J. Cancer* 9: 374–382.

12. Diengdoh, J. V., and Booth, A. E. 1976. Postirradiation necrosis of the temporal lobe presenting as a glioma. *J. Neurosurg.* 44(No. 6): 732–734.

13. Ellman, L., and Green, G. 1971. L2C guinea pig leukemia: Immunoprotection and immunotherapy. *Cancer* 28: 647–654.

14. Evans, C. A., Weiser, R. S., and Ito, Y. 1962. Antiviral and antitumor immunologic mechanisms operative in slope papilloma-carcinoma system. *Cold Spring Harbor. Symp. Quant. Biol.* 27: 453–462.

15. Everson, T. C., and Cole, W. H. 1966. *Spontaneous Regression of Cancer.* W. B. Saunders Co., Phildelphia.

16. Fass, L., and Fefer, A. 1972. Studies of adoptive chemo-immunotherapy of a Friend virus-induced lymphoma. *Cancer Res.* 32: 997–1001.

17. Fefer, A. 1971. Adoptive chemoimmunotherapy of a Moloney lymphoma. *Int. J. Cancer* 8: 364–373.

18. Ferrer, J. F. 1968. Role of the spleen in passive immunological enhancement. *Transplantation* 6: 167–172.

19. Fewer, D., Wilson, C. B., Boldrey, E. B., Enot, K. J., and Powel, M. R. 1972. The chemotherapy of brain tumors. *JAMA* 222(No. 5): 549–552.

20. Fox, J. L. 1964. Development of recent thoughts in intracranial pressure and the blood-brain barrier. *J. Neurosurg.* 21: 909–967.

21. Frankel, S. A., and German, W. I. 1958. Glioblastoma multiforme. Review of 219 cases with regard to natural history, pathology, diagnostic methods, and treatment. *J. Neurosurg.* 15: 489–503.

22. Gowans, J. L. 1959. The recirculation of lymphocytes from blood to lymph in the rat. *J. Physiol.* 146: 54–68.

23. Grace, J. T., Perese, D. M., Metzgar, R. S., Sasabe, T., and Holdridige, B. 1961. Tumor autograft responses in patients with glioblastoma multiforme. *J. Neurosurg.* 18: 159–167.

24. Greene, H. S. N. 1951. Transplantation of tumors to brain of heterologous species. *Cancer Res.* 11: 529–534.

25. Greene, H. S. N. 1957. Heterotransplantation of tumors. *Ann. N.Y. Acad. Sci.* 69: 818–829.

26. Harrison, R. G. 1910. The outgrowth of the nerve fiber as a mode of protoplasmic movement. *J. Exp. Zool.* 9: 787–847.

27. Hellström, I., Sjögren, H. O., and Werner, G. 1971. Blocking of cell-mediated immunity by sera from patients with growing neoplasms. *Int. J. Cancer* 7: 226–237.

28. Israel, L., Mannoni, P., Delobel, J., Mawas, C., Gross, B., *et al.* 1967. Notes sur les résultats des intradermo-reactions de lymphocytes viables, homologues et heterologues chez des receveurs cancereux et des témoins. *Path. Biol.* 15: 593–595.

29. Israel, L., Mannoni, P., Mawas, C., Gineste, J., Gross, B., and Sors, C. 1967. 70 perfusions de lymphocytes homologues dans 25 cas de cancers avances. *Path. Biol.* 15: 603–606.

30. Jelsma, R., and Bucy, P. C. 1967. The treatment of glioblastoma multiforme of the brain. *J. Neurosurg.* 27: 388–400.

31. Kaplan, H. I., and Streilein, J. W. 1974. Do immunologically privileged sites require a functioning spleen? *Nature* 251: 553–554.

32. Kornblith, P. L., Dohan, F. C., Wood, W. C., and Whitman, B. O. 1974. Human astrocytoma: Serum-modiated response. *Cancer* 33: 1513–1519.

33. Kredel, F. E. 1928. Tissue culture of intracranial tumors. *Amer. J. Path.* 4: 337–340.

34. Krementz, E. T., and Samuels, M. S. 1967. Tumor cross transplantation and cross transfusion in the treatment of abnormal malignant disease. *Bull. Tulane Univ. Med. Faculty* 26: 263–270.

35. Krementz, E. T., Samuels, M., Wallace, J. H., and Benes, E. N. 1970. Clinical experiences in the immunotherapy of cancer. *Abstr. Tenth Int. Cancer Cong.* p. 203.

36. Kumar, S., Taylor, G., Steward, J. K., Waghe, M. A., and Morris, J. P. 1973. Cell-mediated immunity and blocking factors in patients with tumors of the central nervous system. *Int. J. Cancer* 12: 194–205.

37. Kumar, S., and Taylor, G. 1973. Specific lymphocytotoxicity and blocking factors in tumors of the central nervous system. *Brit. J. Cancer* 28(Suppl. 1): 135–141.

38. Levy, N. L., Mahaley, M. S., and Day, E. D. 1972. In vitro demonstration of cell-mediated immunity to human brain tumors. *Cancer Res.* 32: 477–482.

39. Lim, R., and Kluskens, L. 1972. Immunological specificity of astrocytoma antigens. *Cancer Res.* 32: 1667–1670.

40. Mahaley, M. S., Jr., and Day, E. D. 1965. Immunological studies of human gliomas. *J. Neurosurg.* 23: 363–370.

41. Mahaley, M. S., Jr. 1968. Immunological considerations and the malignant glioma problem. *Clin. Neurosurg.* 15: 175–189.

42. Mahaley, M. S., Jr. 1971. Immunological studies with human gliomas. *J. Neurosurg.* 34: 458–459.

43. Mahaley, M. S., Jr. 1972. Immunological aspects of the growth and development of human and experimental brain tumors. *In* Kirsch, W. M., Grossi-Paolletti, E., and Paoletti, P. (eds.), *Experimental Biology of Brain Tumors.* Charles C Thomas Co., 561–547.

44. Medewar, P. B. 1948. Immunity to homologous grafted skin: III. The fate of skin homografts transplanted to the brain, to subcutaneous tissues and anterior chamber of the eye. *Brit. J. Exp. Pathol.* 29: 58–69.

45. Morley, T. D. 1959. The recovery of tumor cells from venous blood draining cerebral gliomas. *Canad. J. Surg.* 2: 363–365.

46. Murphy, J. B., and Sturm, E. 1923. Conditions determining transplantability of tissue to brain. *J. Exp. Med.* 38: 183–197.

47. Nadler, S. H., and Moore, G. E. 1966. Clinical immunologic study of malignant disease: Response to tumor transplants and transfer of leukocytes. *Ann. Surg.* 164: 482–490.

48. Nakagaki, H., Brunhart, G., Kemper, T. L., and Caveness, W. F. 1976. Monkey brain damage from radiation in the therapeutic range. *J. Neurosurg.* 44: 3–11.

49. Ommaya, A. K. 1976. Immunotherapy of gliomas: A review. *Advances in Neurology* 15: 337–359.

50. Ponten, J., and Macintyre, E. H. 1968. Long term culture of normal and neoplastic human glia. *Acta. Path. Microbiol. Scandinav.* 74: 465–486.

51. Regan, T. J., Bisel, H. F., Childs, D. S., Layton, D. P., Rhoton, A. L., and Taylor, W. F. 1976. Controlled study of CCNU and radiation therapy in malignant astrocytoma. *J. Neurosurg.* 44: 186–190.

52. Ridley, A., and Cavanaugh, J. B. 1971. Lymphocytic infiltration in gliomas evidence of possible host resistance. *Brain* 94: 117–124.

53. Rubenstein, L. J. 1972. Tumors of the central nervous system. AFIP Washington, D.C., p. 1.

54. Russell, D. S., and Bland, J. O. W. 1933. A study of gliomas by the method of tissue culture. *J. Path. Bact.* 36: 273–283.

55. Russell, D. S., and Rubenstein, L. J. 1971. Pathology of tumors of the nervous system. Edward Arnold, pp. 1–4.

56. Scheinberg, L. C., Edelman, F. L., and Levy, W. A. 1964. Is the brain "an immunologically privileged site"? I. Studies based on intracerebral homo-transplantation and isotransplantation to sensitized hosts. Arch. Neurol. 11: 248–264.

57. Scheinberg, L. C., and Taylor, J. M. 1968. Immunologic aspects of brain tumors. Prog. Neurol. Surg. 2: 267 201.

58. Schneck, S. A., Penn, I. 1971. De-novo brain tumor in renal transplant recipients. Lancet 1: 983–986.

59. Shirai, Y. 1971. Transplantations of rat sarcomas in adult heterogenous animals. Japan Med. World 1: 14–15.

60. Shuttleworth, E. C., Jr. 1972. Barrier phenomena in brain tumors. Prog. Exp. Tumor Res. 17: 279–290.

61. Sjögren, H. O., Hellström, I., Bansal, S. C., et al. 1971. Suggestive evidence that the "blocking antibodies" of tumor-bearing individuals may be antigen-antibody complexes. Proc. Natl. Acad. Sci. USA 68: 1372–1375.

62. Takakura, K., Miki, Y., Kubo, O., Ogawa, N., Matsutani, M., and Sano, K. 1972. Adjuvant immunotherapy for malignant brain tumors. Jap. J. Clin. Oncol. 12: 109–120.

63. Taveras, J. M., Thompson, H. G., Jr., Pool, J. L. 1962. Should we treat glioblastoma multiforme? A study of survival in 425 cases. Am. I. Ryentgenol. Radium. Ther. Nucl. Med. 87: 473–479.

64. Thomas, W. G. T., Lannigan, C. B., and Behou, P. O. 1975. Impaired cell-mediated immunity in human brain tumors. Lancet 1: 1389–1390.

65. Trouillas, P., and Lapras, C. L. 1970. Immunotherapie active des tumeurs cérébrales. Neuro-Chirugie 16: 143–170.

66. Trouillas, P. 1973. Immunologie et immunotherapie des tumeurs cérébrales. Revue Neurologique 128: 23–34.

67. Vries, J. K., Becker, D. P., Young, H. F. 1973. A subarachnoid screw for monitoring intracranial pressure. J. Neurosurg. 39: 416–419.

68. Wakamatsu, I., Matsuo, T., Kawauo, S., Ieramato, S., and Matsumera, H. 1971. Glioblastoma with extracranial metastasis through ventriculo-pleurol shunt. J. Neurosurg. 34(No. 5): 697–701.

69. Walker, M. D., and Gehan, E. A. 1972. An evaluation of 1,3-Bis (2-chloroethyl)-1-nitrourea (BCNU) and irradiation alone and in combination for the treatment of malignant gliomas. Proc. Amer. Assoc. Cancer Res. 13: 67 (Abstract).

70. Walker, M. D. 1973. Nitrosureas in central nervous system tumors. Cancer Chemother. Rep. Part 3, 4: 21–26.

71. Walker, M. D. 1975. Malignant brain tumors—A synopsis. Ca-A Cancer J. for Clinician 25(No. 3): 114–115.

72. Weir, B. 1973. The relative significance of factors affecting post-operative survival in astrocytomas, grade 3 and 4. J. Neurosurg. 38: 448–452.

73. Weir, B., Band, P., Urtasun, R., Blain, G., McLean, D., Wilson, F., Mielke, B., and Grace, M. 1976. Radiotherapy and CCNU in the treatment of high-grade supratentorial astrocytomas. J. Neurosurg. 45: 129–134.

74. Wickremesinghe, H. R., and Yates, P. O. 1971. Immunological properties of neoplastic neural tissues. *Brit. J. Cancer* 25: 711–720.

75. Wolf, A., Cawen, W., Stewart, W. B. 1954. Glioblastoma with extracranial metastasis byway of a ventriculopleurol anastomasis. *Trans. Amer. Neurol. Ass.* 79: 140–142.

76. Young, H. F., Sakalas, R., and Kaplan, A. M. 1976. Inhibition of cell-mediated immunity in patients with brain tumor. *Surg. Neurol.* 5: 19–23.

77. Young, H. F., Kaplan, A. M., and Regelson, W. 1977. Immunotherapy with autologous white cell infusions ("lymphocytes") in the treatment of recurrent glioblastomus multiforme. *Cancer* 40: 1037–1044.

78. Young, H. F., Kaplan, A. M. 1976. Cellular immune deficiency in patients with glioblastoma. *Surgical Forum* 27: 476–478.

79. Zimmerman, H. M. 1957. The natural history of intracranial neoplasms, with special reference to the gliomas. *Amer. J. Surg.* 93: 913–924.

80. Zulch, K. J. 1957. *Brain Tumors: Their Biology and Pathology.* Springer Publishing Co., New York.

CHAPTER 14

THE ADOPTIVE IMMUNOTHERAPY OF MURINE LEUKEMIA BY ALLOGENEIC BONE MARROW

Eugene E. Emeson

Department of Pathology
Montefiore Hospital and
Medical Center
Albert Einstein College of Medicine
New York, New York 10467

Bone marrow grafts have recently become a part of the overall therapeutic program of selected human leukemia victims. The spontaneously arising and experimental leukemia-lymphomas of mice provide excellent experimental models for establishing some of the basic therapeutic principles of using bone marrow to treat leukemia.

I. INTRODUCTION

Recent advances in the theory and practice of tissue typing and the techniques of bone marrow transplantation, have provided a new approach to the treatment of selected victims of leukemia. For those few afflicted individuals who are fortunate enough to have an identical twin, the use of isogeneic bone marrow transplants in combination with other anti-leukemic agents, has become an important modality of therapy (21, 95). For another somewhat larger group of leukemia victims with an HL-A matched sibling, the use of bone marrow grafts compatible at the HL-A locus has achieved some degree of success when other modalities of therapy have failed (95). A large number of the latter recipients, however, develop severe graft versus host (GVH) disease (although HL-A matched siblings are compatible at the major histocompatibility complex, they are usually compatible at minor histocompatibility loci).

More than 60% of all leukemia victims (28) do not have identical twins or HL-A matched siblings, and cannot, at present, be offered a marrow transplant as part of their therapy, since engrafted allogeneic marrow almost invariably results in fatal GVH disease (95). While improved matching of unrelated individuals at the major histocompatibility complex (MHC) may partially solve the problem, this approach is not widely available at present. The development of a consistently effective and safe methodology for transplanting allogeneic marrow is thus of current interest.

There are at least three possible reasons why a marrow transplant should be considered as part of the therapeutic regimen for leukemia: (1) The use of a syngeneic or allogeneic marrow transplant might enable the patient to tolerate much higher doses (amounts which are ordinarily lethal) of marrow suppressing antileukemic agents that might more completely eradicate his clonogenic leukemia cells; (2) the use of a syngeneic marrow transplant might also reconstitute an immunologic defect in the leukemia victim and, used in combination with chemoradiotherapy, might enable the patient to mount a more effective graft versus leukemia (GVL) response; and (3) the GVH reactivity of allogeneic marrow might potentiate its GVL reactivity.

The following discussion will deal almost exclusively with the use of allogeneic marrow for the treatment of leukemia-lymphomas and will emphasize the mouse as an experimental model.

Among the advantages of using mice in such experiments are that they are readily and cheaply available in a wide variety of inbred strains and that they develop a large variety of well-characterized experimentally induced and naturally occurring leukemia-lymphomas.

One important disadvantage of the use of the mouse as an experimental model is that GVH disease in this animal is less severe and much easier to control or eliminate than in man; therefore, progress achieved in murine models may not always be relevant to man.

II. THE MAJOR PROBLEMS OF TREATING LEUKEMIA WITH ALLOGENEIC MARROW

A. Establishment of the Graft

In the usual model for marrow transplantation in mice, marrow is obtained from one inbred mouse strain (donor) and transplanted to an irradiated recipient of a second inbred strain differing at the MHC (allogeneic model). F_1 hybrids of the donor strain and another inbred strain are frequently used as recipients to minimize a potential host versus graft (HVG) reaction (semi-allogeneic model).

In the allogeneic model, since the marrow recipient is fully capable of rejecting allogeneic marrow by a HVG reaction, it is essential to use immunosuppressive agents to suppress the recipient's immune response. Total body irradiation, cyclophosphamide, anti-lymphocyte serum (ALS), or combinations of the three are most commonly used for this purpose. The amount of immunosuppression required is strongly influenced by the degree of incompatibility between the donor and recipient (106). Donor: recipient combinations differing at the MHC require the use of much larger amounts of immunosuppression than those compatible at the MHC. The degree of immunogenetic disparity between donor and recipient also strongly influences the number of donor marrow cells required for engraftment. In mice, hematopoietic restoration requires ten to eighty times as many allogeneic marrow cells as isogeneic cells (106). Prior exposure of recipient to a donor's transplantation antigens, either from blood transfusions or prior attempts to graft marrow may seriously jeopardize the success of a graft, although recent experiments in dogs suggest that the presensitized state can be abrogated by the combined use of procarbazine and heterologeus anti-thymocyte serum given prior to the total body irradiation (93). The recipient is also treated with immunosuppressive agents in the semi-allogeneic model in order to reduce the tumor burden and to prevent the possibility of the recipient rejecting the marrow graft by attacking the surface membrane recognition receptors of the donor lymphocytes (81).

Immunosuppressive agents used to condition marrow recipients should also have marked activity against tumors and "space" making properties. The anti-tumor activity is required because adoptive immunotherapy is usually only effective against a small tumor burden (31, 36, 113). The concept of "space" required for marrow engraftment includes not only physical space, but other poorly defined factors of the marrow microenvironment that are required for successful engraftment (87). In mice, allogeneic marrow transplants are subject to at least one additional restriction that is determined by a class of noncodominant genes designated Hh for hematopoietic-histocompatibility (22, 23, 64). Donor marrow grafts that differ from the recipient at this locus are subject to an unusually radioresistant HVG. The recipient cells responsible for this reaction are extremely radioresistant and are thought to consist of a subpopulation of silica-sensitive macrophages and another nonthymic lymphoid cell (64). It is not presently known for certain if an analogous genetic system occurs in man. There is some evidence that this genetic resistance to bone marrow transplantation represents a natural lymphoma-leukemia defense mechanism (38, 56).

B. Prevention of GVH Disease

The most important obstacle to the successful transplantation of allogeneic marrow at present is GVH disease. In this disease donor lymphocytes with specific GVH reactivity to recipient alloantigens launch an active immunological assault against the recipient. This attack, primarily launched at the recipients' lymphoid organs, skin, gastrointestinal tract and liver, impairs the function of these organs, thereby rendering the recipient extremely susceptible to infection. This immunological assault is predominantly cell-mediated with T-lymphocytes assuming the role of principal aggressors. (For recent reveiws of the biology of GVH reactions, see 27, 45). GVH disease presents itself in both an acute and chronic or delayed form. Acute symptoms appear within the first two or three weeks after grafting and are generally severe. The chronic form of the disease is more insidious and appears from one to three months following engraftment. Both forms of the disease are associated with a high mortality.

Allogeneic marrow grafts (mismatched at the MHC) cause the acute form of GVH disease in humans, other primates, and dogs, and the chronic form in mice. This difference is thought to be due to the fact that there are far fewer immunocompetent T-cells in mouse marrow than in human marrow. The delay in onset of the disease in mice may represent the time required for T-cell precursors to multiply and reach maturity.

Measures that have been employed to prevent GVH reactivity of adoptively transferred marrow can be classified into one of two general categories: nonspecific and immunospecific. Both can be directed at the marrow donor prior to obtaining the marrow, or at the marrow cells in vitro, or at the recipient following the transplant. A wide variety of pharmacological, biological and physical agents have been used in all categories.

The following agents have been used with variable degrees of success to nonspecifically treat bone marrow donors. Anti-lymphocytic serum (ALS) (17, 57, 59, 89), FAB fragment of ALS (40), lymphoid cell chalones (41), recipient alloantigens (72), recipient alloantigens plus cyclophosphamide (37), a variety of antigens other than alloantigens (61), and bacterial endotoxin (84). The treatment of marrow donors by neonatal thymectomy and/or lethal total body irradiation (7, 27, 74) can also substantially reduce GVH reactivity of marrow, but these measures are far too damaging to the donor to be considered for clinical use. Alloantigens plus cyclophosphamide (37, 108), killed Corynebacterium parvum (88), phytohemaglutinin, and hemocyanin (49) have been used to treat donors of lymphoid cells other than marrow.

Among the large variety of nonspecific agents that have been used to treat donor lymphoid cells in vitro to reduce GVH reactivity are ASL (17, 59, 89, 97), FAB fragment of ALS (39, 82), anti-TL serum (96), anti-Thy-l serum (20, 90, 102), lymphoid cell chalones (41, 55), phytohemaglutinin (67), Concanavalin A (58, 103), mitomicin C (60), neuraminidase (2, 50), ultraviolet light (48) and differential centrifugation (19, 26, 42). Culturing marrow cells at 37C (71) with or without the presence of recipient alloantigen (15, 68) has also been successfully employed to eliminate GVH reactivity. In general, agents that can be used to treat the marrow in vitro are preferable to those requiring treatment of donor or recipient, since they present no additional hazards to the donor or recipient.

The ability to control GVH disease in marrow recipients depends upon the severity of the reaction. The severest reactions, occurring when donors and recipients are mismatched at the MHC, are extremely difficult to control, while the somewhat milder reactions, resulting when they are matched at the MHC, may be curbed by immunosuppressive agents. Cyclophosphamide (77, 107), methotrexate (91, 107), ALS (57), or combinations of these agents have been used to suppress GVH reactions with variable degrees of success. Mathé et al. (72) have recently demonstrated a reduction of GVH reactivity in murine marrow recipients treated with thymic chalone.

The important pitfall of using nonspecific measures to suppress GVH disease is that they suppress a broad spectrum of bone marrow activities and often make an immunological cripple out of the recipient. Immunospecific measures attempt to selectively suppress only those donor cells with specific reactivity to the recipient's alloantigens and at the same time attempt to preserve donor cells with reactivity against the rest of the immunological universe.

Immunospecific measures generally act by directly eliminating or inactivating lymphocytes with specific GVH reactivity or by activation of suppressor mechanisms involving serum blocking factors (24, 46, 109, 114, 116), lymphocyte factors (35), or cell-to-cell interactions (43).

Several recently developed immunospecific methods to suppress the GVH reactivity of transplanted lymphoid cells deserve special mention. Bonavida and Kedar (10), Mage et al. (66), and Lonai et al. (63) have succeeded in depleting allogeneic lymphoid cells of specific GVH reactivity by absorbing them onto cultured allogeneic cell monolayers. This method has not as yet, to my knowledge, been used successfully to graft allogeneic marrow in either rodents or man. There is also recent evidence that one can prevent significant recipient GVH disease by using donor lymphoid cells free of post-thymic T-lymphocytes. This approach has proven to be successful in rodents by Sprent et al. (90) who used anti-Thy-l treated parental marrow cells to reconstitute lethally irradiated F_1 recipients and by several groups of investigators (65, 101, 104) who used allogeneic fetal liver cells to reconstitute lethally irradiated recipient mice. These studies suggest that prethymic T-cells are susceptible to tolerance induction to alloantigen even when in an adult environment. The prethymic T-cells with specific reactivity to antigens other than the alloantigens of the recipients apparently achieve a relatively normal state of immune competence when they mature. More recently fetal liver cells have been used to successfully reconstitute three patients with severe combined immunodeficiency (18, 53).

Two approaches for deleting GVH reactivity from lymphoid cells from sites other than marrow may prove to be effective with those from marrow. In both approaches radioactive isotopes with high specific activity were used to render lymphocytes with specific GVH reactivity inactive. In the first approach lymphocytes with specific GVH reactivity were destroyed in vitro by the damaging effects of ^{3}H-thymidine of high specific activity, which they incorporated following their exposure in vitro to the recipient's alloantigens ("burn out" method) (85). In the second approach, the purified alloantigens of the recipient, labeled with isotope of high specific activity, were added to lymphocytes in vitro to selectively seek out and kill those lymphocytes with specific antirecipient GVH reactivity (antigen suicide) (1). Both of these latter approaches are immunospecific, but neither has been used successfully, to my knowledge, to eliminate GVH reactivity from marrow. And finally, Binz (8) and Joller (51) have used specific anti-idiotypic antibody in vivo and in vitro to selectively reduce specific GVH reactions in mice. It is unlikely that the appropriate anti-idiotypic antibodies to human lymphocytes will be available in the near future. In fact, of all the methods discussed in this section, none have proven to be consistently reliable in humans.

C. Potentiation of GVL Reactivity

Since available conditioning regimens cannot completely irradicate the tumor cells of leukemic mice, marrow transplants must not only enable the animal to survive the immediate post-conditioning period, but must assist the animal's efforts to eliminate those tumor cells which survive the conditioning regimen. While allogeneic lymphoid cells, including allogeneic bone marrow, have been demonstrated to have a considerable degree of GVL reactivity (Reviewed in 31, 33), syngeneic or H-2 matched lymphoid cells have little or no demonstrable GVL reactivity unless preimmunized against the recipient's tumor cells (14, 30, 34, 44, 105). Evidence has been recently provided that engrafted lymphoid cells must contain T-lymphocytes (6) and must persist, at least transiently, in the recipient to have a GVL effect (54).

At least three general approaches are available to potentiate the GVL reactivity of adoptively transferred marrow cells: (1) Syngeneic or MHC-matched marrow can be preimmunized to the tumor specific antigens (TSA) of the recipients' leukemia cells in vitro, (2) recipients of syngeneic or allogeneic marrow can be actively immunized with the TSA of their own tumor cells and adjuvants after the transplant (active immunotherapy plus adoptive immunotherapy), and (3) the GVH reactivity of allogeneic marrow can be utilized.

In regard to the first approach, several groups of investigators have presented evidence that lymphoid cells can be preimmunized to TSA in vitro (47, 52, 98, 110). Of these, the methods of Treves et al. (98) and Hellström and Hellström (47) appear to be the ones that could be most readily applicable to humans. These investigators demonstrated that murine splenic or lymph node lymphocytes could be sensitized in vitro to TSA by culturing them with syngeneic macrophages that had been previously fed with a cell-free antigen preparation of syngeneic tumor cells. These sensitized cells displayed specific anti-tumor reactivity both in vitro and in vivo. None of the above investigators used bone marrow cells. The fact that bone marrow contains but a small proportion of mature T-lymphocytes (111, 115) suggests that the task of preimmunizing it to TSA in vitro would be a formidable one. The addition of donor peripheral blood leukocytes to the marrow culture to increase its proportion of

T-lymphocytes and/or the modification of the antigenicity of the TSA to make them more immunogenic (11, 62, 80, 83) might make the in vitro approach more feasible with bone marrow cells.

The second approach, that of actively immunizing the recipient, surprisingly enough, has not been previously utilized in combination with allogeneic marrow.

The third approach, use of a GVH reaction to potentiate GVL reactivity has received considerable attention in the past 20 years and will be discussed in detail in Section III.

D. Restoration of Normal Immunological Competence in the Recipient

Thus far I have dealt primarily with the marrow recipient's ability to respond immunologically to the few residual leukemia-lymphoma cells remaining after the conditioning regimen. It is also important that the recipient be able to recover immunological competence in general. Lethally irradiated mice saved with bone marrow, whether syngeneic or allogeneic, have markedly impaired or absent humoral or cell mediated immunity for a variable period of time after transplantation, depending on the immune parameter tested, the dose of the antigen used for testing and, to a lesser extent, the strain of mouse studied (Reviewed in 29, 76, 95). Mice reconstituted with syngeneic marrow ultimately regain relatively normal immune reactivity while those that survive GVH disease after reconstitution with allogeneic marrow, recover reactivity at a slower rate, and more often than not, exhibit residual immunological defects. The slower recovery of immune reactivity in allogeneic chimeras as compared to syngeneic chimeras is thought to be due to the destructive effects of the GVH reaction on donor lymphoid cells, the immunosuppressive effects of agents used to condition the host and/or prevent GVH disease, and the immunodeficiency that may result from a GVH induced malabsorption syndrome (95). Long-term human survivors of allogeneic marrow grafts also exhibit long-lasting selective immunological defects such as inability to be sensitized to dinitrochlorobenzene (29) and increased susceptibility to interstitial pneumonias due to Pneumocytis carinei, cytomegalic virus, varicella zoster, as well as other infectious agents (75). Bacterial and candidal infections are frequent and especially serious in marrow recipients with agranulocytosis (9). In contrast to both rodents and humans, canine recipients of allogeneic marrow show almost complete recovery of both cellular and humoral immunity if they survive at least 200 days after grafting (76).

One additional complication of marrow transplantation for the treatment of leukemia which may or may not be due to the recipients' suppressed immune response is that of recurrent leukemia in which the leukemic cells are apparently of donor origin. Evidence in favor of malignant transformation of donor cells in two female patients with childhood acute lymphoblastic leukemia has been presented (36, 94).

It may be possible to accelerate and/or improve normal immunologic competence in allogeneic marrow recipients by the use of transfer factor, immune RNA, or non-specific immunopotentiators such as thymopoetin, levamisole, BCG, or C. parvum.

III. REVIEW OF PREVIOUS ATTEMPTS AT USING ALLOGENEIC MARROW FOR THE ADOPTIVE IMMUNOTHERAPY OF MURINE LEUKEMIA

As previously indicated, neither in vivo or in vitro methods have as yet been developed to preimmunize bone marrow against the TSA of leukemic cells. Furthermore, since syngeneic or MHC-matched marrow has little or no capacity to generate GVL reactivity, allogeneic marrow has most often been utilized in animal research. This approach dates back to the studies of Barnes et al. (4) and Barnes and Loutit (5) who showed that CBA mice, injected with a transplantable syngeneic irradiation-induced leukemia and treated with lethal irradiation plus syngeneic or allogeneic marrow have a slightly prolonged survival as compared to untreated controls. Those mice that received syngeneic marrow died with overt leukemia while mice that received allogeneic marrow died of a chronic wasting disease (which we now know to be GVH disease). Many of the latter mice were found to be free of leukemia. Similar results were obtained by de Vries and Vos (25) when treating a transplantable spontaneous lymphosarcoma of C57Bl/6 origin, Mathé et al. (70) when treating the L1210 leukemia with allogeneic marrow and/or lymph node cells in (DBA × C57Bl/6)F$_1$ mice, and Boranić (12) when using allogeneic marrow and spleen cells in a RF myeloid leukemia model and a lymphoid leukemia of A-strain mice. Wallis et al. (112) demonstrated a marked decrease in the incidence of radiation induced leukemia in F$_1$ mice receiving parental marrow or spleen cells.

The convincing evidence that a GVH reaction could eradicate leukemia cells led to the next important problem, how to rescue the recipient from the deadly GVH disease which almost invariably followed successful destruction of leukemia cells. Would it be possible to dissociate the desirable GVL effects from the dreaded GVH effect or were the two effects inseparable? These problems were first explored by Mathé et al. (69) in a L1210 tumor model in (DBA × C51Bl/6)F$_1$ mice. Mice were treated with 850R and bone marrow from normal C57Bl/6 donors and then started on a regimen of methotrexate or cyclophosphamide two weeks later. The addition of methotrexate or cyclophosphamide regimen to control GVH disease resulted in an increased number of long-term cures. In the previously mentioned model of Boranić (12), the use of cyclophosphamide and anti-lymphocyte serum to control GVH disease resulted in a prolonged survival of mice treated with these agents, although only one mouse survived over 100 days. Most of these animals were allegedly free of leukemia. The dosage and time schedule of the cyclophosphamide administration was later shown to be critical for obtaining these results (13). Mice rescued from GVH disease by cyclophosphamide and syngeneic hematopoietic cells showed the most prolonged survival times with 75% surviving two months or more and 36% surviving more than 100 days. Of the 14 animals that died between days 60 and 90, 12 were thought to be free of leukemia.

Bortin et al. (16) used an approach similar to that of Boranić to rescue leukemic AKR mice from the GVH effects of DBA/2 marrow. They used sublethal doses of total body irradiation in combination with sublethal doses of cyclophosphamide to condition the marrow recipients. This conditioning regimen had a marked anti-tumor effect and permitted engraftment of the marrow. The sequential use of cyclophosphamide, a potential anti-DBA/2 serum (to eliminate the aggressor DBA cells) and a second marrow graft from H-2-compatible CBA or RF donors (to restore the animals' hematopoietic tissue) was then used to rescue the mice from GVH disease. The marrow of the two H-2-compatible strains, especially that of the RF strain caused far less GVH mortality than the H-2-incompatible DBA/2 marrow. These investigators (14) also provided evidence that GVH and GVL reactions can be separated. Their observations, if valid in other experimental leukemia models (and humans), are extremely important in that they are among the first to suggest that allogeneic cells can be used to effectively destroy residual tumor cells without demolishing the recipient in the process. Kende et al. (54), on the other hand, were unable to separate the GVH and GVL reactions by alloantiserum in their studies of a transplantable Moloney leukemia in Balb/C mice. The fact that their studies involved a different tumor model, and more importantly, the fact that they utilized immunized allogeneic spleen cells for the adoptive transfer, may account for the discrepancies in these two studies. Similar attempts at rescuing dogs (92) and monkeys (73) from GVH disease have encountered little success.

Two additional methods of preventing fatal GVH disease in murine leukemia-lymphoma models treated with allogeneic lymphoid cells are of considerable interest. Pollard and his co-workers at the University of

Notre Dame have exploited the fact that irradiated germ-free mice reconstituted with allogeneic bone marrow survive without clinical evidence of
GVH disease to successfully treat two leukemia-lymphoma models in
mice. These investigators (78) were able to prevent the development of
spontaneous leukemia in germ-free AKR mice by treating them at 11
weeks of age with 1000R total body irradiation followed 24 hours later
with a marrow graft from germ-free DBA/2 mice. Conventional AKR mice
normally begin to develop leukemia at 6 months of age with 90% being
affected by 9 months of age. When a similar therapeutic regimen was used
to treat mice that had already developed clinical evidence of leukemia, 11
of 12 mice survived the 60-day observation period (100). Untreated AKR
mice die within 10 days after the appearance of leukemia symptoms.
There was also a high 60-day survival (14 of 17) among identically treated
conventional mice which were decontaminated of bacteria and fungi by
12 or more weeks of antibiotic therapy. The prevention and treatment of
the reticular cell sarcoma in SJL mice by similar means was also successful (79, 99). In contrast, most of the conventional mice (not decontaminated) or irradiated mice receiving syngeneic marrow died of GVH disease and/or recurrence of leukemia in both the AKR and SJL models.
While these studies are obviously of great importance, since they suggest
that it may be possible to avoid the GVH disease of allogeneic marrow by
bacterial decontamination of the recipient, Thomas et al. (95) have recently stated that "As yet there is no objective evidence that a protective
environment is of value in human marrow transplantation."

And finally, Fefer (32) has provided evidence that the fatal consequences of GVH disease can be circumvented by the use of a "sneak
through" procedure. In these experiments, Fefer showed that H-2 incompatible spleen cells in numbers inadequate to produce clinically evident
GVH disease, in conjunction with cyclophosphamide were more effective
against a Moloney virus-induced lymphoma than cyclophosphamide
alone. Whether or not this approach can be effectively utilized with bone
marrow is not currently known.

IV. FUTURE PROSPECTS

The successful use of bone marrow to treat murine leukemia and,
by extrapolation, human leukemia requires: (1) Potent anti-cancer agents
to reduce the tumor burden; (2) the adequate engraftment and, to some
extent, survival of the marrow; (3) the presence of GVL reactivity within
the marrow; and (4) the avoidance of lethal GVH disease by the marrow.
While advances in our understanding of these requirements are accruing

at a rapid rate, huge gaps in our knowledge persist, rendering the use of allogeneic marrow more or less a last resort measure for the treatment of most leukemia victims.

As I view these requirements, several general approaches seem most fruitful. One approach depends primarily on the development of anti-cancer agents capable of completely eradicating the clonogenic leukemia cells of the leukemia victim or at least rendering them susceptible to immunologic destruction. Bone marrow transplants would then be required only to the extent that these anti-cancer agents inadvertently destroyed the patient's immunologic and hematopoietic capacity and would not be required for their GVL potentiality. If successful in this endeavor, I believe that added investigative efforts could then be directed toward using syngeneic marrow when available and improving our methods of matching marrow donors and recipients when syngeneic marrow is not available. In this regard much of the methodology for matching donor and recipient MHC is currently at hand (reviewed in 3). As these methods improve and become more widely available throughout the world, it is conceivable that, with the help of modern computer technology, properly matched donors will be readily available within the next few years. The use of syngeneic or matched marrow has the added benefit in that it avoids many of the problems of marrow engraftment failure and GVH disease.

If completely effective anti-cancer agents cannot be developed, then syngeneic or MHC-matched marrow cannot be relied upon by themselves as adequate immunotherapy, since as previously pointed out, syngeneic or MHC-matched marrow is not very effective against leukemia cells unless preimmunized to their TSA. An alternative approach, therefore, is to develop the means to preimmunize syngeneic or MHC-matched marrow. In vitro methods would be preferable to other methods since they could be most readily adapted for use with humans. It is currently possible to preimmunize spleen or lymph node cells of rodents in vitro. The task of preimmunizing bone marrow cells which contain meager numbers of T-lymphocytes will undoubtedly turn out to be a far more difficult undertaking. The addition of donor peripheral blood leukocytes to the culture might improve the chances of achieving adequate in vitro preimmunization by virtue of the added T-lymphocytes, but may alternatively aggravate the problem of GVH disease if the donor and recipient are not adequately matched.

A third approach, the utilization of the GVH reactivity of MHC-incompatible allogeneic marrow to potentiate GVL reactivity, has proven to be extremely successful in wiping out residual clonogeneic leukemia cells in experimental animal models, but requires bold and effective new measures for dealing with the devastating effects of GVH disease, especially in humans. While I am certain that such measures can be developed in the not-too-distant future, one enormous question mark regarding the use of allogeneic marrow freed of GVH reactivity persists. Can the GVL effects of the marrow be retained when the GVH effects are eliminated, i.e., are the two effects in fact separable? The effectiveness of allogeneic marrow might also be further improved by preimmunizing it in vitro to the TSA of the leukemia cells, although it might be necessary to use TSA freed of their associated alloantigens for this purpose lest the marrow cells also develop increased GVH reactivity.

One final comment should be made in regard to suppressor T-cells. A further understanding of this exciting new target of research could conceivably provide methods of manipulating the reactivity of donor and recipient cell populations making it feasible to bolster GVL reactivity and/or reduce GVH reactivity of transplanted marrow by radically different approaches.

In conclusion, the problems associated with the use of allogeneic marrow for the treatment of murine leukemia have been dealt with in detail. Some of the solutions to these problems will not only be applicable to a wide variety of non-neoplastic diseases such as immuno-deficiency diseases, aplastic anemias, and genetic blood diseases, but will also further our understanding of the immunobiology of the lymphocyte.

ACKNOWLEDGMENTS

This work was supported by Grant CA 1746-02 awarded by the National Cancer Institute, DHEW. The author gratefully acknowledges the assistance of Jean Emeson for editing the manuscript and Elda Brown for typing it.

REFERENCES

1. Ada, G. L., and Byrt, P. 1969. Specific inactivation of antigen reactive cells with ^{125}I-labeled antigen. Nature 22: 1291–1292.

2. Adolphs, H. D. 1973. Humoral antibody response and GVH reactivity with neuraminidase treated murine lymphocytes as donor cells. Z. Immunitaetsforsch. Exp. Immunol. 146: 45–54.

3. Bach, F. H., and van Rood, J. J. 1976. The major histocompatibility complex—genetics and biology. N. Engl. J. Med. 295: 806–813, 872–878, 927–936.

4. Barnes, D. W. H., Corp, M. J., and Loutit, J. F. 1956. Treatment of murine leukaemia with x-rays and homologous bone marrow. Brit. Med. J. 2: 626–627.

5. Barnes, D. W. H., and Loutit, J. F. 1957. Treatment of murine leukemia with x-rays and homologous bone marrow: II. Brit. J. Haemat. 3: 241–252.

6. Berenson, J. R., Einstein, A. B., Jr., and Fefer, A. 1975. Syngeneic adoptive immunotherapy and chemoimmunotherapy of a Friend leukemia: Requirement for T cells. J. Immunol. 115: 234–238.

7. Billingham, R. E. 1968. The biology of graft-versus-host reactions. Harvey Lect. 62: 21–78.

8. Binz, H. 1975. Local graft-versus-host reaction in mice specifically inhibited by anti-receptor antibodies. Scand. J. Immunol. 4: 79–87.

9. Bodey, G. P. 1973. Infections in patients with cancer, in J. F. Holland and E. Frei (eds.), Cancer Medicine 1973, p. 1135–1165. Lea and Febiger, Philadelphia, Pa.

10. Bonavida, B., and Kedar, F. 1974. Transplantation of allogeneic lymphoid cells specifically depleted of graft versus host reactive cells. Nature 249: 658–659.

11. Boone, C., and Blackman, K. 1972. Augmented immunogenicity of tumor cells homogenates infected with influenza virus. Cancer Res. 32: 1018–1022.

12. Boranić, M. 1968. Transient graft-versus-host reaction in the treatment of leukemia in mice. J. Natl. Cancer Inst. 41: 421–433.

13. Boranić, M., and Tonković, I. 1971. Time pattern of the antileukemic effect of graft-versus-host reaction in mice. Cancer Res. 31: 1140–1147.

14. Bortin, M. M., Rimm, A. A., Rose, W. C., and Saltzstein, E. C. 1974. Graft-versus-leukemia. V. Absence of antileukemic effect using allogeneic H-2-identical immunocompetent cells. Transplantation 18: 280–283.

15. Bortin, M. M., Rimm, A. A., and Saltzstein, E. C. 1971. Graft-versus-host inhibition. IV. Production of allogeneic radiation chimeras using incubated spleen and liver cell mixtures. J. Immunol. 107: 1063–1070.

16. Bortin, M. M., Rose, W. C., Truitt, R. L., Rimm, A. A., Saltzstein, E. C., and Rodey, G. E. 1975. Brief communication: Graft versus leukemia. VI. Adoptive immunotherapy in combination with chemoradiotherapy for spontaneous leukemia-lymphoma in AKR mice. J. Natl. Cancer Inst. 55: 1277–1229.

17. Brent, L., Courtenay, T., and Gowland, G. 1967. Immunological reactivity of lymphoid cells after treatment with antilymphocytic serum. Nature 215: 1461–1464.

18. Buckley, R. H., Whisnant, J. K., Schiff, R. I., Gilbersten, R. B., Huong, A. T., and Platt, M. S. 1976. Correction of severe combined immunodeficiency by fetal liver cells. N. Engl. J. Med. 294: 1076–1081.

19. Burleson, R., and Levey, R. H. 1972. Studies on the isolation of lymphocytes active in cell-mediated immune responses. I. Demonstration of an active population of thymus-derived cells in mouse bone marrow. Cell. Immunol. 4: 305–315.

20. Cantor, H. 1972. The effects of anti-theta antiserum upon graft-versus-host activity of spleen and lymph node cells. Cell. Immunol. 3: 461–469.

21. Cline, M. J., Gale, R. P., Stiehm, E. R., Opelz, G., Young, L. S., Feig, S. A., and Fahey, J. L. 1975. Bone marrow transplantation in man. Ann. Intern. Med. 83: 691–708.

22. Cudkowicz, G., and Bennett, M. 1971. Peculiar immunobiology of bone marrow allografts. I. Graft rejection by irradiated responder mice. J. Exp. Med. 134: 83–102.

23. Cudkowicz, G., and Bennett, M. 1971. Peculiar immunobiology of bone marrow allografts. II. Rejections of parental grafts by resistant F_1 hybrid mice. *J. Exp. Med.* 134: 1513–1528.

24. Currie, G. A., and Basham, C. 1972. Serum mediated inhibition of the immunological reactions of the patient to his own tumour: A possible role for circulating antigen. *Brit. J. Cancer* 26: 427–438.

25. de Vries, M. J., and Vos, O. 1958. Treatment of mouse lymphosarcoma by total-body X irradiation and by injection of bone marrow and lymph node cells. *J. Natl. Cancer Inst.* 21: 1117–1129.

26. Dicke, K. A., Tridente, G., van Bekkum, D. W. 1969. The selective elimination of immunologically competent cells from bone marrow and lymphocyte cell mixtures. *Transplantation* 8: 422–434.

27. Elkins, W. L. 1971. Cellular immunology and the pathogenesis of graft versus host reactions. *Progr. Allergy* 15: 78–222.

28. Fahey, J. L., Mann, D. L., Asofsky, R., and Rogentine, G. N. 1969. Recent progress in human transplantation. *Ann. Intern. Med.* 71: 1177–1196.

29. Fass, L., Ochs, H. D., Thomas, E. D., Mickelson, E., Storb, R., and Fefer, A. 1973. Studies of immunological reactivity following syngeneic or allogeneic marrow grafts in man. *Transplantation* 16: 630–640.

30. Fefer, A. 1971. Adoptive chemoimmunotherapy of a Moloney lymphoma. *Int. J. Cancer* 8: 364–373.

31. Fefer, A. 1973. Adoptive tumor immunotherapy in mice as an adjunct to whole body X-irradiation or chemotherapy: A review. *Israel J. Med. Sci.* 9: 350–365.

32. Fefer, A. 1973. Treatment of a Moloney lymphoma with cyclophosphamide and H-2 incompatible spleen cells. *Cancer Res.* 33: 641–644.

33. Fefer, A., Einstein, A. B., Jr., and Cheever, M. A. 1976. Adoptive chemoimmunotherapy of cancer in animals: A review of results, principles and problems. *Ann. N.Y. Acad. Sci.* 277: 492–504.

34. Fefer, A., Einstein, A. B., Jr., Cheever, M. A., and Berenson, J. R. 1976. Models for syngeneic adoptive chemoimmunotherapy of murine leukemias. *Ann. N.Y. Acad. Sci.* 276: 573–583.

35. Feldman, M. 1974. Antigen specific T-cell factors and their role in the regulation of T-B interaction, in E. Sercarz, A. R. Williamson, and C. F. Fox (eds.), *The Immune System: Genes, Receptors, Signals 1974*, pp. 497–510. Academic Press, New York.

36. Fialkow, P. J., Thomas, E. D., Bryant, J. I., and Neiman, P. E. 1971. Leukaemic transformation of engrafted human marrow cells in vivo. *Lancet* 1: 251–255.

37. Fink, M. P., and Cloud, C. L. 1974. Graft-versus-host disease in rats after donor treatment with cyclophosphamide and spleen cells of host origin. *Transplantation* 17: 508–512.

38. Gallagher, M. T., Lotzová, E., and Trentin, J. J. 1976. Genetic resistance to marrow transplantation as a leukemia defense mechanism. *Biomed.* 25: 1–3.

39. Gallagher, M. T., Richie, E. R., Heim, L. R., Judd, K., Trentin, J. J. 1972. Inhibition of the graft-versus-host reaction. I. Reduction of the graft-versus-host

potential of mouse spleen cells (with a sparing of stem cells) by treatment with antilymphocyte globulin derived Fab fragments. *Transplantation* 14: 597–602.

40. Gallagher, M. T., Richie, E. R., and Trentin, J. J. 1973. Inhibition of allograft reactivity *in vitro* and *in vivo* by Fab fragments obtained from ALG. *Transpl. Proc.* 5: 869–872.

41. Garcia-Giralt, E., Morales, V. H., Lasalvia, E., and Mathé, G. 1972. Suppression of graft-versus-host reaction by a spleen extract. *J. Immunol.* 109: 878–880.

42. Gelfand, E. W., Phillips, R. A., Miller, R. G., McCulloch, E. A., and Rosen, F. S. 1974. The use of cell separation techniques and isoantibody to host antigens in the treatment of severe combined immunodeficiency disease with HLA incompatible maternal marrow. *Exp. Hematol.* 2: 122–130.

43. Gershon, R. K. 1974. T-cell control of antibody production, *in* M. D. Cooper and N. L. Warner (eds.), *Contemporary Topics in Immunobiology 1970*, 3: 1–40. Plenum Press, New York.

44. Glynn, J. P., and Kende, M. 1971. Treatment of Moloney virus-induced leukemia with cyclophosphamide and specifically sensitized allogeneic cells. *Cancer Res.* 31: 1383–1388.

45. Grebe, S. C., and Streilein, J. W. 1976. Graft-versus-host reactions: A review. *Adv. Immunol.* 22: 119–221.

46. Hellström, K. E., and Hellström, I. 1974. Lymphocyte-mediated cytotoxicity and blocking serum activity to tumour antigens. *Adv. Immunol.* 18: 209–277.

47. Hellström, I., and Hellström, K. E. 1976. Specific sensitization of lymphocytes to tumor antigens by co-cultivation with peritoneal cells exposed to such antigens. *Int. J. Cancer* 17: 748–754.

48. Horowitz, S., Cripps, D., and Hong, R. 1974. Selective T-cell killing of human lymphocytes by ultraviolet radiation. *Cell. Immunol.* 14: 80–86.

49. Hunter, R. L., Millman, R. B., and Lerner, E. M., II. 1969. Suppression of graft-versus-host disease and antibody formation by phytohemaglutinin. *Transplantation* 8: 413–421.

50. Im, H. M., and Simmons, R. L. 1971. Modification of graft-versus-host disease by neuraminidase treatment of donor cells. Decreased tolerogenicity of neuraminidase treatment of donor cells. *Transplantation* 12: 472–478.

51. Joller, P. W. 1972. Graft-versus-host reactivity of lymphoid cells inhibited by anti-recognition serum. *Nature New Biol.* 240: 214–215.

52. Kall, M. A., and Hellström, I. 1975. Specific stimulatory and cytotoxic effects of lymphocytes sensitized *in vitro* to either alloantigens or tumor antigens. *J. Immunol.* 114: 1083–1088.

53. Keightley, R. G., Lawton, A. R., and Cooper, M. D. 1975. Successful fetal liver transplantation in a child with severe combined immunodeficiency. *Lancet* 2: 850–853.

54. Kende, M., Keys, L. D., Gaston, M., and Goldin, A. 1975. Immunochemotherapy of transplantable Moloney leukemia with cyclophosphamide and allogeneic spleen lymphocytes and reversal of graft-versus-host disease with alloantiserum. *Cancer Res.* 35: 346–351.

55. Kiger, N., Florentin, I., and Mathé, G. 1973. Inhibition of graft-versus-host reaction by preincubation of the graft with a thymic extract (lymphocyte chalone). *Transplantation* 16: 393–397.

56. Kumar, V., Bennett, M., and Eckner, R. J. 1974. Mechanism of genetic resistance to Friend virus leukemia in mice. I. Role of ^{89}Sr-sensitive effector cells responsible for rejection of bone marrow allograft. *J. Exp. Med.* 139: 1093–1109.

57. Ledney, G. D. 1969. Antilymphocyte serum in the therapy and prevention of acute secondary disease in mice. *Transplantation* 8: 127–140.

58. Ledney, G. D. 1972. Secondary disease in mice after *in vitro* exposure of hematopoietic cells to concanavalin A. *Transplantation* 14: 671–682.

59. Ledney, G. D., and van Bekkum, D. W. 1968. Suppression of acute secondary disease in the mouse with antilymphocyte serum, *in* J. Dausset, J. Hamburger, and G. Mathé (eds.), *Advances in Transplantation 1968*, pp. 441–447. Williams and Wilkins, Baltimore.

60. Lemmel, E. M., and Good, R. 1969. Immunsuppressive action of mitomycin C on lymphoid cells. I. Effect on cell-mediated immunity after *in vitro* treatment, tolerance induction, and recovery *in vivo*. *Int. Arch. Allergy Appl. Immunol.* 36: 554–565.

61. Liacopopoulos, P., Merchant, B., and Harrell, B. E. 1967. Inhibition of graft-versus-host reactions by pretreatment of donors with various antigens. *Transplantation* 5: 1423–1435.

62. Lindenmann, J., and Klein, P. A. 1967. Viral oncolysis: Increased immunogeneicity of host cell antigen associated with influenza virus. *J. Exp. Med.* 126: 93–108.

63. Lonai, P., Eliraz, A., Wekerle, H., and Feldman, M. 1973. Depletion of specific graft-versus-host reactivity following adsorption of nonsensitized lymphocytes on allogeneic fibroblasts. *Transplantation* 15: 368–374.

64. Lotzová, E., Gallagher, M. T., and Trentin, J. J. 1976. Macrophage involvement in genetic resistance to bone marrow transplantation. *Transpl. Proc.* 8: 477–482.

65. Lowenberg, B. 1975. Fetal liver cell transplantation: Role and nature of the fetal haematopoietic stem cell. Doctoral Thesis, Erasmus University (Rotterdam) Rijswijk (A.H.), The Netherlands, Publication of the Radiobiological Institute, pp. 1–142.

66. Mage, M. G., McHugh, L. L., and Rothstein, T. L. 1976. Separation of graft-versus-host antigen reactive cells *in vitro*. *Transpl. Proc.* 8: 399–401.

67. Marcus, Z., Rigas, D., Siegel, B. V. 1968. Suppression of graft-versus-host reaction by phytohemagglutinin. *Experientia* 24: 836–837.

68. Marcus, Z. 1969. Suppression of graft-versus-host phenomenon by specific antigen. *Transplantation* 8: 80–83.

69. Mathé, G., Amiel, J. L., and Niemetz, J. 1962. Greffe de moelle osseuse après irradiation totale chez des souris leucémiques suivie d l'administralion d'un antimitotique pour reduire l'effet antileucémique. *C.R. Acad. Sci. (Paris)* 254: 3603.

70. Mathé, G., Amiel, J. L., Schwarzenberg, L., Cattan, A., and Schneider, M. 1965. Adoptive immunotherapy of acute leukemia: Experimental and clinical results. *Cancer Res.* 25: 1525–1531.

71. Mathé, G., Amiel, J. L., Schwarzenberg, L., and Merz, A. M. 1963. A method of reducing the incidence of the secondary syndrome in allogeneic marrow transplantation. *Blood* 22: 44–52.

72. Mathé, G., Kiger, N., Florentin, I., Garcia-Giralt, E., Martyre, M. C.,

Halle-Pannenko, O. H., and Schwartzenberg, L. 1973. Progress in the prevention of GVH: Bone marrow grafts after ALG conditioning with lymphocyte split chimerism, use of a lymphocyte "chalone T" and soluble histocompatibility antigens. *Transpl. Proc.* 5: 933–939.

73. Merritt, C. B., Darrow, C. C., II, Vaal, L., Herzig, G. P., and Rogentine, G. N., Jr. 1973. Rescue of rhesus monkeys from acute lethal graft-versus-host disease using cyclophosphamide and frozen autologous bone marrow. *Transplantation* 15: 154–159.

74. Miller, J. F. A. P., and Osoba, D. 1967. Current concepts of the immunological function of the thymus. *Physiol. Rev.* 47: 437–520.

75. Neiman, P., Wasserman, P. B., Wentworth, B. B., Kao, G. F., Lerner, R., Storb, R., Buckner, C. D., Clift, R. A., Fefer, A., Fass, L., Glucksberg, H., and Thomas, E. D. 1973. Interstitial pneumonia and cytomegalovirus infection as complications of human marrow transplantation. *Transplantation* 15: 478–485.

76. Ochs, H. D., Storb, R., Thomas, E. D., Kolk, H. V., Graham, T. C., Mickelson, E., Parr, M., and Rudolph, R. H. 1974. Immunologic reactivity in canine marrow graft recipients. *J. Immunol.* 113: 1039–1057.

77. Owens, A. H., and Santos, G. W. 1971. The effect of cytotoxic drugs on graft-versus-host disease in mice. *Transplantation* 11: 318–382.

78. Pollard, M., and Truitt, R. L. 1973. Allogeneic bone marrow chimerism in germfree mice. I. Prevention of spontaneous leukemia in AKR mice. *Proc. Soc. Exp. Biol. Med.* 144: 659–665.

79. Pollard, M., and Truitt, R. L. 1974. Allogeneic bone marrow chimerism in germ-free mice. II. Prevention of reticulum cell sarcomas in SJL/J mice. *Proc. Soc. Exp. Biol. Med.* 145: 488–492.

80. Prager, M. D., and Baechtel, F. S. 1973. Methods for modification of cancer cells to enhance their antigenicity, *in* H. Busch (ed.), *Methods in Cancer Research 1973*, Vol. 9, p. 399. Academic Press, New York.

81. Ramseier, H., and Lindenmann, J. 1972. Aliotypic antibodies. *Transpl. Rev.* 10: 57–96.

82. Richie, E. R., Gallagher, M. T., and Trentin, J. J. 1973. Inhibition of the graft-versus-host reaction. II. Prevention of acute graft-versus-host mortality by FAB fragments of antilymphocytic globulin. *Transplantation* 15: 486–491.

83. Rios, A., and Simmons, R. L. 1976. Experimental cancer immunotherapy: modification of tumor cells to increase immunogenicity. *Ann. N.Y. Acad. Sci.* 276: 45–60.

84. Rose, W. C., Rodey, G. E., Rimm, A. A., Truitt, R. L., and Bortin, M. M. 1976. Mitigation of graft-versus-host disease in mice by treatment of donors with bacterial endotoxin. *Exp. Hemat.* 4: 90–96.

85. Salmon, S. E., Krakauer, R. S., and Whitmore, W. F. 1971. Lymphocyte stimulation: Selective destruction of cells during blastogenic response to transplantation antigens. *Science* 172: 490–492.

86. Saltzstein, E. C., Glasspiegel, J. S., Rimm, A. A., Giller, R. H., and Bortin, M. M. 1972. Graft versus leukemia for "cell cure" of long-passage AKR leukemia after chemoradiotherapy. *Cancer Res.* 32: 1658–1662.

87. Santos, G. W. 1974. Immunosuppression for clinical marrow transplantation. *Seminars in Haemat.* 11: 341–351.

88. Scott, M. T. 1972. Biological effects of the adjuvant *Corynebacterium parvum*. I. Inhibition of PHA, mixed lymphocyte and GVH reactivity. *Cell. Immunol.* 5: 459–468.

89. Shaffer, C. F., Streilein, J. W., Freedberg, P. S., and Sherman, J. 1971. Studies on antilymphocyte serum and transplantation immunity in Syrian hamsters. *Transplantation* 11: 396–403.

90. Sprent, J., von Boehmer, H., and Nabholz, M. 1975. Association of immunity and tolerance to host H-2 determinants in irradiated F₁ hybrid mice reconstituted with bone marrow cells from one parental strain. *J. Exp. Med.* 142: 321–331.

91. Storb, R., Epstein, R. B., and Graham, T. C. 1970. Methotrexate regimens for control of graft-versus-host disease in dogs with allogeneic marrow grafts. *Transplantation* 9: 240–246.

92. Storb, R., Epstein, R. B., Graham, T. C., Kolb, H. J., Kobb, H., and Thomas, E. D. 1973. Rescue from canine graft-versus-host reaction by autologous or DL-A-compatible marrow. *Transplantation* 18: 357–367.

93. Storb, R., Floersheim, G. L., Weinden, P. L., Graham, T. C., Kolb, H. J., Lerner, K. G., Shroeder, M. L., and Thomas, E. D. 1974. Effect of prior blood transfusions on marrow grafts: abrogation of sensitization by procarbazine and antithymocyte serum. *J. Immunol.* 112: 1508–1516.

94. Thomas, E. D., Bryant, J. I., Buckner, C. D., Clift, R. A., Fefer, A., Johnson, F. L., Neiman, P., Ramberg, R. E., and Storb, R. 1972. Leukaemic transformation of engrafted human marrow cells *in vivo*. II. *Lancet* 1: 1310–1313.

95. Thomas, E. D., Storb, R., Clift, R. A., Fefer, A., Johnson, L. Neiman, P. E., Lerner, K. G., Glucksberg, H., and Buckner, C. D. 1975. Bone marrow transplantation. *N. Engl. J. Med.* 292: 831–843, 895–902.

96. Tigelaar, R. E., Gershon, R. K., and Asofsky, R. 1975. Graft-versus-host reactivity of mouse thymocytes: Effect of *in vitro* treatment with anti-TL serum. *Cell. Immunol.* 19: 58–64.

97. Trentin, J. J., and Judd, K. P. 1973. Prevention of acute graft-versus-host (GVH) mortality with spleen-absorbed antithymocyte globulin (ATG). *Transpl. Proc.* 5: 865–868.

98. Treves, A. J., Schechter, B., Cohen, I. R., and Feldman, M. 1976. Sensitization of T-lymphocytes *in vitro* by syngeneic macrophages fed with tumor antigens. *J. Immunol.* 116: 1059–1064, 1976.

99. Truitt, R. L., and Pollard, M. 1976. Allogeneic bone marrow chimerism in germ-free mice. IV. Therapy of "Hodgkin's-like" reticulum cell sarcoma in SJL mice. *Transplantation* 21: 12–16.

100. Truitt, R. L., Pollard, M., and Srivastata, K. K. 1974. Allogeneic bone marrow chimerism in germ-free mice. III. Therapy of leukemic AKR mice. *Proc. Soc. Exp. Biol. Med.* 146: 153–158.

101. Tschetter, P. N., Githens, J. H., Moscovici, M. G. 1961. Studies of the irradiation protection effect of fetal liver in mice. I. Influence of the gestational age of the donor tissue. *Blood* 18: 182–186.

102. Tyan, M. L. 1973. Modification of severe graft-versus-host disease with antisera to the θ antigen or to whole serum. *Transplantation* 15: 601–604.

103. Tyan, M. L. 1974. Graft-versus-host disease. Modification with con-

canavalin A. *Transplantation* 18: 305–311.

104. Uphoff, D. E. 1958. Preclusion of secondary phase of irradiation syndrome by inoculation of fetal hematopoietic tissue following lethal total body X-irradiation. *J. Natl. Cancer Inst.* 20: 625–632.

105. Vadlamudi, S., Padarathsingh, M., Bonmassar, E., and Goldin, A. 1971. Effect of combination treatment with cyclophosphamide and isogeneic or allogeneic spleen and bone marrow cells in leukemic (L1210) mice. *Int. J. Cancer* 7: 160–166.

106. van Bekkum, D. W. 1974. The double barrier in bone marrow transplantation. *Seminars Hemat.* 11: 325–340.

107. van Bekkum, D. W., and De Vries, M. J. 1967. *Radiation Chimaeras.* pp. 1–277. Logos, London, Academic Press, New York.

108. van Winkle, M. G. 1971. Cyclophosphamide-induced graft-versus-host immunotolerance. *J. Reticuloendothel. Soc.* 10: 403–417.

109. Voisin, G. A., Kinsky, R., and Maillard, P. 1968. Protection against homologous disease in hybrid mice by passive and active immunological enhancement-facilitation. *Transplantation* 6: 187–202.

110. Wagner, H., and Röllinghoff, M. 1973. *In vitro* induction of tumor specific immunity. I. Parameters of activation and cytotoxic reactivity of mouse lymphoid cells immunized *in vitro* against syngeneic and allogeneic plasma cell tumors. *J. Exp. Med.* 138: 1–5.

111. Waksman, B. H., Raff, M. C., and East, J. 1972. T and B lymphocytes in New Zealand Black Mice. *Clin. Exp. Immunol.* 11: 1–11.

112. Wallis, V., Davies, A. J. S., and Koller, P. C. 1966. Inhibition of radiation-induced haematopoietic tissue: A study of chimaerism. *Nature* 210: 500–504.

113. Woodruff, M. F. A. 1970. Immunotherapy of cancer. *Brit. Med. J.* 4: 486–487.

114. Wright, P. W., Hargreaves, R. E., Bansal, S. C., Bernstein, I. D., and Hellström, K. E. 1973. Allograft tolerance: Presumptive evidence that serum factors from tolerant animals that block lymphocytes-mediated immunity *in vitro* are soluble antigen-antibody complexes. *Proc. Natl. Acad. Sci.* 70: 2539–2543.

115. Youdim, S., Stutman, O., and Good, R. A. 1973. Thymus dependency of cells involved in transfer of delayed hypersensitivity to *Listeria monocytogenes* in mice. *Cell. Immunol.* 8: 395–402.

116. Zighelboim, J., Bonavida, B., Rao, V. S., and Fahey, J. L. 1974. Blocking activity induced by solubilized alloantigens. *J. Immunol.* 112: 433–435.

CHAPTER 15

NONSPECIFIC ADOPTIVE IMMUNOTHERAPY OF T CELL ACUTE LYMPHOBLASTIC LEUKEMIA IN AKR MICE: A Model for the Treatment of T Cell Leukemia in Man

Mortimer M. Bortin
Robert L. Truitt
Alfred A. Rimm

May and Sigmund Winter
Research Laboratory
Mount Sinai Medical Center
and Departments of Medicine
and Biostatistics
Medical College of Wisconsin
Milwaukee, Wisconsin 53233

Human T cell leukemia accounts for 20–30% of all cases of acute lymphoblastic leukemia and its response to chemotherapy is poor. The spontaneous T cell leukemia of AKR mice represents an excellent counterpart of the human disease and serves as an experimental model in which to test innovative treatment strategies. Nonspecific adoptive immunotherapy in combination with chemoradiotherapy for AKR T cell leukemia resulted in survival data which surpassed that obtained with chemotherapy alone. The rapidly improving results in clinical marrow transplantation suggest that adoptive immunotherapy has very real potential as a treatment for T cell leukemia in man.

I. THE PROBLEM

Despite recent remarkable advances in the treatment of human acute leukemia, less than 15% of the patients survive 5 years (58). Of all cases of acute lymphoblastic leukemia, the T cell* form accounts for 20–30% (18, 36, 59, 68). The T cell disease responds poorly to chemotherapy and the duration of remissions is significantly shorter than in childhood non-T cell acute lymphoblastic leukemia with a dismal probability for 5-year survival (18, 36, 59, 68). A formidable problem confronting hematologists and oncologists is how to treat those patients whose leukemia becomes refractory to sublethal doses of chemotherapeutic agents. Described in this chapter are the results of our studies investigating a treatment strategy using chemotherapy, radiotherapy and adoptive immunotherapy for T cell acute lymphoblastic leukemia in AKR mice. This experimental leukemia was selected for study because it represents an excellent counterpart for the human disease.

II. THE EXPERIMENTAL TUMOR SYSTEM

Approximately 90% of AKR mice develop and die of spontaneous acute lymphoblastic leukemia between 6 and 12 months of age (28, 44, 57). The cytokinetic characteristics of the leukemic cells have been described by Lin and Bruce (41) and by Schabel et al. (57) who estimated that the number present at the time of death was 1 to 1.5×10^9. The growth characteristics suggested that one viable (clonogenic) leukemia cell multiplied to the lethal number in less than 60 days. AKR spontaneous leukemia can be diagnosed accurately by means of physical examination: splenomegaly, plus axillary or brachial and inguinal lymphadenopathy, all more than three times normal size. Using these diagnostic criteria during 1974–1976 the median survival time (MST) for 630 untreated AKR control mice in our laboratory was 19.8 days; only two (0.3%) survived 60 days after clinical diagnosis.

We believe that AKR spontaneous leukemia represents an excellent animal model for human T cell acute lymphoblastic leukemia because of the many features shared by the two diseases. Shown in Table 1 is a comparison between the human and AKR leukemias.

*Abbreviations are explained at the end of the article.

Table 1. Comparison of human and AKR T cell acute lymphoblastic leukemias

Factors[a]	Human T Cell Leukemia[b]	AKR T Cell Leukemia
1. Origin in thymus	+	+
2. Viral etiology	?	+
3. Theta antigen	+	+
4. TL antigen	+[c]	+
5. B cell markers	−	−
6. Surface immunoglobulins	−	−
7. Complement receptors	−	−
8. Age at onset	>6 years	>6 months
9. Higher incidence in males	±	−
10. Very high WBC counts	+	+
11. Mediastinal mass	+	+
12. Lymphadenopathy	+	+
13. Hepatomegaly	+	+
14. Splenomegaly	+	+
15. Inhibition of MLC reactions	+	+
16. Brief response to chemotherapy	+	+

a. Factors with an incidence of 50% or higher.

b. These factors (except for 5–7) are significantly different from non-T cell acute lymphoblastic leukemia of childhood.

c. Thymus leukemia-like antigen.

Both the human (60) and AKR (37, 71) diseases are believed to arise from malignant transformation of thymus cells. Although the Gross murine leukemia virus (GMuLV) is fairly well established as the etiologic agent for the disease in AKR mice (32), evidence linking a virus to the human disease is lacking. Malignant cells from both the human (18, 36, 59, 68) and murine (37, 71) forms of the disease express theta antigen. Also, human marrow lymphoblasts form spontaneous rosettes when cultures with sheep erythrocytes, a T cell characteristic (18, 36, 59, 68). The thymus leukemia (TL) antigen on AKR leukemic lymphoblasts has been known for some years (17, 37); recently a TL-like antigen has been identified on leukemic blasts from children with T cell leukemia (60). B cell markers, surface immunoglobulins and complement receptors are rarely found on human (36) or AKR (37) T cell leukemic lymphoblasts.

Most cases of non-T cell acute lymphoblastic leukemia of childhood appear within the first five years of life, whereas the median age at the time of diagnosis of T cell leukemia is nine years (59). Similarly the T cell spontaneous leukemia of AKR mice appears well after infancy and the median age at the time of death for untreated mice is nine months (57). The incidence of the disease in humans was significantly higher in males according to some authors (59, 68), but there was no significant difference in sex distribution according to others (18); the frequency of the disease in male and female AKR mice is equal (57). Median white blood cells (WBC) counts were over 50,000 per mm³ (59) and counts of 100,000 per mm³ were not unusual in children with the T cell disease (36, 59). According to recent studies by Borella (personal communication) WBC counts exceeded 100,000 per mm³ in 50% of children with T cell leukemia, while counts in that range occurred in only 8% of children with non-T cell acute lymphoblastic leukemia. At the time of diagnosis of AKR T cell leukemia, WBC counts exceeded 30,000 per mm³ in more than 50% of the mice (57). A mediastinal mass, marked lymphadenopathy and hepatosplenomegaly occurred with a frequency greater than 50% in both the human (18, 36, 59, 68) and murine (35, 37, 57, 71) diseases. Both human (68) and AKR (65) leukemic lymphoblasts that were irradiated or treated with mitomycin-C inhibited normal allogeneic responder cells in mixed leukocyte cultures. Finally, as measured by median time until relapse and the proportion of long-term survivors, both the human (36, 59, 68) and murine (27, 35, 56) T cell leukemias respond poorly to chemotherapy.

III. ADOPTIVE IMMUNOTHERAPY AS A TREATMENT STRATEGY

A. Conceptual Considerations

New insights in immunobiology have caused a resurgence of interest in immunotherapy as an adjunct to currently available leukemia therapy. Many reasons exist which make it difficult to manipulate a patient's own immune system (i.e., active immunotherapy) so it can become decisively effective against his own malignancy. Transplantation of immunocompetent cells from a normal individual to the leukemic patients (i.e., adoptive immunotherapy) offers an alternative immunotherapeutic approach. The concept of adoptive immunotherapy utilizes a transplant of foreign bone marrow cells, not merely to restore hematopoiesis after doses of drugs or radiation which cause severe damage to normal hematopoietic tissues, but also as an aggressive antileukemic treatment.

Barnes et al. (6) first proposed that the transplantation of allogeneic immunocompetent cells might be capable of killing residual leukemia cells following unsuccessful chemoradiotherapy. Since the early 1900's it has been known that normal individuals given injections of viable cancer cells rarely developed the malignancy (33). The concept of adoptive immunotherapy is based on those observations. Cells from the immunological defense apparatus of normal recipients are thought to recognize and react against foreign histocompatibility antigens and tumor associated antigens on the surface of the injected tumor cells and reject them. To apply adoptive immunotherapy, the leukemic host must be prepared with vigorous immunosuppressive treatments in order to prevent rejection of the transplanted killer cells, thereby giving them time to react against residual tumor cells. We use the term graft-versus-leukemia (GVL) reaction to signify the adoptive immunotherapeutic effect of transplanted immunocompetent cells against leukemia cells.

Unfortunately, the transplanted immunocompetent cells also attack normal tissues of the host, causing potentially lethal graft-versus-host (GVH) disease. The term GVH disease is used to signify the consequences of an attack by transplanted immunocompetent cells against the normal tissues of a vulnerable host. GVH disease is one of the major stumbling blocks preventing widespread use of adoptive immunotherapy for the treatment of cancer in man.

Application of adoptive immunotherapy for human hematological malignancy (and perhaps other forms of cancer) should be possible if clinical bone marrow transplantation can be carried out with a high probability of success and if GVH disease can be circumvented without loss of the GVL reaction.

B. Current Status of Clinical Bone Marrow Transplantation

A review of 200 human bone marrow transplants performed prior to 1968 disclosed that only 2 were successful (10). In 1968, a significant advance was made when Bach et al. (5) and Gatti et al. (29) first demonstrated that marrow transplantation could be used successfully in man when the donor and recipient were closely matched at the major histocompatibility complex (MHC). Since then, improvements in immunosuppressive regimens to ensure engraftment, measures to prevent and treat GVH disease, histocompatibility testing techniques, and new methods to prevent and treat infections have all contributed to the progressively rising success rate of clinical marrow transplantation. For example, in patients with severe aplastic anemia, 43% of 75 patients who received marrow transplants from HLA (the MHC in man) identical donors are currently alive with functioning grafts (1). The probability for "cure" exceeded 90% when fewer than 15 pretransplant transfusions were given and transplantation was performed within nine months of diagnosis (1). Bone marrow transplantation has resulted in a 63% "cure" rate for children with severe combined immunodeficiency disease when donors and recipients were HLA genotypically identical (3). This disease, characterized by an absence of functional B and T cells, was uniformly fatal prior to 1968 and almost all children died in the first year of life.

Allogeneic marrow transplants have been less effective in the treatment of acute leukemia; however, several teams recently reported encouraging results when marrow transplantation from HLA compatible siblings was used as a last resort to treat patients with terminal acute leukemia who failed to respond to chemotherapy (23, 64). As currently employed, marrow from HLA compatible donors is given to restore hematopoietic function following massive doses of antileukemic agents in patients whose disease has become refractory to conventional doses of antileukemic agents. It is noteworthy that Storb et al. (62) found that recurrent leukemia was the most common cause for failure in their patients who were treated with marrow transplants from HLA identical siblings. There has been no convincing evidence that marrow from HLA identical donors had detectable antileukemic reactivity (63, 64). This observation correlates with our own finding in a mouse model that no detectable GVL effect was observed when marrow from donors that were phenotypically identical with AKR hosts at H-2 (the MHC in mice) was tested against AKR long-passage (13) or spontaneous T cell leukemias (see section IV C).

In summary, clinical marrow transplantation has shown steadily improving results over the past few years and is now considered by many to be the primary treatment for severe aplastic anemia and severe combined immunodeficiency disease. With respect to leukemia, HLA compatible marrow transplantation has been used to restore hematopoiesis after otherwise lethal doses of chemoradiotherapeutic agents, but the transplanted cells have not had an antileukemic effect.

C. Strategies to Circumvent GVH Disease Without Losing the Antileukemic Reaction

Numerous investigators have used experimental tumors in rodents to demonstrate (after chemotherapy and/or surgery) that the transplantation of allogeneic immunocompetent cells from unprimed donors induced an antitumor effect which destroyed residual malignant cells (e.g., 9, 22, 43, 45, 70). However, to obtain the desired adoptive immunotherapeutic effect immunocompetent cells from H-2 incompatible donors had to be engrafted and the resultant GVH disease proved to be a formidable problem in each of these studies. Several measures have been used or suggested in an effort to avoid GVH disease without losing the antitumor reaction.

Intensive treatment of GVH disease was used by Owens (45) among others; however, treatment could not be started within 6 days post-transplant without losing the desired GVL reaction. Chester et al. (22) reported some success using a graft-versus-graft reaction to terminate both the GVII and GVL reactions in AKR mice bearing a long-passage lymphoblastic leukemia. On the premise that separate subpopulations of T lymphocytes exist, one reactive against histocompatibility antigens and another reactive against tumor-associated antigens, Bortin (11) proposed application of cell separation techniques such as immunoadsorbents (69), bromodeoxyuridine-light (72), or ^{3}H-thymidine suicide (54) to selectively eliminate GVH reactive cells while sparing other immunocompetent cells (including those responsible for the GVL reaction).

Some workers have demonstrated that treatment of donor mice with bacterial lipopolysaccharide (endotoxin) resulted in amelioration of GVH disease (24, 39). We have confirmed these reports in nonleukemic AKR mice transplanted with cells from H-2 incompatible DBA/2 donors that had been treated with endotoxin (52). Transplantation of immunocompetent cells from endotoxin-treated donors for treatment of a long-passage AKR T cell leukemia resulted in survival rates significantly higher than those found when nonendotoxin treated donors were used (67). In an accompanying chapter in this volume, Truitt describes his work indicating that GVH disease in mice can be circumvented without loss of the GVL effect by using gnotobiotic techniques.

To avoid fatal GVH disease, Boranić (9) used spleen cells from H-2 incompatible donors in a transient GVL reaction; following completion of the antileukemic attack, the incompatible effector cells were killed, and spleen cells from syngeneic donors were transplanted to restore hematopoietic and lymphoid function to the "cured" hosts. Boranić reasoned that "if there was a margin of time between eradication of the leukemia and irreparable damage to the host, this interregnum should allow termination of the GVH reaction without recurrence of the leukemia" (8).

In recent years, a major research effort of our laboratory has centered on the application of a transient GVL reaction to studies of adoptive immunotherapy of AKR long-passage and spontaneous T cell leukemias. In an effort to increase the clinical relevance of the model proposed by Boranić, we modified his treatment plan by administering histoincompatible bone marrow plus lymph node cells instead of spleen cells for the GVL reaction (first transplant). The histoincompatible cells were killed after they had fulfilled their antileukemic mission; then, bone marrow and lymph node cells from allogeneic donors that were compatible with the host at H-2 (instead of spleen cells from syngeneic donors) were administered to restore hematopoiesis (second transplant).

Present methods for collection of human marrow for transplantation inevitably result in contamination of the marrow cells with large numbers of peripheral blood T lymphocytes with a resultant increase in the intensity of the GVH reaction (46). On the other hand, mouse marrow has few T cells (65), can be collected without significant peripheral blood contamination and, in general, causes delayed rather than acute GVH disease. Adding lymph node cells to marrow markedly intensifies the GVH reaction in mice and mimics the acute GVH reaction seen in man when histoincompatible marrow is transplanted. Furthermore, there is little or no detectable GVL reactivity in mouse marrow alone and the addition of lymph node cells provides T cells in the transplant with resultant increased GVL reactivity (unpublished observations). Our successful application of a transient GVL reaction for cure of a long-passage AKR T cell leukemia (12) encouraged us to expand our work to the more difficult AKR spontaneous T cell leukemia. Several of the key findings in both experimental tumor systems are described in the following sections.

IV. EXPERIMENTAL BASES FOR THE TREATMENT STRATEGY

A. Overview of the Treatment Model

The treatment model is diagramed in Fig. 1. In Step I, AKR mice bearing advanced spontaneous T cell leukemia were given chemoradiotherapy (A, Fig. 1). The chemoradiotherapy was designed to be: (1) sublethal when followed by a bone marrow transplant; (2) sufficiently cytoreductive to decrease the tumor load to the level of "minimal residual cancer" but, to mimic the clinical problem, resulted in infrequent cures by itself; and (3) sufficiently immunosuppressive to prevent rejection of the GVL reactive cells. In Step II, the AKR mice were given bone marrow and lymph node cells i.v. from histoincompatible donors (B, first transplant, Fig. 1). These cells initiated the desired GVL reaction (and the concomitant undesired GVH reaction). The GVL reaction was permitted to proceed for six days (C, Fig. 1). In Step III, the AKR hosts were "rescued" from a potentially lethal GVH reaction by killing the first transplant with combination chemotherapy (D, Fig. 1). Hematopoietic and immune functions were restored by administering marrow and lymph node cells (second transplant) from a donor that is allogeneic, but phenotypically identical with AKR at H-2 (E, Fig. 1).

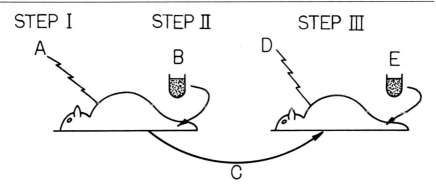

Fig. 1.   Three-step chemoradioimmunotherapeutic model for the treatment of AKR spontaneous T cell leukemia:

Step I.   Combined chemoradiotherapy for tumor cell reduction and immunosuppression (*A*).

Step II.   Administration of immunocompetent cells from mismatched donors to initiate the GVL reaction (*B*). Time for GVL reaction (*C*).

Step III.   Combination chemotherapy to inactivate the mismatched (GVL and GVH reactive) cells (*D*) and reconstitution of the hematopoietic and lymphoid systems with a marrow transplant from an allogeneic, but histocompatible donor (*E*).

B. Chemoradiotherapy for Immunosuppression and Leukemia Cytoreduction

In our work with BW5147, an AKR long-passage T cell leukemia, we found that 185 mg/kg cyclophosphamide (CY) plus 400r total body radiation (TBR) was sublethal, immunosuppressive and markedly antileukemic but not curative (12). However, this chemoradiotherapeutic regimen proved to be unsatisfactory in AKR mice bearing spontaneous T cell leukemia due to severe toxicity (51). We investigated 42 regimens for Step I of the treatment model (Fig. 1) employing chemotherapy, combination chemotherapy, radiotherapy and chemoradiotherapy. Mortality in the first 24 hours exceeded 40%, and 70–100% of the mice died within 2 weeks when the initial treatment was a high dose of chemotherapy, radiotherapy or chemoradiotherapy (51). When low dose chemotherapy was given first, mortality in the first 24 hours was minimal and, most significantly, no deaths occurred in the 24 hours after subsequent high dose treatments. From these results we concluded that chemotherapeutic and chemoradiotherapeutic regimens for AKR spontaneous T cell leukemia should be designed so that low, minimally lethal doses precede

Table 2.   Details of treatment plan for AKR mice bearing spontaneous leukemia-lymphoma[a]

Step:	I			II			III			
Day:	0		2	8			14			
	AmB	MeC	CY	TBR	BM	LN	CY	PCZ	BM	LN
	10	16	175	300	10^7	2×10^6	150	100	10^7	5×10^5

a. Steps are from Fig. 1. Day zero represents day of diagnosis. Abbreviations used: Am-B = amphotericin B; MeC = methyl cyclohexylnitrosourea; CY = cyclophosphamide; TBR = total body radiation; PCZ = procarbazine; BM = bone marrow cells; and LN = lymph node cells. Drug doses are expressed in mg/kg of body weight, and TBR exposure is expressed in Roentgens.

higher doses (51). Shown in Table 2 are dose and schedule information for the regimen which has provided our best results to date.

C. Donor Selection for Adoptive Immunotherapy

The chemoradiotherapy regimen shown in Table 2 (when administered without transplants on days 8 and 14) induced a remission in the spontaneous T cell leukemia as evidenced by modest prolongation of the MST and 60-day survival of about one-fourth of the mice. Therefore, transplantation of immunocompetent cells was incorporated into the treatment plan to eliminate residual leukemia cells by means of a GVL reaction.

Ideally, the optimal donor for use in adoptive immunotherapy would show great antileukemic reactivity and no reactivity against the normal tissues of the host. Functionally separate subpopulations of T lymphocytes are known to exist (20, 21, 30) and experimental evidence indicates that a different subpopulation of effector cells attack tumor cells than those which attack normal host cells (26, 34). Several investigators have reported that immunization across MHC differences resulted in increased cell-mediated cytotoxicity against tumor targets with little or no increase in GVH reactivity (19, 53, 61) and antitumor reactivity could be separated from antihost reactivity by incubating the effector cells on allogeneic fibroblasts (42).

Similarly, we reported evidence suggesting that GVH and GVL reactions were functions of different subpopulations of effector cells (13, 15, 38). In these experiments immunocompetent cells from 16 donor strains of mice with a wide range of histocompatibility differences from AKR were tested in vivo against nonleukemic AKR mice for GVH reactivity and in AKR mice bearing BW5147, a long-passage T cell leukemia, for GVL reactivity (13, 15, 38). GVH reactivity was measured by MST and 30- and 100-day survival rates of immunosuppressed nonleukemic AKR mice given cells from the panel of donors. GVL reactivity was evaluated in a bioassay system which has been described in detail (14) and is depicted in Fig. 2. Briefly, leukemia cells were inoculated into irradiated normal AKR mice; one day later, the leukemic hosts were given immunocompetent cells from the panel of donors; then, after a 6-day GVL reaction, the spleen of each AKR primary host was removed and injected i.p. into an individual AKR secondary recipient. The assumption was made that transfer of one viable leukemia cell would cause death of the secondary recipient

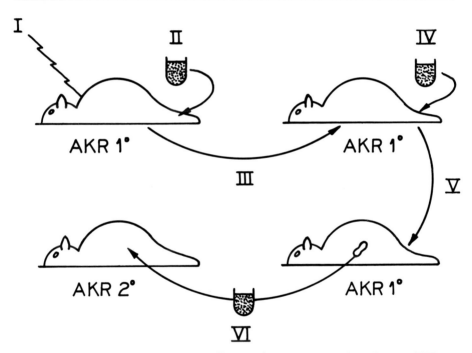

Fig. 2. Bioassay model to measure efficacy of GVL reaction. Step I, 800 r TBR to AKR mice on morning of day 0. Step II, administration of leukemia cells on afternoon of day 0. Step III, time for leukemia cells to establish residence and resume multiplication (1 day). Step IV, day 1 administration of 2 × 10⁷ bone marrow cells and 10⁷ lymph node cells from donors with varying degrees of histoincompatibility to initiate GVL reaction. Step V, time for GVL reaction (6 days). Step VI, transfer of spleen cells to AKR secondary recipients (bioassay) on day 7.

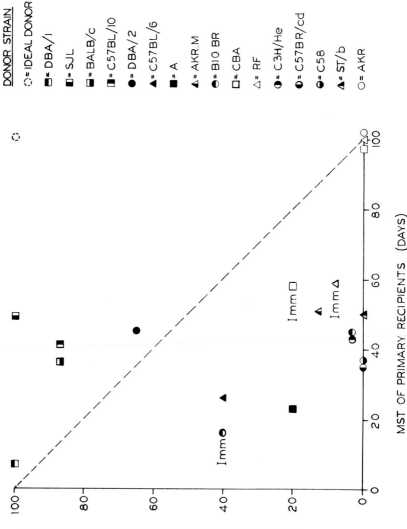

DONOR STRAIN	H-2	H-2 SPECIFICITIES
◌ = IDEAL DONOR	?	?
◨ = DBA/1	q	qqqqqq
◧ = SJL	s	ssssss
▣ = BALB/c	d	dddddd
◩ = C57BL/10	b	bbbbbb
● = DBA/2	d	dddddd
▲ = C57BL/6	b	bbbbbb
■ = A	a	kkkddd
△ = AKR.M	m	kkkkkkq
◑ = B10 BR	k	kkkkkk
□ = CBA	k	kkkkkk
△ = RF	k	kkkkkk
◓ = C3H/He	k	kkkkkk
◕ = C57BR/cd	k	kkkkkk
◒ = C58	k	kkkkkk
▲ = ST/b	k	kkkkkk
○ = AKR	k	kkkkkk

GRAFT VERSUS LEUKEMIA REACTIVITY

PERCENT SURVIVAL OF SECONDARY RECIPIENTS AT 60 DAYS

MST OF PRIMARY RECIPIENTS (DAYS)

GRAFT VERSUS HOST REACTIVITY

due to leukemia within 60 days. The theoretical and experimental bases for this assumption and the rationale for the use of the spleen as the most sensitive bioassay organ have been described (14). Survival of secondary recipients was interpreted to indicate that all leukemic cells had been eliminated from (at least the spleens of) the primary recipients by an immunologic reaction of the transplanted donor cells.

Shown in Figure 3 are the results of the GVH and GVL assays in AKR mice. GVH reactivity is expressed on the abscissa as the MST post-transplant; GVL reactivity against BW5147 is shown on the ordinate as the percent survival of the secondary recipients. The dashed circle in the upper right-hand corner is the data point for the hypothetical ideal donor. The dashed diagonal line is where all data points would fail if a positive correlation existed between GVH and GVL reactivity.

All donors differed from AKR at minor histocompatibility loci except AKR.M which is cogenic and differs only at the H-2D subregion of the MHC. Other donors had varying degrees of compatible within the MCH (shown in Fig. 3). In addition, three H-2 compatible donor strains were primed by multiple injections of irradiated BW5147 leukemia cells and tested for GVH and GVL reactivity.

Immunosuppressed nonleukemic AKR mice that received transplants from unprimed H-2 compatibility donors demonstrated a wide range in the severity of GVH disease, yet the same donor strains had no significant GVL reactivity when tested in leukemic AKR hosts (Fig. 3). Also, no significant GVL reactivity was found when cells from syngeneic AKR or congenic AKR.M donors were administered. H-2 compatible donors that were immunized with γ-irradiated AKR leukemic spleen cells showed modest GVL reactivity, but associated with the immunization was a disproportionate increase in acute and delayed GVH mortality. Mice that were incompatible with AKR at H-2 also exhibited considerable variation in the severity of GVH disease produced but they also demonstrated a wide range in GVL reactivity (Fig. 3). A-strain mice, which are matched with AKR at H-2K, IA and IB of the MHC, caused intense GVH disease (23-day MST and no survivors at 60 days) but were relatively ineffectual against the leukemia (80% of the secondary recipients died of leukemia). Among the H-2 incompatible donors, mice of the SJL strain appeared to most closely approach the ideal because of least intense GVH reactivity and maximal GVL reactivity against BW5147 (38).

Fig. 3. Comparison of GVH reactivity of immunocompetent cells in immunosuppressed normal AKR mice and GVL reactivity in AKR mice bearing BW5147 T cell leukemia. Dashed line represents a perfect correlation between GVH and GVL reactivity.

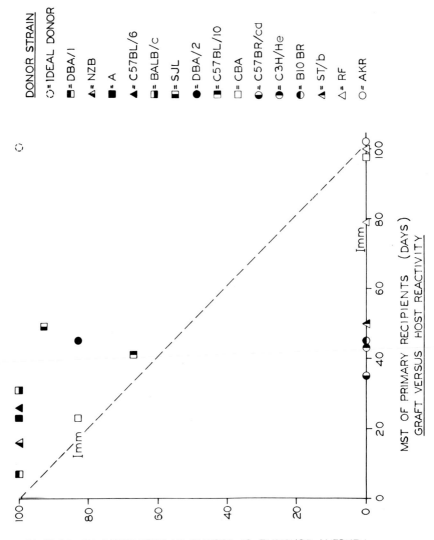

DONOR STRAIN

		H-2	H-2 SPECIFICITIES
○= IDEAL DONOR		?	?
▣= DBA/1		q	qqqqqq
▲= NZB		d	dddddd
■= A		a	kkkddd
▲= C57BL/6		b	bbbbbb
▣= BALB/c		d	dddddd
▣= SJL		s	ssssss
●= DBA/2		d	dddddd
◨= C57BL/10		b	bbbbbb
□= CBA		k	kkkkkk
◑= C57BR/cd		k	kkkkkk
◔= C3H/He		k	kkkkkk
◑= BIO BR		k	kkkkkk
▲= ST/b		k	kkkkkk
△= RF		k	kkkkkk
○= AKR		k	kkkkkk

MST OF PRIMARY RECIPIENTS (DAYS)
GRAFT VERSUS HOST REACTIVITY

PERCENT SURVIVAL OF SECONDARY RECIPIENTS AT 60 DAYS
GRAFT VERSUS LEUKEMIA REACTIVITY

Tests of GVL reactivity using a panel of 15 allogeneic donor strains against AKR spontaneous T cell leukemia again demonstrated that cells from H-2 compatible donors had no detectable antileukemic effect (Fig. 4). Furthermore, immunization of H-2 compatible RF donors with irradiated spontaneous leukemia cells failed to induce GVL reactivity. Although immunization of H-2 compatible CBA donors markedly increased their GVL reactivity, their GVH reactivity changed from delayed (MST > 100 days) to acute (MST = 23 days). A-strain mice which had little GVL reactivity against BW5147 were able to eliminate spontaneous leukemia cells from 100% of the AKR primary hosts. We believe that differences in the level of GVL reactivity against the AKR long-passage and spontaneous T cell leukemias by individual strains of mice may have been due to differences in antigenicity of the two leukemias—the spontaneous leukemia perhaps being more antigenic. Also, the data shown for GVL reactivity of H-2 incompatible donors against AKR spontaneous T cell leukemia are preliminary and based upon small group sizes (7–28 mice). Additional studies using higher doses of spontaneous leukemia cells need to be performed to determine which of the H-2 incompatible strains have the most effective GVL reaction. However, for the purpose of selecting a donor for use in adoptive immunotherapy, most H-2 incompatible strains can be removed from consideration because of unacceptably high GVH reactivity. As tested in these preliminary experiments mice of the SJL or DAB/2 strains appear to most closely approximate the ideal donor because of least intense GVH disease with moderate to marked GVL reactivity against AKR spontaneous T cell leukemia.

D. Duration of the Graft-versus-Leukemia Reaction

To apply nonspecific adoptive immunotherapy successfully, sufficient time must be allowed for the transplanted effector cells to kill all residual leukemia cells; but, to avoid lethal GVH disease, the graft must be terminated as early as possible. Using DBA/2 donors with known high reactivity against AKR T cell leukemias, we found that 2-day and 4-day GVL reactions failed to eradicate the leukemia (55 and unpublished). Other investigators have shown in a variety of murine experimental leukemias that 6 days is the minimal time necessary for an effective GVL

Fig. 4. Comparison of GVH reactivity of immunocompetent cells in immunosuppressed normal AKR mice and GVL reactivity in AKR mice bearing spontaneous T cell leukemia. Dashed line represents a perfect correlation between GVH and GVL reactivity.

reaction (8, 9, 22, 45); we have confirmed these observations in both long-passage and spontaneous AKR T cell leukemias (55 and unpublished).

E. Rescue from Graft-versus-Host Disease

Successful treatment of an established GVH reaction is exceedingly difficult and achieved infrequently (31, 64). Perhaps the most effective way is to kill the transplanted cells; however, killing the graft leaves the host without functional hematopoietic or lymphoid tissues making it necessary to restore hematopoietic and lymphoid function with a second transplant. We have tested 108 different treatments to kill a graft without killing the host (12, 55 and unpublished). Thus far, two regimens have proved to be most effective in eliminating the histoincompatible killer cells. A combination of CY plus an antiserum directed at histocompatibility antigens of the killer cells has worked well in some experiments, but not in others. The difference in results was probably due to variability in the potency of different lots of antiserum (12). More recently, as suggested by the work of Glucksberg and Fefer (31), we have had considerable success using a combination of CY and procarbazine (16 and Table 2). Based upon the studies of GVH reactivity following transplantation of immunocompetent cells from H-2 compatible donors (Figs. 3 and 4), mice of the RF and CBA strains were selected as donors to restore hematopoietic and lymphoid function after terminating the graft of histoincompatible cells.

V. RESULTS OF TREATMENT

Described below are the results in AKR mice bearing spontaneous T cell leukemia employing the treatment plan diagramed in Fig. 1. The survival data for control and experimental groups are shown in Table 3. DBA/2 mice were used as donors for adoptive immunotherapy in the experimental groups (Groups 7–9). A remission was induced by chemoradiotherapy alone (Group 2) as evidenced by an increase in the MST (calculated from day 14, the last day of treatment) of treated mice over untreated mice (Group 1, Table 3, calculated from day 0, day of diagnosis) and by the proportion of long-term survivors. Many deaths in the chemoradiotherapy controls were attributed to drug and/or radiation toxicity since most mice that died within 14 days following completion of treatment were leukemia-free on gross examination. Some of the early toxicity could be overcome by transplanting syngeneic bone marrow plus lymph node cells (Group 3). The transplant of AKR cells provided hematopoietic support but had no detectable antileukemic effect, and most mice died with overt leukemia. Thus, the MST and survival rates for syngeneic controls were not significantly better than chemoradiotherapy controls.

Cells from AKR donors were given on day 8 (providing hematopoietic support, but no GVL effect) and cells from RF donors were administered on day 14 to evaluate a possible adoptive immunotherapeutic contribution of the RF cells ("rescue controls," Group 4, Table 3). Any improvement in survival of this group over the syngeneic control group (Group 3) could be ascribed to an antileukemic (or other beneficial) effect of the RF cells. However, there were no significant differences between the rescue controls, syngeneic controls or chemoradiotherapy controls as measured by MST and proportion surviving 60, 90 and 120 days.

Allogeneic, H-2 compatible controls were used to evaluate the effect of a double transplant of cells from H-2 matched RF and CBA donors in combination with chemoradiotherapy (Groups 5 and 6, Table 3). Treatment of AKR mice bearing spontaneous T cell leukemia with double

Table 3. Survival data for control and experimental AKR mice bearing spontaneous leukemia-lymphoma that were "rescued" from graft-versus-host disease after treatment with chemoradiotherapy and adoptive immunotherapy[a]

Group	N	BM+LN Cells Given on Day 8	14	MST (days)[b]	Percent Surviving[b] 60 Days	90 Days	120 Days
1	630	—	—	20[c]	0.3[c]	0[c]	0
2	80	—	—	26	26	14	9
3	30	AKR	AKR	39	13	3	0
4	29	AKR	RF	31	28	21	10
5	27	RF	RF	6	7	7	4
6	30	CBA	CBA[d]	6	7	7	0
7	29	DBA/2	CBA	18	21	21	10
8	30	DBA/2	CBA[d]	15	10	0[e]	0
9	38	DBA/2	RF	64	53	40	29

a. All AKR hosts (except Group 1, concommitant and historical untreated controls) were treated with the regimen shown in Table 1.

b. Calculated from day 14, the last day of treatment for all mice entered into the experiment on day 0.

c. Calculated from day of diagnosis.

d. Bone marrow cells without lymph node cells were given on day 14.

e. Surviving mice were sacrificed before day-90 for tests of chimerism.

transplants of cells from RF or CBA donors resulted in shortened MST's and failed to improve the survival rates when compared with the other control groups.

A temporary graft of immunocompetent cells from H-2 incompatible DBA/2 donors resulted in improved survival data when cells from RF donors (Group 9, Table 3) were used to restore hematopoiesis on day 14, but not when CBA cells were used in the second transplant (Groups 7 and 8). The 64 day MST for mice treated with DBA/2 cells for adoptive immunotherapy and rescued with RF cells (Group 9) was significantly longer ($P < 0.01$ to < 0.001) than all groups except the rescue controls (Group 4). Similarly, the 53%, 40% and 29% survival rates at 60, 90 and 120 days following completion of treatment respectively were superior to the survival rates in the control groups ($P < 0.06$ to < 0.01), except for the rescue controls at 90 and 120 days.

Although significant prolongation of the survival time of AKR mice was achieved by combining transient adoptive immunotherapy with chemoradiotherapy, some of the mice in Group 9, Table 3 that died more than 2 weeks after completion of therapy had gross and histologic evidence of leukemia. The overall incidence of recurrent leukemia in mice that lived more than two weeks following completion of therapy is shown in Table 4. The 35% incidence of leukemic deaths found in mice from Group 9 was significantly lower ($P < 0.001$) than the 91% incidence of recurrent leukemia in the syngeneic controls (Group 3). Deaths without overt leukemia were attributed to infectious complications, toxicity of the treatment regimen or to GVH disease. It is not known whether recurrent leukemia was a result of a relapse of the original disease or whether a new disease episode was induced in residual AKR cells or in rescue cells from H-2 compatible donors that are known to be susceptible to leukemogenesis by GMuLV (32, 40).

We found in related studies that adoptive immunotherapy of AKR spontaneous T cell leukemia using DBA/2 donors failed to reduce the tissue concentration of GMuLV (66 and Truitt, this volume). Relative susceptibility of H-2 compatible strains to AKR leukemia may explain why the incidence of recurrent leukemia was greater in those animals rescued with cells from RF donors than those rescued with cells from CBA donors. We found that 19/30 (63%) of RF mice developed and died of leukemia within 30 days following an i.v. dose of 2×10^7 AKR spontaneous leukemia cells, whereas 30/30 CBA mice survived more than 100 days after an i.v. dose of 5×10^7 AKR spontaneous leukemia cells (unpublished).

In an effort to improve the survival rates in AKR mice bearing spontaneous T cell leukemia, we varied the dose of TBR and GVL effector (DBA/2 lymph node) cells. The basic chemoradiotherapy treatment reg-

Table 4.   Incidence of recurrent
leukemia in control and experimental
groups

Group[a]	N at Risk[b]	N Deaths with Leukemia (%)[c]
1		630(100)[d]
2	51	27(53)
3	23	21(91)
4	21	10(48)
5	7	1(14)
6	12	3(25)
7	15	2(13)
8	13	5(38)
9	31	11(35)

a. From Table 3.
b. Alive 14 days after completion of treatment (28 days after diagnosis).
c. Percent leukemia deaths = (N leukemic at 90 days post-treatment × 100)/N mice at risk 14 days post-treatment.
d. Number of untreated controls dead of leukemia 90 days after diagnosis.

imen outlined in Table 2 was used and all variables were kept constant except for the dose of TBR and lymph node cells. We found a deleterious effect on survival as the dose of TBR was increased above 300r and the dose of DBA/2 lymph node cells was decreased below 2×10^6. Highest survival rates were achieved when the TBR dose was 200 to 300r and the lymph node dose was 2 to 4×10^6 cells (16).

In other experiments (data not shown) using similar chemoradiotherapy regimens, a 9-day GVL reaction resulted in lower survival rates than found with a 6-day GVL reaction. All of these experiments were associated with high mortality rates due to GVH disease.

VI. COMPARISON WITH RESULTS USING OTHER APPROACHES

Of particular relevance to the research described in this chapter are the experiments of Mathé et al. (43), Alexander (4) and Denton and Symes (25) who reported failures due to fatal GVH disease in their trials of adoptive immunotherapy for AKR spontaneous T cell leukemia. The inev-

Table 5. Survival data following treatment of AKR spontaneous T cell leukemia as described in published reports and from Table 3[a]

Study	Mice	MST	60-Day Survival (%)
Schabel et al. (56)	29	38	28
Frei et al. (27)	34	28	6
Kende et al. (35)	17	2	0
Bekesi et al. (7)	>40	48	44
Bortin et al. (Table 3)	38	64	53

a. Median survival times computed from last day of treatment for all mice entered into each experiment; percent survival at 60 days computed from last day of treatment for all mice entered into each experiment. Some data from published reports have been adjusted in order to present uniform endpoints.

itable complication of GVH disease must be dealt with when applying adoptive immunotherapy; the main difference between the results of these investigators (4, 25, 43) and those reported in this chapter was our use of a transient GVL reaction. In the accompanying chapter in this volume, Truitt also found a high incidence of fatal GVH disease as a major complication of adoptive immunotherapy, but was able to prevent it by using gnotobiotic techniques.

In Table 5 is a comparison of the survival data presented here using chemoradiotherapy plus transient nonspecific adoptive immunotherapy with the survival data of others testing chemotherapy or chemotherapy plus active specific immunotherapy and antiviral agents for AKR spontaneous T cell leukemia. The data show that combination chemotherapy (27, 35, 56) was less effective than specific active immunotherapy plus interferon (7) or our results with adoptive immunotherapy.

VII. CLINICAL IMPLICATIONS AND FUTURE DIRECTIONS FOR RESEARCH

We firmly believe that animal models of human disease are needed in which innovative treatment strategies can be tested and perfected before clinical trials. Implicit in basic research is the assumption that most findings are based upon biological principles which transcend species differences. In the following discussion we accept that tacit assumption in order to extrapolate from mouse to man.

From the data presented in Section II it appears that the AKR spontaneous T cell leukemia is an ideal animal counterpart for human T cell acute lymphoblastic leukemia, a disease for which currently available treatments are largely unsuccessful. Using this animal model to investigate the therapeutic potential of allogeneic bone marrow transplantation, we described several observations which may be relevant for the treatment of patients with T cell leukemia.

First, remission induction should start with low doses and can then be followed by very high doses.

Second, significant GVL reactivity was not detected when donor and leukemic recipient were compatible at the MHC; no antileukemic effect was found even when the transplanted cells caused moderately severe GVH disease. This finding conforms with the clinical observation that even in the presence of severe GVH disease, there is no convincing evidence of an antileukemic effect when HLA identical siblings were used as donors.

Third, GVL reactivity in unprimed donors was always associated with incompatibility at the MHC. These results suggest that different subpopulations of killer cells may be responsible for GVH and GVL reactions. Since one would anticipate a wide range in the levels of naturally occurring GVH and GVL reactivity against a specific leukemic patient, it would be unwise to select a marrow donor for adoptive immunotherapy merely on the basis of differences at the MHC.

Finally, the increase in GVL reactivity obtained by immunizing MHC identical donors was offset by the increase in the severity of the ensuing GVH reaction; repeated injections of histocompatible donors with irradiated AKR leukemic spleen cells appeared to sensitize the donors not only against leukemia associated antigens but also against minor histocompatibility antigens. Thus, in vivo or in vitro sensitization of HLA compatible donors or their cells with irradiated leukemia cells is an approach which seems unlikely to succeed.

The treatment plan described in this chapter (chemoradiotherapy plus transient nonspecific adoptive immunotherapy) took the above experimental findings into account and resulted in a level of success which surpassed that achieved with conventional combination chemotherapy alone. To apply this strategy in man, in vitro tests need to be available which will predict accurately among a group of donors the level of GVH and GVL activity that will appear in vivo. However, despite advances in histocompatibility testing techniques, the hard fact is that marrow transplants from HLA genotypically identical donors still result in severe GVH disease in approximately half of leukemia patients, with death ascribed to GVH disease in 25%. Methods to improve the predictive value of histocompatibility testing are under intensive study in transplantation centers throughout the world. We, and others, are investigating in vitro tests which hopefully will exhibit a close correlation with in vivo GVL reactivity. As methods improve, it should be possible to select a donor with naturally occurring relatively high GVL and relatively low GVH reactivity.

The therapeutic approach to AKR T cell leukemia described here demonstrated that H-2 incompatible marrow transplantation plus chemotherapy not only killed additional malignant cells, but also provided survival results superior to those obtained with chemotherapy alone. Although this strategy has the potential for clinical trial, we believe it is far from the final solution to T cell leukemia. The need for two transplants, the high risk of damage or death due to GVH disease, and the late attrition due to recurrent leukemia make it obvious that other tactics need to be tested in the AKR T cell model. Summarized below are several strategies which we believe deserve investigation.

There are two basic approaches which we propose for further investigation to improve the safety of adoptive immunotherapy. One entails the use of histoincompatible donors (to ensure an antileukemic effect) followed by measures to avoid GVH disease such as a transient GVL reaction. Also, in this volume, Truitt describes his work using gnotobiotic techniques to avoid GVH disease following histoincompatible marrow transplantation. Cell separation techniques to selectively eliminate GVH reactive cells while maintaining the functional integrity of all other immunocompetent cells was cited in Section III C. The work of Mage and McHugh (cited in Section IV C) in which cells with antitumor reactivity were separated from those with antihost reactivity by incubation of lymphocytes on host fibroblasts raises the intriguing possibility of transplanting only GVL reactive cells. Finally, the observation that cells from endotoxin-treated donors exhibited reduced GVH reactivity without loss of GVL reactivity suggests that in vitro methods to treat donor cells before transplantation should be investigated.

An alternative approach might use histocompatible donors whose cells were specifically sensitized in vitro against the leukemia but not the host. We believe that in vitro, rather than in vivo sensitization is an ethical requisite to avoid exposure of normal individuals to potentially oncogenic material. Based upon current knowledge, we believe that highly purified solubilized tumor antigens (with histocompatibility antigens removed) or xenogeneic immune RNA are the two most promising agents for in vitro priming of donor cells.

The experimental results presented here offer hope that T cell leukemia in man may be vulnerable to adoptive immunotherapy, and that this treatment strategy may prove useful for other malignancies which are, or become refractory to more conventional therapy.

ACKNOWLEDGMENTS

We thank Gail Abendroth, Elizabeth Allen, Dr. Fritz Bach, Lynn Crandall, Roger Giller, John Glasspiegel, Susan Goelzer, Kathleen Kohut, Marcia Hilger, Mark Jacobson, Anita Lapp, William LeFeber, Peter McIver, LaVerne Milewski, Jesse Miller, Marc Rasansky, Ann Rhodes, Dr. Glenn Rodey, Dr. William Rose, Dr. Edward Saltzstein, James Seltzer, Rafaat Shalaby and Barbara Stephan whose participation in the research reported here is gratefully acknowledged. Special thanks are extended to Mrs. Evangeline Reynolds whose supervision of all experiments assured technical excellence.

Drugs used in this study were provided by the Drug Synthesis and Chemistry Branch, Division of Cancer Treatment, National Cancer Institute.

This work was supported by Public Health Service Research Contract N01-CB-33853 and Grant CA-20484 from the National Cancer Institute; American Cancer Society Grant ET-55; and grants from the Briggs and Stratton Corporation Foundation, the Patrick and Anna M. Cudahy Fund, the Leukemia Research Foundation, Inc., the Margaret and Fred Loock Foundation, the Milwaukee Division of the American Cancer Society, Northwestern Mutual Life Insurance Co., the Order of the Eastern Star, the Stackner Family Foundation, a Memorial to Frederick P. Stratton, the Margaret Elizabeth Stratton Memorial Foundation, and the Board of Trustees, Mount Sinai Medical Center.

ABBREVIATIONS

BW5147   a long passage AKR T cell acute lymphoblastic leukemia
CY   cyclophosphamide
GMuLV   Gross murine leukemia virus
GVH   graft-versus-host
GVL   graft-versus-leukemia
H-2   the MHC of mice
HLA   the MHC of man
MHC   major histocompatibility complex
MST   median survival time
TBR   total body radiation
T cell   thymus derived lymphocyte expressing theta antigen and, in humans, forming spontaneous rosettes when incubated with sheep erythrocytes
TL   thymus leukemia

REFERENCES

1. Advisory Committee of the International Bone Marrow Transplant Registry. 1976. Bone marrow transplantation from histocompatible, allogeneic donors for aplastic anemia. JAMA 236: 1131.

2. Advisory Committee of the International Bone Marrow Transplant Reg-

istry. 1975. Report from the ACS/NIH Bone Marrow Transplant Registry. *Exp. Hematol.* 3: 149.

3. Advisory Committee of the International Bone Marrow Transplant Registry. 1977. Severe combined immunodeficiency disease: Characterization of the disease and results of transplantation. *JAMA* 238: 591.

4. Alexander, P. 1967. Immunotherapy of leukemia: The use of different classes of immune lymphocytes. *Cancer Res.* 27: 2521.

5. Bach, F. H., Albertini, R. J., Joo, P., Anderson, J. J., and Bortin, M. M. 1968. Bone marrow transplantation in a patient with Wiskott-Aldrich syndrome. *Lancet* 2: 1364.

6. Barnes, D. W. H., Corp, M. J., Loutit, J. F., and Neal, F. E. 1956. Treatment of murine leukaemia with x-rays and homologous bone marrow. *Brit. Med. J.* 2: 626.

7. Bekesi, J. G., Roboz, J. P., Zimmerman, E., and Holland, J. F. 1976. Treatment of spontaneous leukemia in AKR mice with chemotherapy, immunotherapy or interferon. *Cancer Res.* 36: 631.

8. Boranić, M. 1971. Time-pattern of the antileukemic effect of the graft-versus-host reaction in mice. *Transplant. Proc.* 3: 394.

9. Boranić, M. 1968. Transient graft versus host reaction in the treatment of leukemia in mice. *J. Natl. Cancer Inst.* 4: 421.

10. Bortin, M. M. 1970. A compendium of reported human bone marrow transplants. *Transplantation* 9: 571.

11. Bortin, M. M. 1974. Graft-versus-leukemia, *in* F. H. Bach and R. A. Good (eds.), *Clinical Immunobiology* Vol. II, p. 287. Academic Press, New York.

12. Bortin, M. M., Rimm, A. A., Rodey, G. E., Giller, R. H., and Saltzstein, E. C. 1974. Prolonged survival in long-passage AKR leukemia using chemotherapy, radiotherapy and adoptive immunotherapy. *Cancer Res.* 34: 1851.

13. Bortin, M. M., Rimm, A. A., Rose, W. C., and Saltzstein, E. C. 1974. Graft-versus-leukemia. V. Absence of antileukemic effect using allogeneic, H-2 identical immunocompetent cells. *Transplantation* 18: 280.

14. Bortin, M. M., Rimm, A. A., and Saltzstein, E. C. 1973. Graft-versus-leukemia: Quantification of adoptive immunotherapy in murine leukemia. *Science* 179: 811.

15. Bortin, M. M., Rimm, A. A., Saltzstein, E. C., and Rodey, G. E. 1973. Graft-versus-leukemia. III. Apparent independent antihost and antileukemic activity of transplanted immunocompetent cells. *Transplantation* 16: 182.

16. Bortin, M. M., Truitt, R. L., Rose, W. C., Rimm, A. A., and Saltzstein, E. C. 1976. Adoptive immunotherapy of spontaneous leukemia-lymphoma in AKR mice, *in* H. Friedman, M. R. Escobar and S. M. Reichard (eds.), *Advances in Experimental Medicine and Biology, The Reticuloendothelial System in Health and Disease, Immunologic and Pathologic Aspects.* Vol. 73B, p. 331. Plenum Press, New York.

17. Boyse, E. A., Old, L. J., and Stockert, E. 1966. The TL (thymus leukemia) antigen: A review, *in* P. Grabar and P. A. Miescher (eds.), *Immunopathology. IV. the International Symposium,* p. 23. Schwabe and Co., Basel.

18. Brouet, J.-C, Valensi, F., Daniel, M.-T., Flandrin, G., Preud homme, J.-L., and Seligmann, M. 1976. Immunological classification of acute lymphoblastic leukaemias: Evaluation of its clinical significance in 100 patients. *Brit. J. Haematol.* 33: 319.

19. Brunner, K. T., Mariel, J., Rudolf, H., and Chapuis, B. 1970. Studies of allograft immunity in mice. I. Induction, development and in vitro assay of cellular immunity. Immunology 18: 501.

20. Cantor, H., and Asofsky, R. 1972. Synergy among lymphoid cells mediating the graft-versus-host response. III. Evidence for interaction between two types of thymus derived cells. J. Exp. Med. 135: 764.

21. Cerrotini, J. C., and Brunner, K. T. 1974. Cell-mediated cytotoxicity, allograft rejection and tumor immunity. Adv. Immunol. 18: 67.

22. Chester, S. J., Esparza, A. R., and Albala, M. M. 1975. Graft-versus-leukemia without fatal graft-versus-host disease in AKR mice. Cancer Res. 35: 637.

23. Cline, M. J., Gale, R. P., Stiehm, E. R., Opelz, G., Young, L. W., Feig, S. A., and Fahey, J. L. 1975. Bone marrow transplantation in man. Ann. Intern. Med. 83: 691.

24. Damais, C., Lamensans, A., and Chedid, L. 1972. Endotoxines bactériennes et maladie homologue du nouveau-né. C.R. Acad. Sci. 274: 1113.

25. Denton, P. M., and Symes, M. D. 1969. Attempts to induce a graft-versus-tumor reaction against AKR lymphomata in isogeneic mice, by injection of melphalan and foreign immunologically competent cells. Brit. J. Cancer 23: 95.

26. Fernandes, G., Yunis, E. J., and Good, R. A. 1975. Depression of cytotoxic T cell subpopulations in mice by hydrocortisone treatment. Clin. Immunol. Immunopathol. 4: 304.

27. Frei, E., III, Schabel, F. M., Jr., and Goldin, A. 1974. Comparative chemotherapy of AKR lymphoma and human hematological neoplasia. Cancer Res. 34: 184.

28. Furth, J., Seibold, H. R., and Rathbone, P. R. 1933. Experimental studies on lymphomatosis of mice. Amer. J. Cancer 19: 521.

29. Gatti, R. A., Allen, H. D., Meuwissen, H. J., Hong, R., and Good, R. A. 1968. Immunological reconstitution of sex-linked lymphopenic immunological deficiency. Lancet 2: 1366.

30. Gershon, R. K. 1975. A disquisition on suppressor T cells. Transplant. Rev. 26: 170.

31. Glucksberg, H., and Fefer, A. 1973. Combination chemotherapy for clinically established graft-versus-host disease in mice. Cancer Res. 33: 859.

32. Gross, L. 1970. Oncogenic Viruses, 2nd ed., p. 1991. Pergamon Press, Oxford.

33. Gross, L. 1971. Tentative guidelines referring to inoculation of homologous cancer extracts in man. Int. J. Cancer 7: 182.

34. Kedar, E., and Bonavida, B. 1975. Studies on the induction and expression of T cell-mediated immunity. IV. Non-overlapping populations of alloimmune cytotoxic lymphocytes with specificity for tumor-associated antigens and transplantation antigens. J. Immunol. 115: 1301.

35. Kende, M., Goldberg, A. I., Glynn, J. P., Mantel, N., and Goldin, A. 1972. Relationship between white blood cell count and diagnosis and therapeutic response in AKR mice with spontaneous leukemia (lymphoma). Cancer Chemother. Rep. 56: 73.

36. Kersey, J., Nesbit, M., Hallgren, H., Sabad, A., Yunis, E., and Gajl-Peczalska, K. 1975. Evidence for origin of certain childhood acute lymphoblastic leukemias and lymphomas in thymus derived lymphocytes. Cancer 36: 1348.

37. Krammer, P. H., Citronbaum, R., Read, S. E., Forni, L., and Lang, R. 1976. Murine thymic lymphomas as model tumors for T-cell studies, T-cell markers, immunoglobulin and F_c receptors on AKR thymomas. *Cell. Immunol.* 21: 97.

38. LeFeber, W. P., Truitt, R. L., Rose, W. C., and Bortin, M. M. 1977. Graft-versus-leukemia. VII. Donor selection for adoptive immunotherapy in mice, *in* S. Baum (ed.), *Experimental Hematology Today*, p. 239. Springer-Verlag, New York.

39. Liacopoulos, P., and Merchant, B. 1969. Effet du traitement des donneurs avec des endotoxines sur la maladie homologue des réceveurs adultes irradiés, *in* L. Chedid (ed.), *Coll. Intern. sur les Endotoxines*, CNRS no. 174, p. 341, Paris.

40. Lilly, F., and Pincus, T. 1973. Genetic control of murine viral leukemogenesis. *Adv. Cancer Res.* 17: 231.

41. Lin, H., and Bruce, W. R. 1972. A cellular approach to the chemotherapy of spontaneous leukemia of AKR mice. *Ser. Haematol.* 5: 73.

42. Mage, M. C., and McHugh, L. L. 1973. Retention of graft-vs-host activity in nonadherent spleen cells after depletion of cytotoxic activity by incubation on allogeneic target cells. *J. Immunol.* 111: 652.

43. Mathé, G., Amiel, J. L., Schwarzenberg, L., Cattan, A., and Schneider, M. 1965. Adoptive immunotherapy of acute leukemia: Experimental and clinical results. *Cancer Res.* 25: 1525.

44. Metcalf, D., and Brumby, M. 1967. Coulter counter analysis of lymphoma differentiation patterns in AKR mice with lymphoid leukemia. *Int. J. Cancer* 2: 37.

45. Owens, A. H., Jr. 1970. The effect of cyclophosphamide and graft-versus-host disease on two mouse tumors. *Proc. Amer. Assoc. Cancer Res.* 2: 62.

46. Park, B. H., Biggar, W. D., and Good, R. A. 1972. Paucity of thymus-dependent cells in human marrow. *Transplantation* 14: 284.

47. Pauly, J. L., Minowada, J., Han, T., and Moore, G. E. 1975. Disparity of mixed leukocyte reactivity to cultured cells of human T and B lymphoid lines. *J. Natl. Cancer Inst.* 54: 557.

48. Pellis, N. R., and Kahan, B. D. 1977. Methods to demonstrate the immunogenicity of soluble tumor-specific transplantation antigens. I. The immunoprophylaxis assay, *in* H. Busch (ed.), *Methods in Cancer Research*, Vol. 12, Academic Press (in press).

49. Pilch, Y. H., and Kern, D. H. 1977. Immune RNA and tumor immunity, *in* E. P. Conen (ed.), *Immune RNA*. C-R-C Press, Cleveland, Ohio (in press).

50. Rodey, G. E., Sprader, J. C., and Bortin, M. M. 1974. Inhibition of normal allogeneic responder cells in mouse mixed leukocyte culture by long-passage AKR leukemic lymphoblasts. *Cancer Res.* 34: 1289.

51. Rose, W. C., Rimm, A. A., Saltzstein, E. C., Truitt, R. L., and Bortin, M. M. 1975. Low-dose chemotherapy as a prelude to intensive treatment of spontaneous leukemia-lymphoma in AKR mice. *J. Natl. Cancer Inst.* 55: 219.

52. Rose, W. C., Rodey, G. E., Rimm, A. A., Truitt, R. L., and Bortin, M. M. 1976. Mitigation of graft-versus-host disease in mice by treatment of donors with bacterial endotoxin. *Exp. Hematol.* 4: 90.

53. Rouse, B. T., and Wagner, H. 1972. The *in vivo* activity of *in vitro* immunized mouse thymocytes. II. Rejection of skin allografts and graft-vs-host activity. *J. Immunol.* 109: 1282.

54. Salmon, S. E., Krakauer, R. S., and Whitmore, W. F. 1971. Lymphocyte stimulation: Selective destruction of cells during blastogenic response to trans-

plantation antigens. *Science* 172: 490.

55. Saltzstein, E. C., Glasspiegel, J. S., Rimm, A. A., Giller, R. H., and Bortin, M. M. 1972. Graft-versus-leukemia for "cell cure" of long-passage AKR leukemia after chemoradiotherapy. *Cancer Res.* 32: 1658.

56. Schabel, F. M., Jr., Skipper, H. E., Trader, M. W., Laster, W. R., Jr., and Cheeks, J. B. 1974. Combination chemotherapy for spontaneous AKR lymphoma. *Cancer Chemother. Rep.* Part 2, 4: 53.

57. Schabel, F. M., Jr., Skipper, H. E., Trader, M. W., Laster, W. R., Jr., and Simpson-Herren, L. 1969. Spontaneous leukemia (lymphoma) as a model system. *Cancer Chemother. Rep.* 53: 329.

58. Seidman, H., Silverberg, E., and Holleb, A. I. 1976. Cancer statistics, 1976: A comparison of white and black populations. *Ca-A Cancer Journal for Clinicians* 26: 2.

59. Sen, L., and Borella, L. 1975. Clinical importance of lymphoblasts with T markers in childhood acute leukemia. *N. Engl. J. Med.* 296: 828.

60. Sen, L., Mills, B., and Borella, L. 1976. Erythrocyte receptors and thymus-associated antigens on human thymocytes, mitogen-induced blasts and acute leukemia blasts. *Cancer Res.* 36: 2436.

61. Simonsen, M. 1962. Graft-versus-host reactions, their natural history and applicability as tools of research. *Prog. Allergy* 6: 349.

62. Storb, R., Thomas, E. D., Buckner, C. D., Clift, R. A., Fefer, A., Glucksberg, H., and Neiman, P. E. 1974. Transplantation of bone marrow in refractory marrow failure and neoplastic diseases. *Amer. J. Clin. Pathol.* 62: 212.

63. Thomas, E. D., 1976. Marrow transplantation for acute leukemia, *in* H. A. Perkins (ed.), *Human Bone Marrow Transplantation*, p. 19. American Association of Blood Banks, Gunthorp-Warren Printing Co., Chicago.

64. Thomas, E. D., Storb, R., Clift, R. A., Fefer, A., Johnson, F. L., Neiman, P. E., Lerner, K. G., Glucksberg, H., and Buckner, C. D. 1975. Bone marrow transplantation. *N. Engl. J. Med.* 292: 832 and 895.

65. Tridente, G., Collavo, D., Chieco-Bianchi, L., and Fiore-Donati, L. 1969. Thymus-marrow cell interaction *in vitro*: A synergistic effect in PHA response. *Exp. Hematol.* 19: 53.

66. Truitt, R. L. 1976. Allogeneic bone marrow transplantation for the treatment of AKR spontaneous leukemia. *Fed. Proc.* 35: 312.

67. Truitt, R. L., Rose, W. C., Rimm, A. A., and Bortin, M. M. 1976. Antileukemic reactivity of allogeneic immunocompetent cells derived from endotoxin-treated donor mice. *Exp. Hematol.* (Supplement) 4: 191.

68. Tsukimoto, I., Wong, K. Y., and Lampkin, B. C. 1976. Surface markers and prognostic factors in acute lymphoblastic leukemia. *N. Engl. J. Med.* 294: 245.

69. Wigzell, H. 1971. Cellular immunoadsorbents, *in* B. Amos (ed.), *Progress in Immunology*, Vol. I, p. 1105. Academic Press, New York.

70. Woodruff, M. F. A., and Nolan, B. 1963. Preliminary observations on treatment of advanced cancer by injection of allogeneic spleen cells. *Lancet* 2: 426.

71. Zatz, M. M., White, A., Goldstein, A. L. 1973. Lymphocyte populations of AKR/J mice. II. Effect of leukemogenesis on migration patterns, response to PHA, and expression of theta antigen. *J. Immunol.* 111: 1519.

72. Zoschke, D. C., and Bach, F. H. 1971. Specificity of allogeneic cell recognition by human lymphocytes *in vitro*. *Science* 172: 1350.

CHAPTER 16

APPLICATION OF GERMFREE TECHNIQUES TO THE TREATMENT OF LEUKEMIA IN AKR MICE BY ALLOGENEIC BONE MARROW TRANSPLANTATION

Robert L. Truitt

May and Sigmund Winter
Research Laboratory
Mount Sinai Medical Center
Milwaukee, Wisconsin 53233

In this study germfree techniques were applied to the treatment of spontaneous T cell leukemia in AKR mice by adoptive immunotherapy using immunocompetent cells from histoincompatible donors. Secondary disease, the major complication of adoptive immunotherapy, was largely eliminated when the recipient AKR mice were bacteria-free. In addition to decreasing infectious complications, germfree and antibiotic decontamination procedures permitted the use of drug and radiation doses which were not tolerated by leukemic animals maintained in a conventional environment. The combination of intense chemoradiotherapy and histoincompatible marrow transplantation resulted in long-term, disease-free survival in a significant proportion of decontaminated and germfree AKR mice bearing advanced leukemia.

I. Introduction

It is now possible to procure and maintain almost any species of animal, including man, in a germfree environment. A number of infants have been delivered and raised in a completely germfree environment (18); one of the most dramatic recent cases being David, a child with severe combined immunodeficiency disease who has spent all of his six years in protective isolation at Texas Children's Hospital, Houston. Most germfree animals have been Caesarean-derived; however, alternative procedures for eliminating the endogenous microbial flora by high dose antibiotic therapy were developed in rodents (41, 44) and monkeys (42) and recently have been applied to man (16, 26, 43, 45). Just as the development of the flexible film plastic isolator (36) contributed to a vast expansion of germfree research, the development of high-efficiency particulate air or HEPA filters and decontamination procedures have contributed to an expansion of the clinical use of germfree technology thru laminar airflow isolation units. Thus, the science of gnotobiology[1] has advanced beyond the laboratory and reached a point at which it can now be applied with advantage to a number of clinical situations, and as a result, a new field of clinical gnotobiology is developing.

The potential value of germfree technology is most apparent in conditions associated with depressed immune response in which the patient can fall victim to endogenous or exogenous microbes. Immunodeficient states, leukemias and other malignancies, certain renal and gastrointestinal diseases, burns, amyloidosis, transplantation, and open heart surgery are typical situations which have or could benefit from germfree technology (12).

Bone marrow transplantation is frequently considered for the treatment of leukemia which is refractory to conventional therapeutic approaches. In patients undergoing marrow transplantation for the treatment of leukemia the risk of fatal infections is substantial (4, 35). These patients suffer from severe impairment of their immunologic defense capacities because of the malignancy, pre- and post-transplant immunosuppressive conditioning regimens and the immunologic attack by the transplanted cells on the normal tissues of the recipient (i.e., graft-versus-host or GVH disease)[2] (4, 35, 46). Furthermore, experimental evidence has shown that unprimed histocompatible donors are ineffective at eliminating spontaneous T cell leukemia, and an adoptive immunotherapeutic effect[3] can be obtained only when donors that are incompatible at the major histocompatibility complex (MHC) are used (2, and Bortin et al., this volume). The problem, of course, with using MHC-incompatible donors is the severity of the GVH reaction and its potentially lethal complications.

Successful application of bone marrow transplantation to the treatment of leukemia (or any disease) requires resolution of two of the major problems; (a) preventing infections and (b) eliminating fatal GVH disease. In the case of leukemia, the solution to these problems should not interfere with any antitumor effect that the transplanted cells might have. To determine whether the safety of bone marrow transplantation across MHC barriers for the treatment of leukemia could be improved by the use of germfree techniques, we initiated studies in an experimental model using Caesarean-derived germfree, antibiotic decontaminated and conventionally reared AKR mice which spontaneously develop acute T cell lymphoblastic leukemia. This chapter contains a review of the experimental results and a description of our attempts to develop a treatment model which could be applied for the therapy of acute leukemia in man.

II. Secondary Disease in Radiation Chimeras

In early experimental work on marrow transplantation most of the attention was focused on recovery during the first 30 days after transplantation. Eventually, however, workers in the field observed animals that were given allogeneic marrow for longer periods and found that they showed peculiar symptoms such as severe diarrhea, weight lost (wasting), skin lesions, alopecia, dyspnea and kyphosis (39). This syndrome was termed "secondary disease" to distinguish it from "primary disease" (i.e., the acute effects of radiation on hematopoiesis) which resulted in death within the first few days after irradiation. The etiology of secondary disease was and has continued to be the subject of intensive investigation.

Lethally irradiated mice usually develop a delayed form of secondary disease starting about the fourth week after transplantation of allogeneic marrow (39). An acute form of secondary disease which starts within the first week after transplantation can be produced in some strain combinations of mice by grafting post-thymic T cells from lymph nodes or the spleen. Now there seems to be little doubt that secondary disease which develops in allogeneic radiation chimeras[4] is a consequence of GVH disease. However, factors other than the GVH reaction are known to influence the severity and incidence of secondary disease, and subtle distinctions exist between the active immunological attack of donor lymphoid cells against the normal tissues of the host and the consequences of this attack (disturbed organ function, immunodeficiency, infection, etc.).

III. Bone Marrow Transplantation in a Bacteria-Free Environment

In the initial phases of experiments aimed at evaluating the effects of marrow transplantation on a spontaneously developing murine neoplasm, we examined the influence of microbes on secondary disease mortality in young, non-leukemic AKR mice. The AKR strain was developed from an inbred line established by Furth (8). AKR mice develop a high incidence of spontaneous leukemia; 50% of the mice develop and die of leukemia by 9 months of age, and 90% before 12 months of age (38). The leukemia is induced by Gross-type endogenous murine leukemia virus (MuLV) (9) and develops initially in the thymus which becomes engorged with anaplastic cells. Subsequently, there is enlargement of lymph nodes and the spleen followed by leukemic infiltration of non-lymphoid tissues such as the liver, kidney and ovaries.

The AKR mice used in this study were either conventionally reared, Caesarean-derived germfree (20) or conventional mice which have been rendered bacteria-free by continuous treatment with high dose antibiotics per os (Table 1). The procedures for eliminating the microflora of conventional mice (decontamination) were adapted from the methods of van der Waaij (44). Briefly, this involved continuous treatment of the mice with poorly absorbed orally administered antibiotics.[5] At first, Streptomycin, Neomycin, and Bacitracin were given in the drinking water, but later four antibiotic combinations were rotated weekly; Bacitracin plus either Streptomycin, Kanamycin, Gentamicin, or Neomycin. The mice were housed in horizontal laminar airflow hoods and given frequent changes of sterile

Table 1.   Terminology used to describe experimental animals

Terminology	Origin of Mice	Treatment before Transplantation
Germfree (GF)	Caesarean-derived	Bred and maintained in an axenic environment; Trexler-type plastic isolators (closed isolation system).
Decontaminated (DC)	Conventional	Kept in sterile horizontal laminar airflow hoods (open isolation system); high-dose antibiotics in drinking water.
Conventional (CV)	Conventional	Standard mouse facility with open "shoebox" or Isosystem® cages; acidified + chlorinated water.

cages, bedding and food. The intestinal microflora was monitored by culturing fresh feces in thioglycollate broth. No attempt was made to culture fastidious microorganisms; however, extensive bacteriological examinations of mice treated with this decontamination protocol in another study confirmed that all detectable anaerobic and aerobic microorganisms were eliminated (31). Fungal infections were not a problem in our animals.

Four donor strains, incompatible with AKR at the MHC and at minor histocompatibility loci, were selected for study on the basis of variation in the intensity of their secondary disease in AKR mice (15). For the purposes of this chapter, secondary disease has been divided into delayed and acute forms. In delayed secondary disease, the majority of deaths occur more than 30 days after transplantation (i.e., MST > 30 days); in acute secondary disease, the majority of deaths occur within 30 days (i.e., MST < 30 days). With the four donor-recipient combinations chosen, we were able to evaluate the effect of modifications in the microbial environment on delayed and acute secondary disease in allogeneic radiation chimeras. Twenty-four hours prior to transplantation, the AKR hosts were exposed to 1000 r gamma or X-ray total body radiation (TBR) for immunosuppression. The survival data is presented in Table 2.

Caesarean-derived germfree AKR ($H-2^k$) mice which had been bred and maintained in strict axenic isolation for over 20 generations (20) were immunosuppressed and inoculated with marrow cells from DBA/2 ($H-2^d$) mice (Group 1). The use of germfree animals permitted us to evaluate delayed secondary disease mortality under optimal isolation conditions. Germfree mice were housed in Trexler flexible film plastic isolators (36), and were free of all bacteria, yeast and mycoplasma (20). The MST of germfree allogeneic radiation chimeras was greater than 330 days (Group 1) compared with 38 days for chimeras reared and maintained under conventional environmental conditions (Group 3) (P < 0.001). Only two of 14 (14%) conventional allogeneic radiation chimeras survived 100 days post-transplant as compared to 26 of 32 (81%) germfree chimeras (P < 0.001). The DBA/2 mice used as donors in Group 1 were also germfree; however, the use of germfree rather than conventional donors was not essential. In Group 2 cells from conventional donors were transplanted into AKR recipients that were conventionally reared and decontaminated of all bacteria by antibiotic therapy; yet, their MST was 319 post-transplant, and all of the animals survived to 200 days post-transplant. Although the size of Group 2 is small, the results indicated that germfree donors were not essential to decreased mortality in germfree allogeneic radiation chimeras. The MST and survival rate at 100 days for Group 2 was significantly better than Group 3 (P < 0.001 and 0.01, respectively). These results were confirmed in subsequent experiments.

Table 2. Effect of microbial environment on secondary disease mortality in various allogeneic radiation chimeras

Group	Microbial Status of Recipient	N[a]	Donor Strain	Donor Cells (×10[6])	MST[b] (Days)	Percent Survival on Day[b] 30	60	100	200
1	GF	32	DBA/2	BM(>10)[c]	>330[d]	91	84	81	69
2	DC	6	DBA/2	BM(>10)	319	100	100	100	100
3	CV	14	DBA/2	BM(>10)	38	71	14	14	—
4	DC	31	DBA/1	BM(20)	>100[d]	84	68	65	—
5	CV	20	DBA/1	BM(20)	48	75	45	45	—
6	DC	10	DBA/1	BM(20)+LN(10)	9	0	—	—	—
7	CV	20	DBA/1	BM(20)+LN(10)	8	0	—	—	—
8	DC	12	SJL/J	BM(20)+LN(3)	>100[d]	92	75	50	—
9	CV	20	SJL/J	BM(20)+LN(3)	18	45	0	0	—

a. Number of immunosuppressed (1000 r TBR) AKR recipients (approx. 3 mo. of age).

b. Post-transplant.

c. In early experiments donor cells were quantitated as "femur equivalents" and averaged more than 10^7 nucleated cells per recipient.

d. MST not reached.

Conventional AKR mice given DBA/2 bone marrow (Group 3) appeared healthy for a few days, then developed diarrhea, scaly dermatitis, digitigrade and alopecia. The mice were kyphotic, dyspneic and wasted. On autopsy and histological examination, they showed depletion of lymphoid organs, extensive pneumonia, hepatitis and erosion of the intestinal mucosa. In contrast, most of the germfree and decontaminated chimeras (Groups 1 and 2) had no clinical or histological evidence of secondary disease. The lymphoid organs were structurally restored except for some suggestive depletion of thymic dependent areas. Lesions compatible with mild GVH disease were noted in two germfree chimeras. However, the most frequent lesion in long-term surviving germfree chimeras was chronic glomerulonephritis (22). Up to the age of 15 months, spontaneous leukemia was noted in only 3/38 (8%) germfree and decontaminated radiation chimeras as compared with over 90% of untreated AKR mice. Leukemia also developed in AKR mice that were irradiated and reconstituted with syngeneic marrow (22). Thus, the presence of allogeneic DBA/2 cells interfered with the appearance of spontaneous T cell leukemia in the AKR hosts.

Transplantation of marrow from DBA/1 (H-2^q) donors produced delayed secondary disease mortality in both decontaminated and conventional AKR hosts (Groups 4 and 5, Table 2). The MST of decontaminated AKR hosts was longer than that of conventional hosts, and the survival rates at 30, 60, and 100 days exceeded those of conventional animals; however, the differences were not statistically significant with the group sizes tested. Addition of DBA/1 lymph node cells to the marrow inoculum (Groups 6 and 7) resulted in hyperacute secondary disease. Gnotobiotic conditions were incapable of protecting the AKR hosts from such an intense GVH reaction. However, the benefit of antibiotic decontamination and axenic isolation in mice undergoing an acute, but less severe, GVH reaction can be seen in Groups 8 and 9. Administration of bone marrow and lymph node cells from SJL/J (H-2^s) donors to immunosuppressed conventional AKR hosts resulted in an MST of 18 days and 55% mortality within 30 days (Group 9). The MST as well as 30, 60 and 100-day survival rates of decontaminated chimeras (Group 8) were significantly better than those of conventional chimeras ($P < 0.05$ to 0.001).

The results shown in Table 2 clearly demonstrated that mortality commonly attributed to the immunological events associated with GVH reactions is in reality more closely linked to the presence of endogenous and/or exogenous bacteria which act as opportunistic pathogens. Thus, maintaining the hosts in an axenic environment following allogeneic bone marrow transplantation had a significant salutary effect on delayed secondary disease (cf. Groups 1, 2 and 3; Groups 4 and 5) and acute secondary disease (cf. Groups 8 and 9); however, this approach was ineffective against hyperacute secondary disease (cf. Groups 6 and 7).

IV. Demonstration of Chimerism

An important question in these experiments is whether the immunosuppression of 1,000 r TBR was sufficient to permit permanent engraftment of the transplanted tissues, i.e., were the mice truly chimeric? Mixed leukocyte culture (MLC) tests were used to determine if spleen cells from decontaminated AKR mice that received DBA/2 cells had characteristics of AKR or DBA/2 cells. Reciprocal unidirectional MLC tests were done according to modifications of the technique of Bach and Voynow (1) as used in tests for chimerism (3). Assays were performed 90 days after transplant and the results are shown in Table 3. Spleen cells from the experimental mice were stimulated to synthesize DNA when cultured with mitomycin-C treated cells from AKR mice. Conversely, cells from AKR mice were stimulated when cultured with mitomycin-C treated cells from the experimental mice. Reciprocal non-stimulation was found

Table 3.   Results of MLC assays to test for chimerism in decontaminated AKR mice that received 1000 r TBR and a marrow transplant from DBA/2 mice 90 days earlier

Responding Cells ($\times$ 10^6)	Source of Mitomycin C-Treated Stimulator Cells ($\times$ 10^6)					
	AKR$_m$	DBA/2$_m$	X-1$_m$	X-2$_m$	X-3$_m$	X-4$_m$
AKR	2,816[b]	33,364	11,886	26,545	26,191	46,827
DBA/2	70,980	3,241	1,330	2,124	2,486	2,015
X-1[a]	11,829	1,569	662			
X-2	31,252	1,366		1,002		
X-3	29,095	2,032			1,387	
X-4	35,047	1,973				1,768

a. X-1 to X-4 refer to individual AKR mice being tested for chimerism.

b. Counts per minute of ^{3}H-thymidine incorporation by responder cells. Numbers shown are mean values of triplicate cultures.

when cells from the experimental mice were cultured with DBA/2 cells. Thus, the spleen cells from AKR mice that were given transplants from DBA/2 donors more than 90 days earlier had in vitro characteristics of the DBA/2 donors, and the mice were believed to be chimeric. However, the possibility of mixed cell chimerism cannot be excluded on the basis of MLC tests.

V. Bacteria-Free Environments and Adoptive Immunotherapy of Leukemia

Elimination of the microflora of the recipient might be useful in circumventing secondary disease, the major stumbling block which has prevented successful application of adoptive immunotherapy to the treatment of cancer (17). Spontaneous T cell leukemia of AKR mice represents a model tumor system which closely simulates several human malignancies (7, 9, 25, 28), especially the T cell form of acute lymphoblastic leukemia (27, and Bortin et al., this volume). AKR leukemia is extremely resistant to conventional therapeutic approaches (7, 25, 29), carries tumor-associated antigens (10, 19, 47) and provides a rigorous test system in which to evaluate the clinical potential of allogeneic bone marrow transplantation for the treatment of refractory acute leukemias. Our hypothesis in this series of experiments was that the use of a germfree or decontaminated environment would permit transplantation of immuno-competent cells into leukemic AKR recipients across MHC barriers without the occurrence of lethal secondary disease. The use of adoptive immuno-therapy in combination with conventional chemoradiotherapy could result in elimination of the leukemia and cure of a significant proportion of animals.

As in the previous studies, germfree, decontaminated and conventional AKR mice were used. AKR mice were diagnosed as bearing advanced spontaneous T cell leukemia on the basis of palpation of the peripheral lymph nodes and spleen, or in the case of germfree AKR mice on the appearance of the characteristic dyspnea and kyphosis caused by respiratory obstruction by the thymoma. Our diagnostic accuracy during the past two years had been >99; during 1975, the MST of 237 untreated conventional AKR mice diagnosed with leukemia was 20 days, and none of the mice survived beyond 60 days post-diagnosis. The incidence, age at which leukemia developed and the MST post-diagnosis was not significantly affected by germfree or decontaminated status (20, 37 and unpublished results). In these experiments, treatment was not initiated until after the appearance of leukemia; however, the AKR recipients were bacteria-free *before* the disease appeared, either by nature of birth (germfree mice) or through decontamination initiated four to five months prior to the median age at which leukemia usually developed. The results of experiments testing adoptive immunotherapy with chemoradiotherapy are presented in Table 4.

Conventional leukemic AKR mice treated with 185 mg/kg of cyclophosphamide (CY)[6] on day 0 (day of diagnosis) and 1000 r TBR on day 2 were given marrow cells from syngeneic (normal) AKR (Group 1) or allogeneic DBA/2 donors (Group 2). Their respective MSTs were 14 and 10 days post-treatment, and none of the animals survived 100 days. In contrast, when the recipient leukemic AKR mice were germfree, the MST following DBA/2 bone marrow transplantation was 144 days (Group 3). Furthermore, 71% of the animals survived to 100 days post-transplant. The survival data for Group 3 are significantly better than the conventional controls (Groups 1 and 2; $P < 0.05$ to 0.001).

In Groups 4 and 5 conventional and decontaminated leukemic AKR mice were treated with another regimen of CY and TBR. Their survival patterns were similar to those observed for Groups 2 and 3. None of the conventional leukemic mice (Group 4) survived 60 days post-treatment; their MST was 6 days. The MST of six decontaminated leukemic AKR mice (Group 5) treated in the same manner as Group 4 was 162 days. Furthermore, all of the mice in Group 5 survived beyond 60 days, and two (33%) were alive 200 days post-treatment. Four decontaminated leukemic AKR mice were also given chemoradiotherapy and syngeneic (normal)

Table 4. Survival of AKR mice bearing advanced spontaneous T cell leukemia after treatment with chemoradiotherapy and bone marrow transplantation

Group	Microbial Status of Recipient	N[a]	Chemoradiotherapy (day)		Marrow Donor	MST[b] days	Percent Survival on Day[b]			
			CY(mg/kg)	TBR (r)			30	60	100	200
1	CV	14	185 (0)	1000 (2)	AKR	14	36	0	0	0
2	CV	15	185 (0)	1000 (2)	DBA/2	10	47	7	0	0
3	GF	21	185 (0)	1000 (2)	DBA/2	144	90	86	71	29
4	CV	8	100 (0)	1000 (7)	DBA/2	6	13	0	0	0
5	DC	6	100 (0)	1000 (7)	DBA/2	162	100	100	83	33
6	CV	11	—	850 (0)	AKR	42	73	36	18	0
7	DC	31	—	1000 (0)	DBA/2	224	94	81	74	61

a. Number of AKR mice bearing spontaneous T cell leukemia (6–12 mo. of age).
b. Post-transplant.

AKR marrow (not shown in Table 4); all died within 33 days (MST = 22 days), and three had gross evidence of leukemia on autopsy.

Groups 6 and 7 have been included in Table 4 although their treatment regimens were not identical. AKR mice bearing advanced spontaneous T cell leukemia are extremely sensitive to the effects of TBR (23). Fifteen of 20 (75%) conventional leukemic AKR mice died within 24 hours following 1000 r TBR, and many of these died within 4 hours post-irradiation (data not shown). The acute toxic effects of TBR could be overcome if chemotherapy was administered prior to TBR (23) as in Groups 1 through 5. However, if TBR was the only therapy used (other than the marrow transplant), it was necessary to lower the dose given to conventional leukemic mice. Mice in Group 6 were inoculated with marrow from normal AKR donors. These mice were housed in laminar airflow hoods and provided with sterile bedding, food and water in the same manner as decontaminated AKR mice; however, they were not given antibiotics. Thus, they were isolated from exogenous but not endogenous sources of infection. The MST for the syngeneic group (Group 6) was 42 days post-treatment and the 100-day survival rate was 18%. The best survival results for all groups listed in Table 4 were in decontaminated leukemic mice given 1000 r TBR and DBA/2 bone marrow (Group 7). The MST of 31 chimeras was 224 days post-treatment, and 19 (61%) survived beyond 200 days. Some mice in Group 7 were sacrificed more than one year after diagnosis of leukemia when they were more than 20 months of age. The results in Table 4 clearly indicated that absence of microbial flora in leukemic AKR mice permitted the use of therapeutic manipulations which could not be applied successfully to the treatment of conventional animals. Further, transplantation of cells from H-2 incompatible donors resulted in survival data significantly superior to that seen when syngeneic mice were used as donors.

VI. The Problem of Recurrent Leukemia

In evaluating chemotherapeutic treatments for AKR spontaneous T cell leukemia, mice which survived 60 days after the end of therapy without evidence of disease are usually considered to be "cured" (25, 29). Using that criterion, 81% to 100% of the germfree or decontaminated leukemic AKR mice treated with chemoradiotherapy and allogeneic bone marrow transplantation were cured (Table 4). However, when one is dealing with an immunologic treatment procedure such as marrow transplantation, there is the possibility of perturbation in the cytokinetic characteristics of the leukemia, and one must be cautious in extrapolating from cytokinetic patterns developed in untreated mice.

The incidence of recurrent leukemia within 200 days after the end of treatment provides some insight into the actual number of cured mice. Shown in Table 5 is an analysis of the incidence of recurrent leukemia for those groups which had a significant proportion survive more than 200 days after the end of treatment. Group 6 also has been included for comparison purposes. Overall, only 16% (9/58) of the mice treated with allogeneic bone marrow transplantation developed recurrent leukemia within 200 days (Groups 3, 5, and 7). In contrast, of the 11 mice treated with syngeneic marrow and lower TBR (Group 6), all developed recurrent leukemia. Other groups from Table 4 were not included in the analysis because the number of animals surviving beyond 60 days after the end of treatment was not sufficiently high to allow meaningful evaluation of whether recurrent leukemia was a problem.

Most of the mice that survived beyond 200 days post-transplant were sacrificed, and at that time they had no evidence of leukemia. Thus, it is not possible to say whether recurrent leukemia was a significant problem beyond 200 days. In six instances an effort was made to determine whether recurrent leukemia was of donor (DBA/2) or host (AKR) origin using a bioassay procedure. Spleen cells from each of the six treated mice with recurrent leukemia were injected intravenously into young DBA/2 or AKR secondary recipients. The assumption was made that the leukemia would proliferate only in the secondary recipients which were histocompatible with the strain of origin of the leukemia. Adult DBA/2 mice are not susceptible to transplanted AKR spontaneous T cell leukemia (unpublished data). In every instance except one, the leukemia was determined to be of AKR origin. The single exception was a decontaminated allogeneic chimera from Group 7 (Table 4) which was sacrificed 356 days post-transplant and had evidence of recurrent leukemia. All of the DBA/2 secondary recipients showed splenomegaly and lymphadenopathy 30 days after bioassay; none of the AKR recipients showed evidence of leukemia.

Neoplastic transformation of donor cells in leukemic hosts has been reported in both clinical (6, 34) and experimental (14, 32) situations. Although recrudescent leukemia is still a major problem following marrow transplantation in man (35), the frequency with which it occurs in donor cells appears to be low (33). Nevertheless, the threat of leukemogenesis in donor cells poses a serious problem.

The cause of recurrent leukemia in the experiments reported here is not known. It could be simply a failure to eliminate all of the original disease; alternatively, it could be due to induction of a new disease episode in residual host cells or, as seen in the bioassay experiment described above, in donor cells. The possibility of inducing a new disease episode in susceptible normal cells may be enhanced if the leukemia is of

Table 5. Incidence of recurrent leukemia in AKR mice within 200 days after treatment with chemoradiotherapy and bone marrow transplantation

From Table 4	Microbial Status of Recipient	Donor Cells	Number Treated	Number Dead Within 200 Days			Percent Leukemia Within 200 Days
				Leukemia	No Leukemia	Undetermined[a]	
Group 3	GF	DBA/2	21	2	12	1	10
Group 5	DC	DBA/2	6	2	2	0	33
Group 6	CV	AKR	11	11	0	0	100
Group 7	DC	DBA/2	31	5	6	1	17

a. Because of cannibalism or autolysis.
b. (Number dead with leukemia within 200 days × 100)/Number treated − Number of undetermined deaths.

viral origin (6, 9, 14). Therefore, long-term surviving allogeneic chimeras were tested for the presence of endogenous MuLV. The terminal 6-mm section of the tail was collected, a soluble extract prepared and assayed for virus using the XC-plaque assay (24). The results are shown in Table 6. Eighteen mice from Groups 3 and 7 (Table 4) were available for testing $\geq$ 156 days post-transplant. For controls, tail specimens were collected from 13 normal, untreated AKR mice 10 to 12 months of age. The results indicated that chemoradiotherapy plus allogeneic marrow transplantation had no effect on the tissue concentration of MuLV.

The failure of the treatments to eliminate or reduce the leukemia-inducing agent could explain the high incidence of recurrent leukemia which develops late in AKR mice that have their hematopoietic system replaced with syngeneic (Group 6, Table 5) or H-2 compatible marrow after adoptive immunotherapy (see Bortin et al., this volume). If the leukemia virus is not eliminated by the treatments, then restoration of hematopoiesis with cells from MuLV susceptible donors risks viral leukemogenesis in the donor cells. Thus, even though the original disease may have been eliminated, the animal can develop and die of a new leukemia that is the result of induction of the disease in susceptible cells. Presence of MuLV in animals treated with histoincompatible marrow transplantation suggests the possibility that long-term survival of these mice after cell cure was due to the relative lack of susceptibility of DBA/2 cells to endogenous MuLV.

Table 6.   Results of assays for MuLV in tail specimens of untreated, non-leukemic AKR mice and long-term surviving ($\geq$156 days) leukemic AKR mice treated with chemoradiotherapy and allogeneic marrow transplantation

	Microbial Status of Recipient	Marrow Donor	N^a	Log_{10} PFU ($\pm SD$)[b]	
Group 3, Table 4	GF	DBA/2	3	3.43 ($\pm$0.4)	3.39 ($\pm$0.19)
Group 7, Table 4	DC	DBA/2	15	3.38 ($\pm$ 0.1)	
Untreated, Normal	GF	—	9	3.47 ($\pm$0.17)	3.39 ($\pm$0.2)
Untreated, Normal	CV	—	4	3.23 ($\pm$0.08)	

a. Number of mice tested.
b. Plaque-forming units (PFU) per 0.4 ml of 2% extract of 6mm tail specimen.

VII. Recent Experimental Model

Recently, a series of experiments was intiated in which no treatment was started, including decontamination, until after the leukemia had been diagnosed in conventional AKR mice. We have attempted to simulate the clinical situation in which a patient with leukemia, who is being considered for marrow transplantation, is placed on a remission-induction (RI) chemotherapy regimen, and either started on a decontamination protocol or maintained in a conventional environment. The preliminary results in this clinically relevant experimental model are shown in Figure 1.

Conventional AKR mice were diagnosed as bearing advanced T cell leukemia, randomized and entered into control or experimental groups. One group of leukemic control mice (not shown in Figure 1) was placed on high dose antibiotics per os, put into laminar airflow hoods with frequently changed sterile cages, and given no further treatment. The MST for AKR mice that underwent decontamination only was 16 days postdiagnosis, and all of the mice were dead of leukemia within 43 days. Thus, decontamination and axenic isolation alone provided no significant benefit to leukemia-bearing mice. Many of the mice died before their microflora could be eliminated.

In order to simulate the clinical situation and to keep a significant number of leukemic AKR mice alive until decontamination could be accomplished, RI chemotherapy consisting of CY, methyl cyclohexylnitrosourea (MeC) and palmO-cytosine arabinoside (PalmO) was initiated immediately after diagnosis. Experimental mice (see Fig. 1) were given RI chemotherapy simultaneously with decontamination and axenic isolation in laminar airflow hoods. Conventional control mice (see Fig. 1) were also given RI chemotherapy, but they were housed in Isosystem^R cages (Lab Products, Inc., Garfield, N.J.) in a conventional animal facility. Mortality during the 20-day RI chemotherapy was 14% and 16% in the conventional control and decontaminated experimental groups, respectively. Thus, there was no apparent benefit of decontamination and isolation during RI chemotherapy.

Following RI chemotherapy, conventional control and decontaminated experimental mice were given intense cytoreductive and immunosuppressive chemoradiotherapy consisting of 150 mg/kg CY and 700 r TBR. Twenty-four hours later, the immunosuppressed recipients were given a transplant of bone marrow and lymph node cells from H-2 incompatible SJL/J donors (day 0, Fig. 1). Antibiotics and laminar airflow isolation of experimental mice were continued throughout the experiment and follow-up. The MST for decontaminated experimental mice was

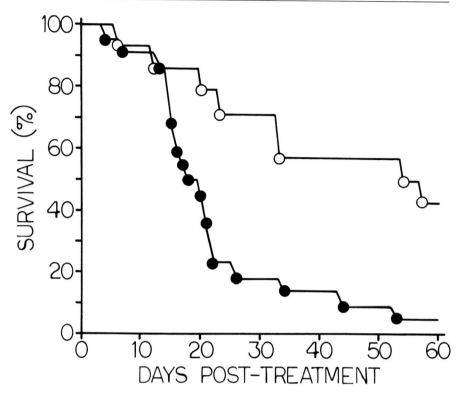

Fig. 1. Survival of AKR mice diagnosed as having spontaneous T cell leukemia on day −22 and given 100 mg/kg CY plus 10 mg/kg MeC (days −22 and −15), 10 mg/kg PalmO (days −9, −7 and −5) and 150 mg/kg CY plus 700 r TBR (day−1) followed by a transplant of 2×10^7 bone marrow and 2×10^6 lymph node cells from H-2 incompatible SJL/J donor mice (day 0): ●, 22 AKR mice maintained in conventional animal room facilities (Isosystem[R] cages); ○, 14 AKR mice started on antibiotic decontamination simultaneously with chemotherapy on day −22 and housed in sterile laminar airflow hoods.

56 days post-treatment compared to 19 days for the conventional control mice ($P < 0.01$), and there was also a significant difference in the survival rates (43% vs. 5%) at 60 days ($P < 0.05$).

    These results are presented as an example of how germfree techniques can be applied to the treatment of leukemia by allogeneic bone marrow transplantation after the disease has been diagnosed. Although the survival data in Figure 1 are not as impressive as when the treatments were applied to spontaneous T cell leukemia in AKR mice that were decontaminated several months before the leukemia developed (Groups 5 and 7,

Table 4), this approach mimics the problem facing physicians treating patients with acute leukemia.

VIII. Restoring Germfree Radiation Chimeras to the Conventional Environment

Due consideration must be given to eventually returning the chimeric animal or patient to a conventional environment following germfree or gnotobiotic isolation. Without this critical final step, clinical application of germfree techniques would not be practical. Jones et al. (13) found that when germfree allogeneic radiation chimeras were removed from protective isolation and placed directly into a conventional animal facility, most of the mice died of secondary disease within a short time. In later studies, we (21) and others (11, 40) avoided secondary disease mortality by step-wise reassociation of germfree or decontaminated chimeras with innocuous bacteria and gradual return to a conventional environment. Van Bekkum et al. (40) found that seeding or colonizing the intestinal tract with nonpathogenic anaerobic bacteria effectively allowed reconventionalization of chimeras as early as 40 days after transplantation.

We have not yet attempted to reconventionalize any of the germfree or decontaminated AKR mice whose leukemia was treated and eliminated by chemoradiotherapy and histoincompatible bone marrow transplantation (Table 4, Figure 1); however, our experience with nonleukemic allogeneic radiation chimeras confirms that intentional introduction of benign bacteria facilitates reconventionalization without appreciable mortality (21 and unpublished results). The microorganisms which bacteria-free chimeras first encounter after removal from protective isolation appears to be a critical factor affecting survival. The introduction of nonpathogenic bacteria which resist colonization of the intestines by pathogens would seem to be the safest was to insure that "friendly" microbes are encountered first.

IX. Clinical Potential of Germfree Techniques for the Treatment of Leukemia by Marrow Transplantation

Infectious complications comprise the leading cause of morbidity and mortality in patients with acute leukemia and lymphoma (16). The toxicity and debility caused by infection can prevent the use of aggressive antileukemic therapy. Isolation and microbial suppression have been tested in several controlled trials using leukemic patients undergoing chemotherapy for remission-induction (26). The decrease in infectious morbidity and mortality was significant.

Several reports have recommended the use of isolation and decontamination in marrow transplant recipients (5, 30, 46). In leukemic patients undergoing bone marrow transplantation, their inordinate susceptibility to infection is compounded by pre- and post-transplant immunosuppressive therapy and immunosuppression caused by GVH disease. The achievement and maintenance of a germfree state might be of significant benefit to these patients. Currently, a prospective study is in progress at the University of Washington, Seattle which is designed to evaluate the effect of isolation or isolation and decontamination on marrow transplantation in patients with leukemia and aplastic anemia (35).

The results of the experiments described in this chapter suggest that the benefits could be significant. The experiments were designed to investigate those factors which are important for successful application of germfree techniques to marrow transplantation for the treatment of acute leukemias which are resistant to conventional therapeutic approaches. By providing a germfree state for the recipient, secondary disease mortality following transplantation of marrow from histoincompatible donors was largely eliminated. In addition to the obvious effect of decreasing infectious complications, use of bacteria-free recipients permitted the use of drug and radiation doses which could not be applied successfully to conventionally reared animals. The combination of more aggressive chemoradiotherapy and incompatible marrow transplantation resulted in long-term, disease-free survival in a significant portion of decontaminated or germfree AKR mice bearing advanced spontaneous T cell leukemia.

ACKNOWLEDGMENTS

This work was supported by United States Public Health Service Research Grant No. CA-18440 from the National Cancer Institute, the Allen-Bradley Foundation and the Board of Trustees, Mount Sinai Medical Center, Milwaukee, Wisconsin.

The author is a Scholar of the Leukemia Society of America, Inc.

The collaboration of Drs. Mortimer M. Bortin, Morris Pollard, Alfred A. Rimm, and Kunwar K. Srivastava during these studies is gratefully acknowledged. Expert technical assistance was provided by Kathleen Kohut, Gail Abendroth, Phyllis Luckert, Evangeline Reynolds, and Barbara Stephan. MuLV assays were kindly provided by Dr. Wallace P. Rowe, NIAID, NIH, and MLC assays by Dr. Glenn E. Rodey, Milwaukee County Medical Complex.

NOTES

1. From the Greek *gnotos* and *biota*, meaning known flora and fauna: the study of animals in which the composition of the flora and fauna, if present, is fully defined by current methodology.

2. Abbreviations used: BM = bone marrow; CV = conventional; CY = cyclophosphamide; DC = decontaminated; GF = germfree; GVH = graft-versus-host; LN = lymph node; MeC = methyl cyclohexylnitrosourea; MHC = major histocompatibility complex; MLC = mixed leukocyte culture; MST = median survival time; MuLV = endogenous murine leukemia virus; PalmO = palmOcytosine arabinoside; RI = remission induction; TBR = total body radiation.

3. When applying adoptive immunotherapy, immunocompetent cells from a normal donor are transplanted, i.e., those cells which would be responsible for rejecting a tumor are adoptively transferred, into the tumor-bearing host. Bone marrow transplantation from nonimmunized donors for the treatment of leukemia is a form of nonspecific adoptive immunotherapy.

4. An animal which carries a foreign hematopoietic system as a result of immunosuppression followed by transplantation of hematopoietic cells obtained from another animal (39).

5. Bulk, veterinary-grade antibiotic powders were generously provided by the following companies: Bacitracin by The Upjohn Co., Kanamycin by Bristol Laboratories; Gentamicin by Schering Corp; and Neomycin by E. R. Squibb and Sons, Inc. Streptomycin was purchased commercially from Calbiochem.

6. Drugs used in this study were provided by the Drug Synthesis and Chemistry Branch, Division of Cancer Treatment, National Cancer Institute.

REFERENCES

1. Bach, F. H., and Voynow, N. K. 1966. One-way stimulation in mixed leukocyte cultures. *Science* 153: 545.

2. Bortin, M. M., Rimm, A. A., Rose, W. C., and Saltzstein, E. C. 1974. Graft-versus-leukemia. V. Absence of antileukemic effect using allogeneic H-2 identical immunocompetent cells. *Transplantation* 18: 280.

3. Bortin, M. M., Rimm, A. A., Saltzstein, E. C., and Rodey, G. E. 1973. Graft-versus-leukemia. III. Apparent independent antihost and antileukemic activity of transplanted immunocompetent cells. *Transplantation* 16: 182.

4. Cline, M. J., Gale, R. P., Stiehm, E. R., Opelz, G., Young, L. S., Feig, S. A., and Fahey, J. L. 1975. Bone marrow transplantation in man. *Ann. Int. Med.* 83: 691.

5. Dooren, L. J., Kamphuis, R. P., de Koning, J., and Vossen, J. M. 1974. Bone marrow transplantation in children. *Sem. Hematol.* 11: 369.

6. Fialkow, P. J., Thomas, E. D., Bryant, J. I., and Neimen, P. 1971. Leukaemic transformation of engrafted human marrow cells *in vivo*. *Lancet* 1: 251.

7. Frei, III, E., Schabel, Jr., F. M., and Goldin, A. 1974. Comparative chemotherapy of AKR lymphoma and human hematological neoplasia. *Cancer Res.* 34: 184.

8. Furth, J., Siebold, H. R., and Rathbone, R. R. 1933. Experimental studies on lymphomatosis in mice. *Amer. J. Cancer* 19: 521.

9. Gross, L. 1970. *Oncogenic Viruses*, 2nd ed., p. 286. Pergamon Press, Oxford.

10. Hays, E. F. 1973. Immune responses in AKR mice: Their relationship to the development of spontaneous leukemia in this strain, *in* W. S. Ceglowski and H. Friedman (eds.), *Virus Tumorigenesis and Immunogenesis*, p. 321. Academic Press, New York.

11. Heit, H., Wilson, R., Fliedner, T. M., and Kohne, E. 1974. Mortality of secondary disease in antibiotic-treated mouse radiation chimeras, *in* J. B. Heneghan (ed.), *Germfree Research: Biological Effects of Gnotobiotic Environment*, p. 477. Academic Press, New York.

12. Herrell, W. E. 1974. Thoughts of the role of gnotobiotics in clinical medicine, *in* J. B. Heneghan (ed.), *Germfree Research: Biological Effects of Gnotobiotic Environment*, p. 9. Academic Press, New York.

13. Jones, J. M., Wilson, R., and Bealmear, P. M. 1971. Mortality and gross pathology of secondary disease in germfree mouse radiation chimeras. *Radiat. Res.* 45: 577.

14. Kuhnert, P. M., Okunewick, J. P., and Erhard, P. 1974. Leukemic transformation of donor spleen cells following their transplantation into supralethally irradiated mice with pre-existing viral leukemia. *Exp. Hematol.* 2: 328.

15. LeFeber, W. P., Truitt, R. L., Rose, W. C., and Bortin, M. M. 1977. Graft-versus-leukemia. VII. Donor Selection for adoptive immunotherapy in mice, *in* S. J. Baum and G. D. Ledney (eds.), *Experimental Hematology Today*, p. 239. Springer-Verlag, New York.

16. Levine, A. S., Graw, R. G., Jr., and Young, R. C. 1972. Management of infections in patients with leukemia and lymphoma: Current concepts and experimental approaches. *Sem. Hematol.* 9: 141.

17. Mathé, G. 1961. Secondary syndrome, a stumbling block in the treatment of leukaemia by whole-body irradiation and transfusion of allogeneic haematopoietic cells, *in Diagnosis and Treatment of Acute Radiation Injury*, p. 191. World Health Organization, Geneva.

18. Medical News. 1971. *J. Amer. Med. Assoc.* 218: 1631.

19. Old, L. F., Boyse, E. A., and Stockert, E. 1965. The G (Gross) leukemia antigen. *Cancer Res.* 25: 813.

20. Pollard, M., Kajima, M., and Teah, B. A. 1965. Spontaneous leukemia in germfree AK mice. *Proc. Soc. Exp. Biol. Med.* 120: 72.

21. Pollard, M., and Truitt, R. L. 1973. Survival of bacteria-contaminated mice with allogeneic bone marrow chimerism. *Fed. Proc.* 32: 83.

22. Pollard, M., and Truitt, R. L. 1973. Allogeneic bone marrow chimerism in germfree mice. I. Prevention of spontaneous leukemia in AKR mice. *Proc. Soc. Exp. Biol. Med.* 144: 659.

23. Rose, W. C., Rimm, A. A., Saltzstein, E. C., Truitt, R. L., and Bortin, M. M. 1975. Low-dose chemotherapy as a prelude to intensive treatment of spontaneous leukemia-lymphoma in AKR mice. *J. Natl. Cancer Inst.* 55: 219.

24. Rowe, W. P., and Pincus, T. 1972. Quantitative studies of naturally occurring murine leukemia virus infection of AKR mice. *J. Exp. Med.* 135: 429.

25. Schabel, F. M., Jr., Skipper, H. E., Trader, M. W., Laster, W. R., Jr., and Cheeks, J. B. 1974. Combination chemotherapy for spontaneous AKR lymphoma. *Cancer Chemother. Rep.* (Part 2) 4: 53.

26. Schimpff, S. C. 1975. Laminar air flow room reverse isolation and microbial suppression to prevent infection in patients with cancer. *Cancer Chemother. Rep.* (Part 1) 59: 1055.

27. Senn, L., and Borella, L. 1975. Clinical importance of lymphoblasts with T markers in childhood acute leukemia. *N Engl. J. Med.* 296: 828.

28. Skipper, H. E., and Shabel, F. M., Jr. 1972. Spontaneous AK leukemia (lymphoma) as a model for human leukemias and lymphomas. *Cancer Chemother. Rep.* (Part 3) 3:3.

29. Skipper, H. E., Schabel, F. M., Jr., Trader, M. W., Laster, W. R., Jr., Simpson-Herren, L., and Lloyd, H. 1972. Basic and therapeutic trial results obtained in the spontaneous AK leukemia (lymphoma) model—End of 1971. *Cancer Chemother. Rep.* (Part 1) 56: 273.

30. Solberg, C. O., Meuwissen, H. J., Needham, R. N., Good, R. A., and Matsen, J. M. 1971. Infectious complications in bone marrow transplant patients. *Brit. Med. J.* 1: 18.

31. Srivastava, K., and Wagner, M. 1974. Decontamination of conventional mice by antimicrobial agents. Abstracts of the Annual Meeting—1974, *Amer. Soc. Micro.* E88.

32. Thiel, E., Baumann, P., and Thierfelder, S. 1975. Leukaemic transformation of F_1-hybrid cells after inoculation of parental leukaemic cells. *Blut* 30: 277.

33. Thomas, E. D. 1976. Progress in marrow transplantation. *JAMA* 235: 611.

34. Thomas, E. D., Bryant, J. I., and Buckner, C. D. 1972. Leukaemic transformation of engrafted human marrow cells. *Lancet* 1: 1310.

35. Thomas, E. D., Storb, R., Clift, R. A., Fefer, A., Johnson, F. L., Neiman, P. E., Lerner, K. G., Glucksberg, H., and Buckner, C. D. 1975. Bone marrow transplantation. *N. Engl. J. Med.* 292: 832 and 895.

36. Trexler, P. C. 1959. The use of plastics in the design of isolator systems. *Ann. N.Y. Acad. Sci.* 78: 29.

37. Truitt, R. L., Pollard, M., and Srivastava, K. K. 1974. Allogeneic bone marrow chimerism in germfree mice. III. Therapy of leukemic AKR mice. *Proc. Soc. Exp. Biol. Med.* 146: 153.

38. Upton, A. C., and Furth, J. 1954. The effects of cortisone on the development of spontaneous leukemia in mice and on its induction by irradiation. *Blood* 9: 686.

39. van Bekkum, D. W., and de Vries, M. J. 1967. *Radiation Chimeras*. Logos Press, London.

40. van Bekkum, D. W., Roodenburg, J., Heidt, P. J., and van der Waaij, D. 1974. Mitigation of secondary disease of allogeneic mouse radiation chimeras by modification of the intestinal microflora. *J. Natl. Cancer Inst.* 52: 401.

41. van der Waaij, D., and Sturm, C. A. 1968. Antibiotic decontamination of the digestive tract of mice. Technical procedures. *Lab. Animal Care* 18: 1.

42. van der Waaij, D., de Vries, J. M., and Lekkerkerk, J. E. C. 1970. Eliminating bacteria from monkeys with antibiotics, in H. Balner and W. I. Beveridge (eds.), *Infection and Immunosuppression in Subhuman Primates*, p. 21.

Munksgaard, Copenhagen.

43. van der Waaij, D., and Dietrich, M. 1974. Evaluative study of patients with acute leukemia under gnotobiotic conditions by the Gnotobiotic Project Group of the European Organization for Research on Treatment of Cancer (E.O.R.T.C.), in J. B. Heneghan (ed.), *Germfree Research: Biological Effects of Gnotobiotic Environment*, p. 49. Academic Press, New York.

44. van der Waaij, D., and Sturm, C. A. 1971. The production of "Bacteria-free" mice. Relationship between fecal flora and bacterial population of the skin. *Antonie van Leeuwenhoek* 37: 139.

45. van der Waaij, D., and Vossen, J. M. 1975. Antibiotic decontamination in animals and in human patients, *in* T. Hasegawa (ed.), *Proceedings of the First Intersectional Congress of IAMS*, p. 233. Science Council of Japan, Tokyo.

46. Vossen, J. M., and van der Waaij, D. 1972. Reverse isolation in bone marrow transplantation: Ultra-clean room compared with laminar flow technique. I. Isolation systems. *Rev. Europ. Etudes Clin. Biol.* 17: 457.

47. Wahren, B. 1966. Demonstration of a tumor specific antigen in spontaneously developing AKR lymphomas. *Int. J. Cancer* 1: 41.

CHAPTER 17

EFFECT OF NEURAMINIDASE ON CELLULAR IMMUNITY

Tin Han

Department of Medicine B
Roswell Park Memorial Institute
New York State Department of Health
Buffalo, New York 14263

Vibrio cholerae neuraminidase (VCN) enhances cell-mediated immunity, in vitro (lymphocyte blastogenic response, "one-way" mixed lymphocyte reaction and E-rosetting assay) and in vivo (skin test response). This enzyme is also capable of enhancing in vitro tumor-specific immune responses in the lymphocytotoxicity test, lymphocyte transformation test, and macrophage or leukocyte migration inhibition test. Enhancement of in vivo immunogenicity of some tumor cells and regression of established tumors in various animal systems have been unequivocally reported.

Vibrio cholerae neuraminidase (VCN) removes sialic acid from the cell surface, causing less negative charge on the cell surface and increased cell deformability (1, 48). Several functional alterations can be induced by removal of cell surface sialic acid. These include rendering cells more easily phagocytosed (29), enhancing the phagocytic activity of monocytes (49), inhibiting viral or mycoplasma-induced hemagglutination (2, 15), inhibiting cell aggregation (28), changing the patterns of cell migration (53) and interfering with amino acid transport across cell membranes (8).

Many conflicting statements have been made about the physiological role of sialic acid moieties bound to the cell periphery and their effect on cellular interactions. Also, of current interest is the modification of cell interactions after removal of cell surface sialic acid by incubation with VCN (51). The detailed biochemistry of sialic acid moieties in the mammalian cell and its periphery is covered in a number of excellent reviews (10, 16, 37, 52). Weiss has discussed the effect of VCN and sialic acid on cell interactions and also traced the background of some of the work and attempted to clarify some apparent contradictions in the literature (51).

This review concerns only the effect of VCN on general cell-mediated immunity and tumor-specific immunity, in vitro as well as in vivo.

IN VITRO GENERAL CELL-MEDIATED IMMUNITY

Mitogen-Induced Lymphocyte Blastogenesis

We have observed that the treatment of human lymphocytes with VCN failed to enhance their blastogenic response to phytohemagglutinin (PHA). In contrast, the lymphocyte response to Concanavalin A (Con A) or pokeweed mitogen (PWM) was significantly enhanced when the cells were treated with VCN (21) (Table 1). Failure of enhancement of PHA response by VCN has been reported (31). It has been shown that PHA is the strongest available mitogen for human peripheral blood lymphocytes (18), inducing blastic transformation in nearly all of them. Con A and PWM are weaker mitogens and induce the blastic transformation of lesser numbers of lymphocytes. Thus, it is possible that VCN can enhance the Con A or PWM response by inducing blastogenesis in higher numbers of lymphocytes. It should be pointed out that the optimal dose of PHA was utilized in our study (21). Enhancement of PHA-induced lymphocyte

Table 1.   Effect of neuraminidase on *in vitro* lymphocyte response to antigens and mitogens (by permission of *Clin. Exp. Immunol.*)

Stimulant	Number of Experiments	Blastogenic Index (Mean $\pm$ S.E.)	
		PBS-treated Cells	VCN-treated Cells
PHA	32	296.3 ± 28.3	291.0 ± 45.3
Con A	32	97.8 ± 20.9^a	147.7 ± 34.4^a
PWM	32	115.7 ± 18.2^a	187.8 ± 22.1^a
PPD	32	38.3 ± 9.7^a	60.2 ± 12.9^a
Varidase	32	75.6 ± 23.0^a	122.5 ± 20.1^a
Monilia	26	7.6 ± 3.4^a	16.0 ± 4.6^a
Mumps	27	12.2 ± 3.1^a	32.4 ± 6.9^a

a. $p < 0.01$.

blastogenesis by VCN treatment has also been described when suboptimal doses of PHA were utilized (30).

Antigen-Induced Lymphocyte Blastogenesis

We have also observed that the human lymphocyte response to purified protein derivative (PPD), Varidase, monilia or mumps antigen was significantly enhanced by VCN treatment (21) (Table 1). Comparison of individual antigen responses between saline-treated and VCN-treated lymphocytes is presented in Figure 1. In 16 of 20 experiments, in which the PPD responses of lymphocytes were significant (Greater than a blastogenic index of 2), the responses were 1.2–27.0-fold greater than those of saline-treated cells; in the remaining 4 experiments, the responses of VCN-treated cells were slightly decreased as compared to those of saline-treated cells. Of the 12 experiments in which the PPD responses of saline-treated lymphocytes were insignificant, five became significantly enhanced after VCN treatment. Similarly, VCN treatment of sensitized lymphocytes enhanced the responses to Varidase, monilia and mumps antigen in all but two of the Varidase, three of the monilia, and two of the mumps experiments (1.1–16.1-fold increase for Varidase or monilia, and 1.2–23.1-fold increase for mumps). Of five experiments, in which the Varidase responses of saline-treated lymphocytes were insignificant, two

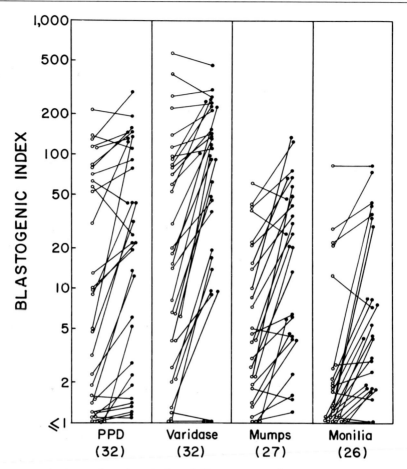

Fig. 1. Comparison of antigen-induced blastogenesis between PBS-treated (O) and VCN-treated (●) lymphocytes. (By permission of *Clin. Exp. Immunol.*)

responses became significantly increased after the cells were treated with VCN. Such an enhancement effect of VCN was noted in five of eight experiments with mumps antigen and in nine of 17 with monilia antigen, in which case the responses of saline-treated lymphocytes were insignificant. It is possible that the lymphocytes, which remained unresponsive to antigen after VCN treatment represented truly unsensitized cells and that the lymphocytes, which became responsive to antigen after VCN treatment, were actually sensitized cells.

To test this hypothesis, we conducted an experiment investigating the effect of VCN on sensitized lymphocytes from the mother (venous blood) and on unsensitized lymphocytes from both mother and child (cord blood). The blastogenic response of sensitized lymphocytes from the mother to Varidase, monilia or mumps antigen was markedly enhanced by VCN treatment (1.3–10.4-fold increase). No enhancement was noted when the unsensitized lymphocytes of the mother (PPD) and of the child (all antigens) were treated with VCN. The blastogenic response of sensitized lymphocytes from guinea pigs to "de novo" antigens (hemocyanins or PPD) was also enhanced by VCN treatment in 21 of 23 instances. In contrast, no effect of VCN on unsensitized guinea pig lymphocytes to these antigens was noted in any of 34 instances. These findings indicate that the enhancement effect of VCN is specific for sensitized lymphocytes (24).

Studies of VCN concentration (1, 4, 16, and 64 units per ml of blood) on the sensitized lymphocyte response to antigen showed a marked enhancement in each concentration. Studies of enhancement of sensitized lymphocytes treated with VCN (4 units per ml of blood) at various doses of antigens indicated that the degree of improvement was greater in cultures containing suboptimal doses (1.9–9.3-fold increase) than in those with optimal doses (1.3–6.3-fold increase).

Heating VCN at 100°C for 10 minutes completely abolished the enhancement effect on the lymphocyte response. VCN treatment did not change the kinetics of antigen-induced blastogenesis. The possibility that enhancement of lymphocyte response may be partly due to mitogenic properties of residual VCN after washing was excluded because we found no difference between the DNA synthesis of VCN-treated cells and that of saline-treated cells (control cultures for both antigen and mitogen). The increased lymphocyte response to antigen could probably be related to unmasking of the antigen receptor sites of the cells, resulting in increased antigen uptake and enhancement of blastogenic response of antigen sensitive cells.

"One-Way" Mixed Lymphocyte Reaction

Lindahl-Kiessling and Peterson first reported that human mixed lymphocyte reaction was enhanced when cells were treated with VCN (30). Lundgren and Simmons reported that the VCN treatment of stimulating cells inactivated by mitomycin C treatment caused a marked increase in their stimulating capacity in human "one-way" mixed lymphocyte reaction as measured by an increase in DNA synthesis of the responding cells; no effect was observed by treating the responding cells (31). On the other hand, we have observed that the "one-way" mixed lymphocyte reaction was greatly enhanced by treating not only stimulating cells, inactivated by X-irradiation, but also responding cells, or both types of cells. The strongest enhancement was seen after VCN treatment of responding lymphocytes (19) (Table 2).

VCN treatment did not change the kinetics of the mixed lymphocyte reaction with the peak response on day 7 of culture. It enhanced responses on days 4, 7 and 9 of culture. The greatest enhancement was observed when the responding lymphocytes were treated with VCN. The increased mixed lymphocyte reaction is probably related to changes in the physical properties of lymphocytes following VCN treatment. Since VCN reduces the negative charge on the cell surface by removing sialic acid from the cell membrane (1), this might result in greater cell-to-cell contact. Also, increased deformability of the cells induced by this enzyme (48) might increase the area of contact between antigenic receptor sites and antigenic determinant sites on the cell membrane of responding lymphocytes and stimulating lymphocytes. A weak stimulation in autologous "one-way" mixed lymphocyte culture, in which the stimulating cells were treated with VCN, has been reported (13, 31). Etheredge et al. (13) suggested that VCN-induced alterations in the cell surface create weak neoantigens. We, on the other hand, found that there was no stimulation in autologous mixed lymphocyte culture and in mixed lymphocyte culture between identical twins, indicating that no weak neoantigens on the cell surface of stimulating cells and no new antigenic receptor sites on the cell surface of responding cells appeared after treating the cells with VCN (19). It has been reported that human lymphocytes treated with VCN are more sus-

Table 2. Enhancement of "one-way" mixed lymphocyte reaction by neuraminidase (by permission of *Transplantation*)

Composition of Culture[a]	^{3}H-Thymidine Incorporation (mean cpm, 10^3, ± S.E.)	Blastogenic Index
RL (PBS)	0.3 ±0.04	
RL (VCN)	0.2 ±0.03	
SL (PBS)[b]	0.3 ±0.06	
SL (VCN)[b]	0.2 ±0.04	
RL (PBS)+SL (PBS)[b]	9.3 ±1.5	27 ± 3.9
RL (PBS)+SL (VCN)[b]	14.6 ±2.7	42 ± 6.0
RL (VCN)+SL (PBS)[b]	18.4 ±3.4	77 ±11.3
RL (VCN)+SL (VCN)[b]	15.9 ±3.4	67 ±14.0

a. RL, responding lymphocytes; SL, stimulating lymphocytes.
b. Indicates that stimulating cells were irradiated with 6000 R.

ceptible to lysis with antisera directed against HLA antigens, indicating the enhancement of antigenicity of lymphocytes by VCN treatment (17).

A similar enhancement of "one-way" mixed lymphocyte reaction, using cultured B cells as stimulators, by VCN treatment has also been reported. It has been reported that "one-way" mixed lymphocyte reactions between normal peripheral blood lymphocytes of human or baboon and inactivated, cultured "leukemic" T cells (MOLT-4) were absent. The treatment of responding lymphocytes and/or the MOLT-4 cells with VCN did not produce a significant reaction (20).

E-Rosette Assay

It has recently been established that E-rosette formation is a useful tool for the identification of human T cells (27, 33). The mechanisms of E-rosette formation of lymphocytes with unsensitized sheep erythrocytes are not fully understood at present. In a recently completed study, investigating the effect of VCN on E-rosette formation of various types of human lymphoid cells (Table 3), we have found E-rosettes significantly increased when the peripheral blood lymphocytes of normal donors were pretreated with VCN. Although the E-rosettes increased following the VCN treatment of other lymphoid cells, the differences were not statistically significant except for spleen cells. The E-rosettes formed by attachment of unsensitized sheep erythrocytes to untreated peripheral blood lymphocytes were easily broken up by incubation at 37°C for 30 minutes or by vigorous shaking. Thus, no stable E-rosettes of untreated lymphocytes were seen. Pre-treatment of lymphocytes with VCN increased the proportion of stable E-rosettes (60–70%) resistant to incubation at 37°C and shaking. Similar findings on the effect of VCN on peripheral blood lymphocytes have been reported by other investigators (6, 14). It has also been reported that the proportion of regular or stable E-rosettes was increased by treating the sheep erythrocytes with VCN (14, 47). We, on the other hand, observed that the regular E-rosette formation was not enhanced by the VCN treatment of sheep erythrocytes or horse erythrocytes.

The exact mechanisms of increased capacity of VCN-treated lymphocytes to form rosettes with unsensitized sheep erythrocytes and of increased stability of E-rosettes are not understood at present. The increased capacity of E-rosette formation is probably related to changes in the cell surface properties of lymphocytes following VCN treatment. It is possible that some of the receptor sites for unsensitized sheep erythrocytes are hidden by sialic acid and that the VCN treatment of those lymphocytes unmasks hidden receptors which then become available for interaction with sheep erythrocytes. An alternative explanation for increased capac-

Table 3.   Effect of neuraminidase treatment of human lymphocytes on E-rosettes[a]

Type of Lymphoid Cells	Number of Experiments	Treatment	E-Rosette % (mean ±S.D.)
Peripheral lymphocytes	25	Untreated	62.0 ± 9.6
	25	VCN-treated	80.1 ± 9.8[b]
PHA-induced blasts	6	Untreated	78.0 ± 9.7
	6	VCN-treated	82.6 ± 8.5
ALL	20	Untreated	44.4 ± 28.8
	20	VCN-treated	56.3 ± 33.3
CLL	12	Untreated	14.2 ± 12.6
	12	VCN-treated	27.5 ± 21.2
Thymus	6	Untreated	79.3 ± 11.2
	6	VCN-treated	91.6 ± 8.4
Spleen	5	Untreated	34.4 ± 14.5
	5	VCN-treated	73.7 ± 8.6[b]
MOLT-4 (T cell line)	3	Untreated	67.7 ± 9.6
	3	VCN-treated	90.2 ± 3.3
B411-4 (B cell line)	1	Untreated	0
	1	VCN-treated	0

a. Various types of lymphoid cells were treated with VCN, 50 U/ml or without VCN at 37°C for 30 min. E-rosetting was then performed.

b. $p < 0.01$.

ity of VCN-treated lymphocytes to form E-rosettes with sheep erythrocytes may be that VCN does not expose hidden receptor sites on the lymphocyte surface but simply reduces its negative charge, resulting in greater and closer contact between the two cell types. Pretreatment by VCN of peripheral blood lymphocytes also significantly enhanced EAC-rosette formation (25).

IN VIVO GENERAL CELL-MEDIATED IMMUNITY

We have recently investigated the effect of VCN on skin test response in patients with a variety of neoplastic diseases and found that delayed hypersensitivity skin test response to specific antigen was enhanced when the antigen was given intradermally with VCN in sensitive subjects (22). Thirty-five of 41 patients had malignant lymphoma (Hodgkin's disease, 18; lymphosarcoma, 12 and reticulum cell sarcoma, 5). Skin test antigens were diluted with equal volumes of normal saline or VCN-containing normal saline. Antigens, 0.2 ml, with or without VCN (5 units) and VCN alone were simultaneously given intradermally on the forearm, and the diameter of skin test response (erythema) was measured in mm at 24 and 48 hours. The results of skin test responses to various antigens with or without VCN are shown in Table 4, indicating that skin test responses were enhanced by VCN. No reaction at the site of VCN was observed in any instance, indicating that VCN was not an irritant and that the enhancement of skin test response by VCN was truly immunological in nature.

The VCN did not change the time course of skin test responses, however, heating the VCN for 10 minutes at 100°C abolished the enhancement effect altogether. It is generally believed that following contact of the sensitized lymphocytes with specific antigen, these cells are activated—resulting in the release of physiologically active substances including skin reactive factors or macrophage inhibition factor (7). VCN-mediated enhancement of delayed skin hypersensitivity to specific antigen is probably related to either an increase in the release of skin reactive factor from activated lymphocytes or to a heightened tissue hypersensitivity response to this skin reactive factor (22).

Table 4. Effect of neuraminidase on delayed skin hypersensitivity (by permission of *Clin. Exp. Immunol.*)

Antigen	Number of Experiments	Skin Test Response[a] (mm) (mean ±S.D.)	
		Normal Saline	VCN
PPD	23	10 ± 3	18 ± 3
KLH	7	12 ± 3	16 ± 4
Varidase	6	10 ± 4	18 ± 6
Mumps	7	20 ± 5	23 ± 6
Monilia	5	10 ± 4	11 ± 6

a. Maximal response at 24 or 48 hours.

IN VITRO TUMOR-SPECIFIC IMMUNITY

In vitro immune response to malignancy can be quantified by (1) measuring the cytotoxic effect of sensitized lymphocytes and macrophages on malignant target cells, (2) by measurement of blastic transformation of host lymphocytes cultured with malignant target cells (inactivated), and (3) by measuring the inhibition of macrophage or leukocyte migration in the presence of tumor antigen.

The cytotoxic effect of sensitized lymphocytes and macrophages on tumor cells appears to involve two steps: (1) a specific adhesion process and (2) killing the target cells. The effect of VCN treatment of P815 mastocytoma target cells on their immunolysis by spleen cells from immunized and nonimmunized mice was investigated by Weiss and Cudney (50). In a highly sensitive in vitro system in which immunolysis was quantitated by measurements of ^{51}Cr release from labeled P815 cells, the VCN treatment of target cells did not increase susceptibility to attack by sensitized spleen cells. Killing proceeded despite a substantial contribution of sialic acid moieties to the net negative surface charge of the untreated P815 cells, and destruction was not enhanced by enzymatic removal of substantial amounts of bound sialic acid, as evidenced by a 60% reduction in anodic electrophoretic mobility. This finding, at least, did not support the suggestion that VCN treatment of tumor cells enhances their contact with, or destruction by, killer cells. We failed to find any published report demonstrating the enhanced tumor cell lysis by sensitized lymphocytes or macrophages following the VCN treatment of target tumor cells. However, in their own in vitro study, Weiss and Cudney (50) showed that in the mastocytoma/sensitized spleen cell interaction, when VCN treatment of the target cells had no effect on immunolysis, enzyme treatment of the spleen cells produced significant enhancement in the killing of target cells. These results were contrary to those of Lundgren and Simmons (31) in suggesting that in their "one-way" mixed lymphocyte culture system, the enhancement of mixed lymphocyte reaction was seen only when the stimulating (target) cells were treated with VCN. In further contrast to Lundgren and Simmons, we have observed that mixed lymphocyte reaction was enhanced by treating not only stimulating cells but also responding cells or both types of cells. In fact, the strongest enhancement was seen when only responding cells were treated with VCN (19). Our findings are then in agreement with those of Weiss and Cudney.

Interactions between tumor cells and macrophages often resulted in destruction and/or phagocytosis of the former (5). Electronmicrographs of interacting target cells and immune macrophages revealed a close apposition between the cells along extremely convoluted, interdigitated margins

(9). At areas of close contact, adherent parts of the target cells were apparently pulled into the macrophage and pinched off. The exact mechanism of target cell kill by macrophages is not known. It is possible that the VCN treatment of macrophages can increase the deformability of these cells which, in turn, increases their ability to phagocytose the target cells. It has been shown that VCN treatment of human monocytes increased their ability to phagocytose negatively charged particles in vitro (49).

Watkins et al. (46) have reported that the lymphoblastic response of rat host peripheral blood leukocytes, cultured with Novikoff hepatoma target cells pretreated with VCN, was accentuated. These authors have also observed a similar response to VCN-treated tumor cells in 8 of 11 human studies. Unfortunately, they did not study the effect of VCN on responding lymphocytes. The possibility that lymphoblastic transformation is due to a non-specific effect of VCN was excluded by the absence of transformation when rat host leukocytes were cultured with syngeneic leukocytes pretreated with VCN. The possibility that transformation might result from stimulation by cryptic tissue-specific antigens exposed by VCN treatment was also excluded by the absence of response when normal homologous hepatocytes were used as the VCN-treated target cells. These observations indicate that the transformation in mixed cell culture was the result of stimulation by tumor-specific antigen (46).

We have recently reported that the migration of leukocytes, obtained from certain patients with lung cancer, was inhibited by tumor-specific antigen extracted from an established culture cell line of undifferentiated lung cancer (23). In a preliminary study, we observed that migration of such leukocytes was further inhibited by lung cancer antigen when the

Table 5. Effect of neuraminidase on migration of leukocytes induced by lung cancer antigen

Experiment Number	Lung Cancer Antigen	Leukocyte Migration Inhibition%[a]	
		Untreated Cells	VCN-Treated Cells
1	100 μg	17.2	27.3
	1000 μg	30.6	37.8
2	100 μg	17.8	34.4
3	100 μg	16.2	25.8

a. Leukocyte migration inhibition of 15% or more is considered a positive result.

leukocytes were exposed to VCN prior to the addition of antigen, suggesting that in vitro tumor-specific immunity was enhanced by VCN (Table 5).

IN VIVO TUMOR-SPECIFIC IMMUNITY

Sanford first reported that fewer tumors developed in mice receiving VCN-treated tumor cells than in those receiving untreated tumor cells. She interpreted that the reduced transplantability of VCN-treated tumor (TA3) cells was due to "unmasking" of histocompatibility antigens (38). Similar findings with Landschutz ascites tumors in mice were reported by Currie and Bagshawe (11, 12). Hauschka et al. (26), on the other hand, failed to observe any effect of VCN treatment on subsequent tumor takes, using the identical TA3 cells and hosts as in Sanford's study. Hauschka et al. found that at low concentrations (e.g., 3×10^4 cells per ml) and in the absence of adequate amounts of protective proteins in the culture medium, cell survival rate was significantly less than at greater concentrations (e.g., 10^6–10^7 cells per ml). Both Sanford, Hauschka, et al. used a 3×10^4 per ml concentration of cells during incubation with VCN. The difference was that Hauschka et al. diluted VCN in phosphate buffered saline, resulting in pH 7.1, whereas Sanford diluted the enzyme in another diluent with a final pH of 5.2. Hauschka et al., however, observed that with the procedures used by Sanford, only 30% of the cells were viable after 30 minute incubation with enzyme at a concentration of 3×10^4 cells per ml. They found no difference in the H-2 antigenic titers of TA3 cells before and after VCN treatment. They concluded that at least in the case examined by them, a decrease of in vivo tumor takes was simply due to a reduction below the LD 100 level in the number of viable cells inoculated and not as the result of an increase in their surface antigenicity.

Bekesi et al. (3) reported that treatment of leukemia L1210 tumor cells with VCN resulted in loss of oncogenicity; 10^7 VCN-treated cells failed to induce leukemia inDBA/2 mice. Immunogenicity of the treated tumor cells was increased since DBA/2 mice were specifically resistant to 10^5 virulent L1210 cells after single immunization. They found that immunogenicity was directly correlated with release of neuraminidase-susceptible N-acetylneuraminic acid. Bekesi et al. have compared the immunogenicity of L1210 tumor cells treated with VCN with those treated with formaldehyde or X-irradiation. They observed that a high degree of immunity was obtained with VCN-treated L1210 tumor cells, with 100% protection against a challenge of 10^5 cells and 40% protection against a 10^6-cell challenge. Formaldehyde-treated cells induced relatively weak immunity, providing complete protection only against 10^2 virulent L1210 cells. When immunization was done with X-irradiated tumor cells, the response was only slightly better, providing 100% protection against 10^3 cells. These observations suggest that the VCN-treated L1210 cells seem 100–1,000-fold more immunogenic than the formaldehyde-treated or X-irradiated tumor cells. In another tumor-host system, Ray et al. (34) found that inoculation of VCN-treated fibrosarcoma (dimethylbenz-dithinnapthrene-induced) in syngeneic Swiss mice resulted in a stronger antitumor immunity than in those inoculated with X-irradiated tumor cells.

Tumor regression experiments in mice by using VCN-treated tumor cells of the same type were first reported by Simmons and his associates (39–41). Syngeneic mice were transplanted with 2 fibrosarcomas, MC-42 and MC-43, originally induced in C_3H/HeJ mice with 3-methylcholan-threne. Firmly established fibrosarcomas in syngeneic mice regressed if the hosts were treated with living tumor cells, pretreated with VCN in vitro. The rejection of the tumor was immunospecific since the MC-42 did not immunize the animals against the MC-43 tumor, or vice versa. Regression of tumor was not induced by inoculation of cells treated with inactivated VCN or by cells incubated with VCN and an excess of free sialic acid.

Regression of established methylcholanthrene-induced fibrosarcomas by intra-tumor injections of VCN was also reported by Simmons et al. (42). Growth of transplanted tumors injected with VCN generally stopped, and a number of the tumors totally regressed. In animals bearing bilateral immunologically identical tumors, injection of one tumor with VCN in-duced the regression not only of the injected tumor, but also of the con-tralateral (uninjected) tumor. When the bilateral tumors were of different types, injection of one did not lead to regression of the other type, but the animals were capable of rejecting the injected tumor while dying of the immunologically different tumor. These observations again indicate the immunospecific effect of VCN.

In contrast, Sparks and Breeding (44) did not observe tumor regres-sion by intratumal injection of VCN in two murine fibrosarcoma systems (BP and MCA-2).

Simmons and Rios (43) also repoted that firmly established trans-plantable C3H/HeJ mammary carcinomas (M-1 and M-2) regressed by host challenge with VCN-treated tumor cells. The effect was totally immuno-specific; even VCN-treated tumors bearing shared mammary tumor virus (MTV) antigen were unable to induce regression. These authors con-cluded that the VCN was capable of increasing the immunogenicity of the private, unique-unshared tumor antigens on mammary carcinomas; VCN was incapable of increasing the immunogenicity of the shared MTV as-sociated tumor antigen (43). In all of these experiments of Simmons et al., the VCN-treated tumor cells were given to the hosts when the established tumors were less than 1 cm in diameter and tumor regression was seen in all instances. However, VCN-treated tumor cells were incapable of regressing established tumors if the challenges were made when the tumors were greater than 1 cm in diameter (35).

Rios and Simmons have also carried out experiments designed to determine if immunotherapy could be more effective if the tumor masses were surgically reduced. They have utilized three tumors (MC-43, M-2 and B16 melanoma) previously shown to be susceptible to active specific immunotherapy in their studies. The combination of subtotal or total excision plus challenge with VCN-treated tumor cells was significantly more effective than either excision or immunotherapy alone. These observations strongly suggest that the reduction in tumor mass by surgical means might allow active specific immunotherapy to become an effective antitumor adjunct (35). The antitumor effect of VCN-treated tumor cells was magnified by the simultaneous administration of a nonspecific immunostimulant, BCG (41).

In a preliminary study, we have investigated the effect of intralesional injection of sensitized spleen cells, untreated or treated with VCN in vitro. Highly antigenic and nonmetastasizing mammary carcinoma cells (0.1 ml of 1:3 diluted tumor cell suspension) were transplanted to inbred rats (W/Fu). Tumors started to grow and were measured 4–5 days after transplantation. At this time, the rats were divided into 4 groups. To groups (a) and (b), intralesional injection of normal untreated and VCN-treated syngeneic spleen cells (6.5×10^7) were made into the tumors, respectively. Similarly, untreated and VCN-treated sensitized spleen cells (from tumor-bearing rats) were intralesionally injected to groups (c) and (d), respectively. Tumor growth patterns showed that tumors injected with VCN-treated sensitized spleen cells grew 25% more slowly than the corresponding tumor injected with untreated sensitized cells. The growth patterns of tumors injected with either untreated or VCN-treated normal spleen cells were quite similar, suggesting that the effect of VCN is specific for sensitized cells (unpublished data).

Although the effectiveness of immunotherapy has unequivocally been demonstrated in a variety of animal tumor systems, immunotherapy of human cancer is still in the experimental state. Immunotherapy in human neoplasms has been attempted sporadically in the past several decades. The results, however, until very recently were very discouraging. This is partly due to lack of knowledge of tumor bioimmunology and partly due to the poor selection of patients, who were far-advanced cases. Mathé et al. (32) first reported the encouraging results of active specific immunotherapy (using allogeneic leukemia cells plus BCG) in children with acute lymphoblastic leukemia. Since then, a number of studies

utilizing nonspecific immunotherapy with BCG, MER-BCG or *C. parvum,*
active specific immunotherapy with autologous or allogeneic tumor cells
plus or minus BCG or passive specific immunotherapy with "immune"
RNA or transfer factor in a variety of neoplastic diseases in man have been
reported.

Bekesi *et al.* (4) recently reported very encouraging results of active
specific immunotherapy with VCN-treated allogeneic myeloid leukemic
cells in patients with acute myeloblastic leukemia. In 10 previously
chemotherapy-treated patients, 6 immunized patients had more than
twice the remission duration of the 4 controls. In previously untreated
patients, a median remission duration on chemotherapy alone was 20
weeks for 7 patients while 5 of 7 patients receiving chemoimmunotherapy
remained in remission from 56 to 97 weeks.

Takita *et al.* (45) demonstrated the usefulness of active specific immunotherapy with Concanavalin A-VCN-treated autologous tumor cells
mixed with Freund's adjuvant, in randomly selected patients with locally
far-advanced bronchogenic carcinoma. Nineteen patients have been followed for more than 12 months. The mean survival of the control group
was 8.1 months with a median of 6 months. Only one of 9 patients was
alive after 18 months. In contrast, the mean survival of the treated group
was 17.4 months and the median was 18 months. Five of 10 patients were
alive from 15 to 26 months. Rosato *et al.* (36) also recently reported a
preliminary study, in which they treated 25 patients with various types of
cancer with VCN-treated autologous tumor cells at monthly intervals.
They observed that the lymphocytotoxicity activity using autologous
target cells was increased in 4 of 5 patients, and that 6 patients who
received the full course of 6 injections were alive without evidence of
progression of disease more than 8 months after the beginning of therapy.

REFERENCES

1. Ambrose, E. J. 1967. Biochemical and biophysical properties of cell membranes, in *Proceedings of the Seventh Canadian Cancer Research Conference,
Toronto,* pp. 247–264. Pergamon Press, New York.

2. Baylor, M. E. 1964. The reaction of receptor glycoprotein with influenza
virus and neuraminidase: An electron miscroscope study. *N.Y. Acad. Sci.* 26:
1103–1111.

3. Bekesi, J. G., St. Arneault, G., and Holland, J. F. 1971. Increase of leukemia
L1210 immunogenicity by Vibrio cholerae neuraminidase treatment. *Cancer Res.*
31: 2130–2132.

4. Bekesi, G., Holland, J. F., Yates, J. W., Henderson, E., and Fleminger, R.
1975. Immunotherapy of acute myelocytic leukemia with neuraminidase-treated
allogeneic leukemic cells. *Proc. Amer. Assoc. Cancer Res. and Amer. Soc. Clin.
Oncol.* 16: 121.

5. Bennett, B. 1965. Phagocytosis of mouse tumor cells in vitro by various homologous and heterologous cells. J. Immunol. 95: 80–86.

6. Bentwich, Z., Douglas, S. D., Skutelsky, E., and Kunkel, H. C. 1973. Sheep red blood cell binding to human lymphocytes treated with neuraminidase enhancement of T cell binding and identification of a subpopulation of B cells. J. Exp. Med. 137: 1532–1537.

7. Bloom, B. R., and Bennett, B. 1971. The assay of inhibition of macrophage and the production of migration inhibition factor and skin reactive factor in the guinea pigs, in B. R. Bloom and P. R. Glade (eds.), In Vitro Methods in Cell-Mediated Immunity, pp. 235–248. Academic Press, New York.

8. Brown, D. M., and Michael, A. F. 1969. Effect of neuraminidase on the accumulation of alpha-aminoisobutyric acid in Hela cells. Proc. Soc. Exp. Biol. Med. 131: 568–570.

9. Chambers, V. C., and Weiser, R. S. 1971. The ultrastructure of target L-cells and immune macrophages during their interaction in vitro. Cancer Res. 31: 2059–2066.

10. Cook, G. M. 1968. Glycoproteins in membranes. Biol. Rev. 43: 363–391.

11. Currie, G. A., and Bagshawe, K. D. 1968. The effect of neuraminidase on the immunogenicity of the Landschutz ascites tumor. Site and mode of action. Brit. J. Cancer 22: 588.

12. Currie, G. A., and Bagshawe, K. D. 1968. The role of sialic acid in antigenic expression: Further studies of Landschutz ascites tumor. Brit. J. Cancer 22: 843–853.

13. Etheredge, E. E., Shons, A. R., and Najarian, J. S. 1972. Neuraminidase-induced autologous stimulation of human leukocyte cultures, in M. R. Schwartz (ed.), Proceedings of the Sixth Leukocyte Culture Conference, pp. 121–135. Academic Press, New York.

14. Galli, U., and Schlesinger, M. 1974. The formation of stable E-rosettes after neuraminidase treatment of either human peripheral blood lymphocytes or of sheep red blood cells. J. Immunol. 112: 1628–1634.

15. Gesner, B., and Thomas, L. 1966. Sialic acid binding sites: Role in hemagglutination by mycoplasma gallisepticum. Science 151: 590–591.

16. Ginsburg, V., and Neufeld, E. F. 1969. Complex heterosaccharides of animals. Ann. Rev. Biochem. 38: 371–388.

17. Grothaus, E. A., Flye, M. W., Yunis, E., and Amos, B. D. 1971. Human lymphocyte antigen reactivity modified by neuraminidase. Science 173: 542–544.

18. Han, T., and Ohnuma, T. 1972. In vitro blastogenesis inhibited by Erwinia carotovora L-asparaginase. Nature New Biol. 239: 50–51.

19. Han, T. 1972. Enhancement of mixed lymphocyte reactivity by neuraminidase. Transplantation 14: 515–517.

20. Han, T., and Minowada, J. 1973. A unique "leukemic" T lymphoid cell line: Absence of stimulating effect in mixed lymphocyte reaction. Clin. Exp. Immunol. 15: 535–541.

21. Han, T. 1973. Enhancement of in vitro lymphocyte response by neuraminidase. Clin. Exp. Immunol. 13: 165–170.

22. Han, T. 1974. Enhancement of delayed skin hypersensitivity by neuraminidase in cancer patients. Clin. Exp. Immunol. 18: 95–100.

23. Han, T., Takita, H., Marabella, P. C., and Mittelman, A. 1975. In vitro transfer of tumor-specific immunity with human "immune" RNA. Clin. Exp. Immunol. 19: 219–221.

24. Han, T. 1975. Specific effect of neuraminidase on blastogenic response of sensitized lymphocytes. Immunology 28: 283–286.

25. Han, T., and Minowada, J. 1976. Enhanced E- and EAC-rosette formation by neuraminidase. J. Immunol. Methods (in press).

26. Hauschka, T. S., Weiss, I., Holdridge, B. A., Cudney, T. L., Zumpft, M., and Planinsek, J. A. 1971. Karyotypic and surface features of murine TA3 carcinoma cells during immunoselection in mice and rats. J. Natl. Cancer Inst. 47: 343–359.

27. Jondal, M., Holm, G., and Wigzell, A. 1972. Surface markers on human T and B lymphocytes. I. A large population of lymphocytes forming nonimmune rosettes with sheep red blood cells. J. Exp. Med. 136: 207–215.

28. Kemp, R. B. 1968. Effect of the removal of cell surface sialic acids on cell aggregation. Nature (Lond.) 218: 1255–1256.

29. Lee, A. 1968. Effect of neuraminidase on the phagocytosis of heterologous red cells by mouse peritoneal macrophages. Proc. Soc. Exp. Biol. Med. 128: 891–894.

30. Luidahl-Kiessling, K., and Peterson, R. D. A. 1969. The mechanism of phytohemagglutinin (PHA) action. Exp. Cell Res. 55: 85–87.

31. Lundgren, G., and Simmons, R. L. 1971. Effect of neuraminidase on the stimulatory capacity of cells in human mixed lymphocyte cultures. Clin. Exp. Immunol. 9: 915–926.

32. Mathé, G., Amiel, J. L., and Schwarzenberg, L. 1969. Active immunotherapy for acute lymphoblastic leukemia. Lancet I: 697–699.

33. Minowada, J., Ohnuma, T., and Moore, G. E. 1972. Rosette-forming human lymphoid cell lines. I. Establishment and evidence for origin of thymus-derived lymphocytes. J. Natl. Cancer Inst. 49: 891–895.

34. Ray, P. K., Thakur, V. S., and Sundaram, K. 1975. Antitumor immunity: I. Differential response of neuraminidase-treated and x-irradiated tumor vaccine. Europ. J. Cancer 11: 1–8.

35. Rios, A., and Simmons, R. L. 1974. Active specific immunotherapy of minimal residual tumor: Excision plus neuraminidase-treated tumor cells. Int. J. Cancer 13: 71–81.

36. Rosato, F. E., Brown, A. S., Miller, E. E., Rosato, E. F., Mullis, W. F., Johnson, J., and Moskovitz, A. 1974. Neuraminidase immunotherapy of tumors in man. Surg. Gyn. Obs. 139: 675–682.

37. Roseman, S. 1970. The synthesis of complex carbohydrates by multiglycosyltransferase systems and their potential function in intercellular adhesion. Chem. Phys. Lipids 5: 270–297.

38. Sanford, B. 1967. An alteration in tumor histocompatability induced by neuraminidase. Transplantation 4: 1273–1279.

39. Simmons, R. L., Rios, A., Lundgren, G., Ray, P. K., McKhann, C. F., and Haywood, G. R. 1971. Immunospecific regression of methylcholanthrene fibrosarcoma using neuraminidase. Surgery 70: 38–46.

40. Simmons, R. L., Rios, A., Ray, P. K., and Lundgren, G. 1971. Effect of

neuraminidase on the growth of a 3-methylcholanthrene-induced fibrosarcoma in normal and immunosuppressed syngeneic mice. *J. Natl. Cancer Inst.* 47: 1087–1094.

41. Simmons, R. L., and Rios, A. 1971. Immunotherapy of cancer: Immuno-specific rejection of tumors in recipients of neuraminidase-treated cells plus BCG. *Science* 174: 591–593.

42. Simmons, R. L., Rios, A., and Ray, P. K. 1972. Regression of established methylcholanthrene tumors by intratumor injections of Vibrio cholerae neuraminidase. *J. Surg. Oncol.* 4: 298–304.

43. Simmons, R. L., and Rios, A. 1973. Differential effect of neuraminidase on the immunogenecity of viral associated and private antigens of mammary car-cinomas. *J. Immunol.* 111: 1820–1825.

44. Sparks, F. C., and Breeding, J. H. 1974. Tumor regression and enhance-ment resulting from immunotherapy with BCG and neuraminidase. *Cancer Res.* 34: 3262–3269.

45. Takita, H., Han, T., and Marabella, P. 1974. Immunotherapy in bron-chogenic carcinoma: Effects on cellular immunity. *Surg. Forum* 25: 235–236.

46. Watkins, E., Jr., Ogata, Y., Anderson, L. L., Watkins, E. III, and Waters, M. F. 1971. Activation of host lymphocytes cultured with cancer cells treated with neuraminidase. *Nature New Biol.* 231: 83–85.

47. Weiner, M. S., Bianco, C., and Nussenzweig, V. 1973. Enhanced binding of neuraminidase-treated sheep erythrocytes to human T lymphocytes. *Blood* 42: 939–945.

48. Weiss, L. 1965. Studies on cell deformability: I. Effect of surface charge. *J. Cell Biol.* 26: 735–739.

49. Weiss, L., Mayhew, E., and Ulrich, K. 1966. The effect of neuraminidase on the phagocytic process in human monocytes. *Lab. Invest.* 15: 1304–1309.

50. Weiss, L., and Cudney, T. L. 1971. Some effects of neuraminidase on the *in vitro* interactions between spleen and mastocytoma (P815) cells. *Int. J. Cancer* 7: 187–197.

51. Weiss, L. 1973. Neuraminidase, sialic acids, and cell interactions. *J. Natl. Cancer Inst.* 50: 3–19.

52. Winzler, R. J. 1970. Carbohydrates in cell surfaces. *Int. Rev. Cytol.* 29: 77–125.

53. Woodruff, J. J., and Gesner, B. M. 1969. The effect of neuraminidase on the fate of transfused lymphocytes. *J. Exp. Med.* 129: 551–567.

INDEX